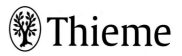

# Periodontology

## The Essentials

2nd Edition

Hans-Peter Mueller, DDS, PhD
Professor of Periodontology
Institute of Clinical Dentistry
Faculty of Health Sciences
UiT–The Arctic University of Norway
Tromsø, Norway

311 illustrations

Thieme
Stuttgart · New York · Delhi · Rio de Janeiro

**Library of Congress Cataloging-in-Publication Data**
Mueller, Hans-Peter, Prof. Dr. med. dent., author.
Periodontology : the essentials / Hans-Peter Mueller. –
2nd edition.
    p. ; cm.
Includes bibliographical references and index.
ISBN 978-3-13-138372-3 (alk. paper) –
ISBN 978313164872-3 (e-book)
I. Mueller, Hans-Peter, Prof. Dr. med. dent. Parodontologie.
3rd edition. Based on (expression): II. Title.
[DNLM: 1.  Periodontal Diseases—Handbooks.  WU 49]
RK361
617.6'32–dc23
                    2015019401

Illustrator: Karin Baum, Paphos, Cyprus

3rd German edition 2012
1st English edition 2005
1st Polish edition 2004
1st Russian edition 2004
1st Spanish edition 2006


© 2005, 2016 Georg Thieme Verlag KG

Thieme Publishers Stuttgart
Rüdigerstrasse 14, 70469 Stuttgart, Germany
+49 [0]711 8931 421, customerservice@thieme.de

Thieme Publishers New York
333 Seventh Avenue, New York, NY 10001, USA
+1-800-782-3488, customerservice@thieme.com

Thieme Publishers Delhi
A-12, Second Floor, Sector-2, Noida-201301
Uttar Pradesh, India
+91 120 45 566 00, customerservice@thieme.in

Thieme Publishers Rio, Thieme Publicações Ltda.
Edifício Rodolpho de Paoli, 25º andar
Av. Nilo Peçanha, 50 – Sala 2508
Rio de Janeiro 20020-906 Brasil
+55 21 3172 2297 / +55 21 3172 1896

Cover design: Thieme Publishing Group
Typesetting by Drückhaus Götz GmbH, Ludwigsburg,
    Germany

Printed in India by Replika Press Pvt. Ltd.

ISBN 978-3-13-138372-3                    5  4  3  2  1

Also available as an e-book:
eISBN 978-3-13-164872-3

**Important note:** Medicine is an ever-changing science undergoing continual development. Research and clinical experience are continually expanding our knowledge, in particular our knowledge of proper treatment and drug therapy. Insofar as this book mentions any dosage or application, readers may rest assured that the authors, editors, and publishers have made every effort to ensure that such references are in accordance with **the state of knowledge at the time of production of the book.**

Nevertheless, this does not involve, imply, or express any guarantee or responsibility on the part of the publishers in respect to any dosage instructions and forms of applications stated in the book. **Every user is requested to examine carefully** the manufacturers' leaflets accompanying each drug and to check, if necessary in consultation with a physician or specialist, whether the dosage schedules mentioned therein or the contraindications stated by the manufacturers differ from the statements made in the present book. Such examination is particularly important with drugs that are either rarely used or have been newly released on the market. Every dosage schedule or every form of application used is entirely at the user's own risk and responsibility. The authors and publishers request every user to report to the publishers any discrepancies or inaccuracies noticed. If errors in this work are found after publication, errata will be posted at www.thieme.com on the product description page.

Some of the product names, patents, and registered designs referred to in this book are in fact registered trademarks or proprietary names even though specific reference to this fact is not always made in the text. Therefore, the appearance of a name without designation as proprietary is not to be construed as a representation by the publisher that it is in the public domain.

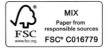

# Contents

# Preface

For half a century, periodontology has spearheaded scientific progress in dentistry. A tiny portion of the vast body of literature that has shaped modern periodontology has recently been listed by the American Academy of Periodontology on the occasion of its centennial.[1] What has kept us clinicians, teachers, and scientists busy was, for example, the discovery that bacteria of the oral cavity, which play a critical role in most periodontal diseases, organize themselves in a biofilm; and that the pathogenesis of periodontitis, like that of any chronic disease, is complex and multifactorial. Opportunities and constraints of guided tissue and other forms of periodontal regeneration have been developed in painstakingly designed animal and clinical experiments, and the somewhat ailing implant dentistry has finally got a firm scientific foundation. Not least, a century-old suspicion that periodontal infections interact, in a bidirectional way, with other systemic diseases and conditions has been revived, and new intervention studies address the possible beneficial effects of periodontal therapy on general health.

The true revolution is, however, the application of well-defined evidence in daily practice. Despite the claim that, in particular, periodontists practice their profession up-to-date, dentists had long been inclined to pursue commercial interests, be it their own or those of providers of new and fancy developments.

That won't be so any longer. Since electronic search engines and, in particular, biomedical data bases are generally available, and electronic access to original articles including all back files is possible, new generations of practitioners will be in the position to quickly identify, critically assess, and filter the exploding amount of new data and retrieve relevant information as regards a specific clinical question or problem, both online and in real time. Dentists are more and more inclined to ask the crucial question, "Is there any evidence?"

The recent surge of systematic reviews of, in particular, well-designed intervention studies has proved that our profession has a sound scientific foundation. The available evidence has to be graded, though, and recommendations should address patient-relevant issues. Real evidence-based medicine does include a strong interpersonal relationship between the patient with chronic disease and the therapist. Thus, continuity of care and emphatic listening is of paramount importance for conjoint decision-making, which does not entirely rely on the available scientific evidence but, to a large extent, also on individual circumstances.

As before, the second edition of *Periodontology—The Essentials* attempts to condense latest developments and concepts in an easily searchable volume. Although undergraduate dentistry and dental hygienist students are again the main target audience for the compendium, general dental practitioners and specialists in other fields of dentistry may benefit from quickly checking specific periodontal details in their daily practice as well.

*Hans-Peter Mueller, DDS, PhD*

---

[1] Kornman KS, Robertson PB, Williams RC. The literature that shaped modern periodontology. J Periodontol 2014; 85: 3–9.

# 1 Anatomy and Physiology

The *periodontium* (from the Greek terms περι, around, and οδονσ, tooth) denotes the soft and hard tissues that anchor the teeth to the bones of the jaws, provide interdental linkage of the teeth within the dental arch, and facilitate epithelial lining of the oral cavity in the region of the erupted tooth.[1-3]

It is a developmental, biological, and functional unit that is comprised of four different types of tissue:

➤ Gingiva—that is, the marginal periodontium
➤ Root cementum
➤ Alveolar bone proper
➤ Periodontal ligament

The *gingiva*, a keratinized soft tissue, surrounds the tooth at the cervical level together with parts of the alveolar process. The *desmodontal fiber apparatus* connects the various mineralized forms of *root cementum*, which are in some ways similar to bone tissue, and the *alveolar bone proper*, which is part of the alveolar process.

The majority of fibers consist of collagen. They insert partly in the inner cortical plate of the alveolar bone and partly in root cementum. The fibers of the periodontal ligament are functionally oriented. During and after tooth eruption they undergo continuous renewal and remodeling, which is mainly controlled by fibroblasts. Those fibers, which are anchored either in root cementum or in alveolar bone proper, are called *Sharpey's fibers*. Oxytalan fiber bundles, which run parallel to the tooth axis, may also be observed. Their function is largely unknown.

## ■ Development

The development of the periodontium is essentially linked to tooth development (**Fig. 1.1**). The number and shape of the teeth are strictly genetically determined. Tooth development is initiated by epithelial thickening of the ectodermal epithelial lining of the primitive oral cavity (stomodeum) between the fifth and sixth week of embryogenesis. This odontogenic epithelium is called the dental plate or *dental lamina*. Originating from the dental lamina, tooth develop-

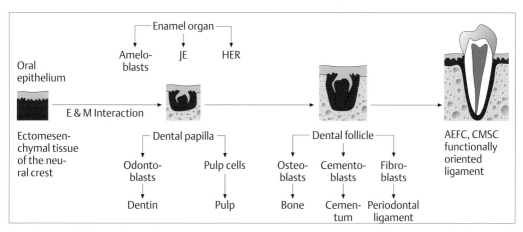

**Fig. 1.1 The development of the periodontium is part of tooth development.** Interactions between epithelium and ectomesenchymal tissue (E & M) of the neural crest beneath lead to the initiation of crown development (enamel, pulp, and dentin). Tissues of the periodontium proper (cementum, alveolar bone proper, periodontal ligament) derive from the dental follicle proper. Proliferation of Hertwig's epithelial root sheath (HER) leads to root formation. JE: junctional epithelium; AEFC: acellular extrinsic fiber cementum; CMSC: cellular mixed stratified cementum. (Adapted from MacNeil and Somerman.[4])

ment is controlled by a chain of cell–cell and cell–matrix interactions. Both ectodermal and ectomesenchymal cells reach increasingly higher degrees of differentiation and eventually develop into highly differentiated ameloblasts and odontoblasts which produce enamel matrix and predentin.

### Crown Development

Between weeks 6 and 8 after ovulation, cells of the dental lamina proliferate in distinct regions (the later positions of deciduous teeth) into the mesenchymal tissue beneath. They induce a condensation of the ectomesenchymal tissue, which derives from the neural crest. This tissue is now called *determinate dental mesenchyme*.

During morphogenesis of the tooth germ, the *tooth bud* develops between the 8th and 12th weeks into the *caplike enamel organ*. The odontogenic mesenchyme divides into two cell lines:
➤ The *dental papilla*, containing progenitor cells of odontoblasts and later the pulp.
➤ The *dental follicle*, which surrounds the tooth germ and develops into the periodontium.

Cells of the enamel organ differentiate into four cytologically and functionally defined strata:
➤ Outer enamel epithelium
➤ Stratum reticulare
➤ Stratum intermedium
➤ Inner enamel epithelium

Finally, the *bell stage* of the tooth germ develops, which already gives an indication of the later shape of the crown. The enamel–dentin border is defined when odontoblasts and later ameloblasts differentiate and start, in the region of the later cusps and incisal edges of the teeth, secreting predentin and enamel matrix, respectively. The dental papilla and enamel organ are surrounded by the dental follicle, which demarcates the dental papilla from the surrounding mesenchyme.

During further odontogenesis the dental lamina of the deciduous molars proliferates distally and becomes committed to the development of the molars of the permanent dentition, which therefore belong to the first dentition.

The tooth germs of the permanent first molars arise between the 13th and 15th week of embryogenesis. The germs of succedaneous teeth arise between the 5th prenatal (central incisors) and 10th postnatal months (second premolars), and develop from an apically prolonged secondary dental lamina lingually and palatally to the deciduous germs.

### Root Development

Root formation starts when dentin and enamel formation reaches the connection between inner and outer enamel epithelium, viz. the later cementoenamel junction. The final shape of the crown has now been determined.

Due to further proliferation of the enamel epithelium, an epithelial root sheath (*Hertwig's root sheath*) develops, which is located between the dental papilla and the dental follicle proper:
➤ Apically, it bends inwards to form the epithelial diaphragm.
➤ The double-layered epithelium (outer and inner stratum) is responsible for differentiation of root dentin-forming odontoblasts.
➤ It thus represents the "mold" for the later tooth root.

Tooth eruption depends on the prolongation of the dentinal tube, while the diaphragm remains in the same location. Coronally, Hertwig's epithelial root sheath loses contact with the root surface. The sheath disintegrates into a loose mesh of epithelial strands, namely the epithelial rests of Malassez.

### Cementogenesis

In contrast to the inner enamel epithelium of the enamel organ, the inner enamel epithelium of Hertwig's root sheath does not differentiate into enamel-producing ameloblasts:
➤ Cell–cell interactions lead to differentiation of cells of the neighboring ectomesenchymal tissue of the dental papilla into odontoblasts, which start forming predentin.
➤ Immediately afterwards an enamel-like material is deposited on the surface of predentin.
➤ This material probably induces differentiation of cementoblasts derived from the dental follicle and mediates anchorage of the cementum to the dentin surface.

Following disintegration of the epithelial root sheath, cells of the dental follicle proper come into contact with the newly formed root surface (cell–matrix interaction). They then start formation of root cementum (**Fig. 1.2**). Cells and fiber bundles of the periodontal ligament and alveolar bone proper are also derived from cells of the dental follicle proper.

These traditional views of cementogenesis have been challenged[5]:

➤ The presence of mesenchymal cells among disintegrated cells of Hertwig's epithelial root sheath is usually interpreted as a sign of cell migration from the dental follicle proper towards the root surface.
➤ Alternatively, cells of the root sheet may have completed epithelial–mesenchymal transformation.
➤ Thus, cementoblasts may originate from Hertwig's epithelial root sheath itself.

In multirooted teeth, shortly after dentin and enamel formation have commenced in the cusp region, two or three epithelial knots are formed in the region of the cervical loop of the enamel epithelium.

➤ Tongues of epithelium proliferate across the dental papilla in a central direction.
➤ While the size of the enamel organ increases, these epithelial tongues meet and fuse in the region of the future fornix of the furcation.

➤ In this way, the future dentin floor of the furcation is created.
➤ This means that the formation of the furcation is part of crown development.

The epithelial root sheath initiates the formation of tooth roots. It determines their shape. In case of multirooted teeth it divides into two or three branching tubes. The presence of enamel epithelium also explains frequent formation of *enamel paraplasias* in the furcation area, such as enamel projections, enamel tongues, and enamel pearls.

Epithelial tongues lie within the connective tissue of the dental papilla and exclude parts of ectomesenchymal tissue from the developing tooth germ. That is why *cementum deposits* (ridges and bulges) are frequently found in the region of fusing epithelial tongues.

## Marginal Periodontium

The epithelial part of the gingiva is of ectodermal origin. Three epithelia can be distinguished:

➤ Junctional epithelium
➤ Oral sulcular epithelium
➤ Oral gingival epithelium

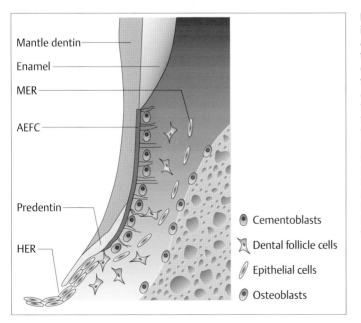

Mantle dentin

Enamel

MER

AEFC

Predentin

HER

◉ Cementoblasts

▱ Dental follicle cells

⬦ Epithelial cells

◎ Osteoblasts

**Fig. 1.2  Traditional view of the initial stages of formation of acellular extrinsic fiber cementum (AEFC).** Fibroblasts of the dental follicle come into contact with predentin in the region of the apical edge after disintegration of the epithelial root sheet, where they attach and, after differentiation into cementoblasts, start to produce collagen fibrils. This results in an initial fiber fringe with maximum fiber density. The mineralization front reaches the base of the fibers and proceeds into the initial fiber fringe. MER: Malassez epithelial rests. (Adapted from MacNeil and Somerman.[4])

The *junctional epithelium* derives from the reduced enamel epithelium which surrounds, in a preeruptive stage, the tooth crown. The reduced enamel epithelium consists of:
➤ ameloblasts, which are reduced in height,
➤ cells of the previous stratum intermedium of the enamel epithelium.

The epithelium attaches to the enamel in a form of *primary epithelial attachment* by hemi-desmosomes. During tooth eruption, reduced enamel epithelium gradually transforms, from coronal to apical, into junctional epithelium (*secondary epithelial attachment*):
➤ Reduced cuboid ameloblasts change shape and become elongated cells of junctional epithelium.
➤ The cells of stratum intermedium regain their ability to divide and become basal cells of junctional epithelium.

Posteruptively, junctional epithelium is a self-renewing tissue with specific structures and functions. In addition, de novo formation of junctional epithelium is facilitated:
➤ Following, for example, a gingivectomy procedure (see Chapter 11), cells of oral gingival epithelium migrate first to the dentogingival region.
➤ Influenced by the underlying connective tissue (i.e., the periodontal ligament), these cells develop characteristics of junctional epithelium:
  – Stratified, two-layered epithelium
  – No keratinization
  – Ability to attach to the tooth surface

## ■ Macroscopic and Microscopic Anatomy

### Oral Mucosa

Traditionally, oral mucosa is classified according to function as lining, specialized, and masticatory mucosa.[6]
  The nonkeratinized *lining mucosa* comprises alveolar mucosa, the mucosa of the oral vestibule, the cheeks and lips, the floor of the mouth and ventral sides of the tongue, and the mucosa of the soft palate. The lining mucosa has a stratified, three-layered epithelium consisting of:

➤ Stratum basale
➤ Stratum filamentosum
➤ Stratum distendum

The lining mucosa contains a distinctive submucosa with a loose arrangement of collagen and elastic fibers.
  The *specialized mucosa* of the dorsum of the tongue mediates touch, temperature, and taste sensations.
  The keratinized *masticatory mucosa* comprises the gingiva and the mucosa of the hard palate:
➤ Gingiva surrounds the teeth at the cementoenamel junction and the alveolar bone and extends to the mucogingival border. Palatally, it consists of a small rim, which continues into the mucosa of the hard palate.
➤ The structural characteristics of the gingival epithelium are essentially the same as those of the mucosa of the hard palate:
  – Gingiva possesses a nonhomogeneous stratum corneum of variable thickness, in which most cells contain a pyknotic nucleus, a sign of *parakeratinization*.
  – Mucosa of the hard palate possesses a regularly *orthokeratinized* epithelium with a uniformly thick stratum corneum without pyknotic cell nuclei.
  – The epithelium of both the gingiva and the mucosa of the hard palate is about 0.3 mm thick, on average.

### Gingiva

Clinically, a healthy gingiva is characterized by certain features of shape, color, and consistency (**Fig. 1.3**):
➤ Its narrow band follows the *scalloped contour* of the necks of the teeth and the cementoenamel junction, which is normally covered by gingival tissue. This gives rise to distinct interdental papillae, their vestibular and oral parts being connected by a saddle-like interdental *col*.
➤ Gingiva of individuals with a northern European heritage is usually pale pink, coral, or mauve in color. In Mediterranean, African, and Asian populations, melanocytes may give a more or less dark color to the gingiva (**Fig. 1.3b**).
➤ Orange-peel-type *stippling* of the surface of the attached gingiva results from indenta-

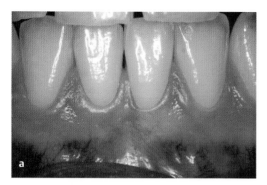 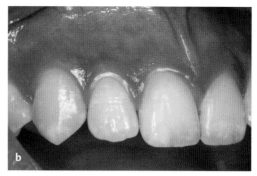

**Fig. 1.3   Clinical characteristics of healthy gingiva.**
**a** Note clinical signs of slight inflammation (cf. Chapter 6) as redness, swelling, and gingival exudate mesio-buccally at tooth 31.
**b** Melanin pigmentation of attached gingiva of a southern European individual.

tions lying at the crossing points of rete ridges of the oral gingival epithelium.
➤ A frequently observed *gingival groove* separates the free gingiva, which adheres to the enamel surface, from the attached gingiva. The free gingiva ends 1 to 2 mm on the enamel surface at a narrow angle.
➤ A small depression at the tooth surface of 0.1 to 0.5 mm is called the gingival sulcus:
  – The sulcus is bordered by the tooth surface, the oral sulcular epithelium, and the junctional epithelium.
  – *Note*: The depth of the gingival sulcus cannot be determined clinically, for example, by using a periodontal probe (see Chapter 6).
➤ The *mucogingival border* demarcates the gingiva apically.

Histologically, three different epithelia may be differentiated:
➤ *Oral gingival epithelium* on the outer surface of the free and attached gingiva.
➤ *Oral sulcular epithelium*, lateral to the gingival sulcus.
➤ Nonkeratinized *junctional epithelium*, which is located at the inner surface of the free gingiva covering enamel and, in certain situations, root cementum.

Oral sulcular epithelium and oral gingival epithelium are keratinized, stratified, four-layered epithelia (**Fig. 1.4a**) comprised of:
➤ Stratum basale
➤ Stratum spinosum
➤ Stratum granulosum
➤ Stratum corneum

Oral gingival epithelium always contains certain nonepithelial cells:
➤ Melanocytes
➤ Antigen-presenting Langerhans cells
➤ Merkel cells, which operate as sensory mechanoreceptors for touch and pressure reception
➤ Small lymphocytes, especially cytotoxic T cells, and to a minor extent T helper cells (see Chapter 3)

Junctional epithelium is not keratinized. It consists of two strata:
➤ Stratum basale
➤ Stratum suprabasale

Oral gingival epithelium and oral sulcular epithelium are as much as 70 to 80% *parakeratinized*; that is, pyknotic cell nuclei are still found in the stratum corneum. In 20 to 30% of cases, the attached gingiva is *orthokeratinized* (**Fig. 1.4a**); that is, the densely packed horny scales do not contain cell nuclei.

Junctional epithelium facilitates epithelial lining of the oral cavity during and after tooth eruption. The mechanism by which junctional epithelium is attached to different structures of the tooth surface (enamel, cementum, dental cuticle) or implant surfaces is mediated by an *internal basal lamina* consisting of glycoproteins and collagen, and *hemidesmosomes*.

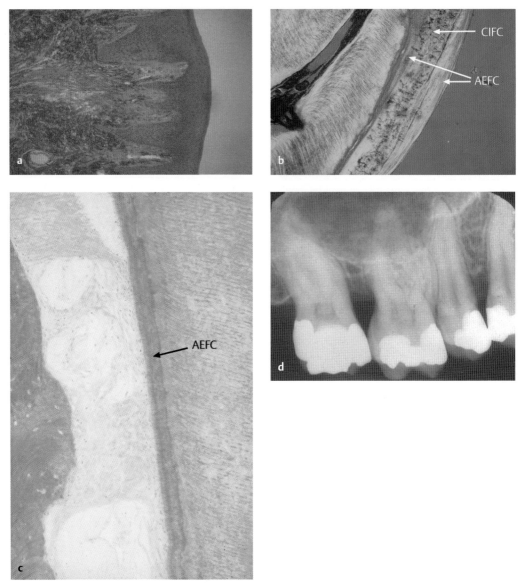

**Fig. 1.4 Tissues of the periodontium.**
**a** Lamina propria (to left) and oral gingival epithelium with stratum basale, stratum spinosum, stratum granulosum, and stratum corneum. In this case, the epithelium is orthokeratinized.
**b** Cellular mixed stratified fiber cementum with layers of cellular intrinsic fiber cementum (CIFC) and acellular extrinsic fiber cementum (AEFC), which covers the surface.
**c** Periodontal ligament between the alveolar bone proper and AEFC.
**d** Alveolar bone proper appears on radiographs as lamina dura (e.g., mesial surface of tooth 17).

**Table 1.1** Composition of the supra-alveolar fiber apparatus of the lamina propria

| Primary fiber apparatus | Secondary fiber apparatus |
|---|---|
| Dentogingival fibers | Transgingival fibers |
| Dentoperiosteal fibers | Intergingival fibers |
| Alveologingival fibers | Interpapillary fibers |
| Circular fibers | Periosteal-gingival fibers |
| Transseptal fibers | Intercircular fibers |
| | Semicircular fibers |

Apart from epithelium, gingiva consists of a firm fibrous connective tissue, the lamina propria. There is no submucosa. The supra-alveolar fiber apparatus of the lamina propria is composed of primary and secondary fibers (**Table 1.1**). The fibers of the secondary fiber apparatus connect primary fiber bundles.

**Peri-implant Mucosa**

The peri-implant mucosa is attached to the surface of titanium implants in two ways:
➤ An epithelial barrier about 2 mm long, which adheres to the implant by hemidesmosomes, corresponding to the junctional epithelium.
➤ Apically, a 1 to 1.5 mm wide zone of fibrous connective tissue can be found. Collagen fibers run *parallel to the implant surface* and insert partly in the periosteum of the alveolar bone.

In the connective tissue, two zones can be differentiated:
➤ A fibroblast-rich zone with few vessels, about 40 µm wide, which is in direct contact with the implant surface.
➤ Laterally, a zone with few cells and dense collagen fibers and more vessels is seen.

Since a periodontal ligament is missing, blood supply is exclusively facilitated by larger supra-periosteal vessels.[7]

**Root Cementum**

Root cementum originates pre-eruptively during root development and throughout life after completion of root growth.[3] Formation of cementum is effected by daughter cells of the ectomesenchymal cells of the dental follicle:
➤ Cementoblasts
➤ Cementocytes
➤ Fibroblasts

Various kinds of root cementum have been described depending on histological features and function (**Table 1.2**):
➤ *Acellular afibrillar cementum* (AAC) is found only on enamel, as tongues or islands, when enamel has come into contact with connective tissue after conclusion of crown development. Its function, if any, is unknown.
➤ The laminar *acellular extrinsic fiber cementum* (AEFC), thickness 20 to 250 µm, is found in the cervical and middle third of the root:
– AEFC consists of densely packed (30,000/mm²), perpendicularly oriented collagen fiber bundles (Sharpey's fibers), each about 4 µm thick.
– Fibers extend into the periodontal ligament and connect the root with the alveolar bone.
– AEFC is produced first by fibroblasts of the dental follicle proper and is thus of ectomesenchymal origin (**Fig. 1.2**).
– Later it is produced by fibroblasts of the periodontal ligament.
– *Note*: AEFC is committed entirely to anchorage of the tooth in its socket.
➤ *Cellular intrinsic fiber cementum* (CIFC) is a product of cementoblasts of the dental follicle proper, the later periodontal ligament:
– CIFC contains cementocytes.
– Collagen fibers run circularly or helically around the root, that is, parallel to the root surface. CIFC does not contain Sharpey's fibers.
– CIFC is repair cementum, but it also forms part of the cellular mixed stratified cementum (CMSC).
➤ *Cellular mixed stratified cementum* (CMSC) is a stratified tissue with alternate layers of AEFC and CIFC/AIFC (**Fig. 1.4b**):
– It is inhomogeneously mineralized, partly porous, and of variable thickness (100 to >600 µm).

**Table 1.2** Different forms of human root cementum. (Adapted from Schroeder[3])

| Type of cementum | Abbreviation | Organic components | Localization | Function |
|---|---|---|---|---|
| Acellular afibrillar cementum | AAC | Homogeneous matrix, no cells, no fibers | At the cemento-enamel junction, on enamel | Unknown |
| Acellular extrinsic fiber cementum | AEFC | Collagen fibrils (Sharpey's fibers), no cells | Cervical up to the middle of the root | Tooth anchoring |
| Cellular intrinsic fiber cementum | CIFC | Intrinsic collagen fibers, cementocytes | Apical and interradicular root surfaces, resorption lacunae, fracture lines | Adaptation, repair |
| Acellular intrinsic fiber cementum | AIFC | Intrinsic collagen fibers, no cells | Apical and interradicular root surfaces | Adaptation |
| Cellular mixed stratified cementum (AEFC + CIFC/AIFC) | CMSC | Intrinsic collagen fibers and collagen fibers as Sharpey's fibers, cementocytes | Apical and interradicular root surfaces | Adaptation, tooth anchoring |

– CMSC is mainly found in the apical third of the root and the furcation area of multi-rooted teeth.
– It is committed to functional adaptation, that is, dynamic change of the outer shape of the root during movements of the tooth, mesial shift, and occlusal drift.
– If it is covered by AEFC, it anchors the tooth in its socket.
– Infrequently, *acellular intrinsic fiber cementum* (AIFC) is found in CMSC.

**Periodontal Ligament**

The periodontal ligament is a cell- and fiber-rich, firm connective tissue which anchors the tooth via root cementum and alveolar bone proper in its socket (**Fig. 1.4c**)[3]:
➤ Developmentally, it derives from ecto-mesenchymal cells of the dental follicle proper.
➤ The periodontal space is narrower in the middle of the root (0.12–0.17 mm) than at the alveolar crest (0.17–0.23 mm) or the tooth apex (0.16–0.24 mm). Higher values are found in adolescents and lower values in older adults.
➤ Functional strain may lead to a widening of the periodontal space and increasing thickness of collagen fiber bundles.

Desmodontal fiber bundles have been described as supracrestal, horizontal, oblique, interradicu-lar, and apical fibers. Cellular elements of the periodontal ligament are:
➤ Fibroblasts
➤ Cementoblasts and dentoclasts
➤ Osteoblasts and osteoclasts
➤ Epithelial cells (Malassez rests)
➤ Immune defense cells and neurovascular elements

The periodontal ligament is heavily vascularized. Blood supply is facilitated via:
➤ the gingival plexus of postcapillary venules, and
➤ a desmodontal blood vessel basket comprised of lateral branches of the alveolar and infraorbital arteries in the maxilla, and the lingual and mental arteries in the mandible.

Lymph vessels form a dense, basketlike network, which anastomoses with lymph vessels of the gingiva and septa of the alveolar bone.
Both sensory and autonomic nerve fibers are found:
➤ Somatosensory, afferent fibers reach the periodontal ligament as terminal branches of the dental nerve. Some of them appear apically as lateral branches of the dental nerve whereas others pass through foramina and the cribriform lamina.
➤ Free nerve endings of sensory fibers are responsible for *pain perception*.

> Ruffini-like endings are *mechanoreceptors* for proprioceptive stimuli, that is, pressure. Pressure sensitivity is extraordinarily refined.
> Nonmyelinated *sympathetic fibers* are responsible for the local regulation of desmodontal vessels.

## Alveolar Bone Proper

Deriving from cells of the dental follicle, the alveolar bone proper is also of ectomesenchymal origin.[3] On radiographs it appears as *lamina dura* (**Fig. 1.4d**). Alveolar bone proper contains *Sharpey's fibers*, which are connected to fibers of the periodontal ligament.

Alveolar bone may be absent on the vestibular aspects of teeth positioned prominently in the jaw. This condition is termed *fenestration* if marginal bone is present and *dehiscensce* if marginal bone is missing.

Three cell types may be distinguished:
> *Osteoblasts*: a mixed population composed of preodontoblasts with large nuclei and fibroblastlike cells with small nuclei and desmodontal progenitor cells of osteoblasts.
> *Osteocytes*, which arise from osteoblasts and become entrapped in their own product, namely bone. Osteocytes are located in bony lacunae and are connected by long cell projections. Young osteocytes are smaller than osteoblasts but have a similar structure. Older osteocytes have a reduced set of organelles.
> *Osteoclasts* are multinucleated giant cells, which are located in surface pits of the bone (Howship's lacunae). They arise by fusion of hematopoietic, mononuclear precursor cells of bone marrow. An organelle-poor, brushlike cytoplasmatic border consisting of microvilli is characteristic. Resorption of bone is facilitated by acidic phosphatases and other hydrolytic enzymes.

## ■ Physiology

Soft (gingiva, periodontal ligament) and hard tissues (root cementum, alveolar bone proper) of the periodontium are committed to various tasks:
> Anchoring of the teeth in their bony sockets
> Keeping teeth together within the jaw as a dental arch

> Adaptation to functional and topographic alterations
> Enabling change in tooth position
> Repair of the effects of traumatic injury
> Maintenance of the epithelial lining of the oral cavity
> Provision of peripheral defense mechanisms against infection
> Perception of pain and pressure, sensing of touch

## Turnover Rates

In *junctional epithelium*, the ratio between the basal cell area and the area of exfoliation results in an extremely high tissue turnover.[3] It is 50 to 100 times higher than for oral gingival epithelium.

Tissue turnover of *gingival connective tissue* is higher than that of dermis:
> Gingival fibroblasts synthesize larger amounts of new collagen than would be necessary for mature collagen replacement.
> The resulting excess seems to be available for tissue repair.

*Cementogenesis*:
> Formation of AEFC is extremely slow. In humans, thickening amounts to about 0.005 to 0.01 µm per day.
> Initial CIFC is formed considerably faster (0.4–3.1 µm per day). Further layers are built up at a rate of 0.1 to 0.5 µm per day, which is still faster than AEFC.
> Growth rates are comparable with those of crown and root dentin, and growth is only slightly slower than the growth of alveolar bone proper.

The turnover rate of the *periodontal ligament* is about twice that of the gingiva and four times that of the dermis. There is a marked capacity for tissue remodeling. Tissue turnover keeps the structural organization of the tissue constant. During *remodeling*, an adaptation of the three-dimensional organization of the desmodontal fiber apparatus to an altered position or functional strain occurs:
> Both processes are accompanied by decomposition and synthesis of collagen fibers and are at times indistinguishable.
> Collagen is removed by *phagocytosing fibroblasts*.

➤ Physiological rates of renewal and removal of collagen fibers are balanced.
➤ Physiologic forces during chewing stimulate these processes. During aging, turnover decreases.

Bony remodeling occurs in the *alveolar process* during growth of the jaw, eruption of the teeth, and during tooth replacement. Apposition of bone predominates:
➤ Growth starts from periosteum and endosteum.
➤ The renewal rate seems to be higher than in other bones.
➤ Remodeling of the alveolar bone proper commences with the tooth's functional period, as soon as it comes into occlusal contact with the antagonist.
➤ Occlusal forces are transferred to the bone by the periodontal ligament.
➤ The direction, frequency, duration, and magnitude of the forces largely determine the extent and rate of remodeling.

The complicated post-eruptive tooth movement is characterized by an oblique tilting with a vertical and horizontal component:
➤ Occlusal drift
➤ Mesial migration
➤ Eruption following extraction of the antagonist

### Defense Mechanism

The gingiva is protected against mechanical, thermal, and chemical injury by the firm consistency of the supra-alveolar fiber apparatus and keratinization of the oral gingival epithelium.

In most circumstances, specific compartments of the peripheral host defense of the gingiva efficiently prohibit bacterial invasion of the dentogingival region (see Chapter 3):
➤ Protection against bacterial infection is provided by both the epithelial and connective tissue components of the gingiva.

➤ Although junctional epithelium does not keratinize, its extreme turnover rate and the presence of resident leukocytes make it relatively resistant to bacterial invasion.
➤ The lamina propria of the gingiva provides cellular and humoral components of the immune system.
➤ Particularly in young individuals, inflammatory cell infiltrates in the gingiva provide some protection against periodontal destruction.

### Possibilities of Repair

Replantation or transplantation of teeth is only successful if cells and fibers of the periodontal ligament on the root surface and the inner surface of the alveolar socket are maintained. Otherwise, ankylosis and/or root resorption will occur. Reparative replacement of desmodontal fibers is carried out by cell populations of the periodontal ligament. The regenerative potential is, however, essentially limited[8]:
➤ Reparative, cellular intrinsic fiber cementum may be formed rapidly during wound healing.
➤ However, this bonelike type of cementum should probably not be regarded as odontogenic tissue.
➤ The true tissues of the tooth-supporting apparatus (i.e., alveolar bone proper, periodontal ligament, acellular extrinsic fiber cementum) all derive from the dental follicle proper, which has its origin in the ectomesenchymal tissue of the neural crest. Differentiation during odontogenesis is dependent on a cascade of genetic signals and growth factors.
➤ Regeneration of the tooth-supporting apparatus in the proper sense of restoration of the normal tissue architecture should therefore not be expected.
➤ *Note*: The mere reparative deposition of cellular cementum has no functional relevance.

# 2 Periodontal Microbiology

## ■ Ecology of the Mouth

### Biodiversity

Whereas the human body consists of about 10 trillion somatic cells ($10^{13}$), 10 times more microorganisms,[1] about 100 trillion ($10^{14}$), colonize the different surfaces of skin, mucous membranes of the oral cavity, the gastrointestinal tract (the vast majority), respiratory and genitourinary tracts, as well as the teeth, dental implants, and dental prostheses.

Currently, the Human Oral Microbiome Database (HOMD) consists of 16S rRNA gene sequences (see below) of more than 700 different taxa of oral bacteria.[2]

➤ Taxa have been assigned to 14 phyla.

➤ About 66% of these taxa have been cultivated in recent years.
➤ For comparison, the proportion of cultivable taxa is less than 1% in most other natural habitats.[3]

More is to be expected.[4] About twice as many taxa could already be identified in the oral cavity. After validation probably more than 400 new taxa will soon be added to the HOMD.[5] The composition of the flora of, in particular, a visceral cavity (e.g., gastrointestinal, genitourinary and respiratory tracts, oral cavity) is remarkably specific:

➤ Between 500 and 1,000 different taxa have been described in the gastrointestinal tract.[6]
➤ However, few (<10%) have been found in both gastrointestinal tract and oral cavity.

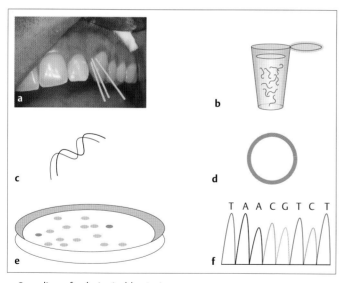

**Fig. 2.1 Cloning and sequencing of bacterial 16S rRNA genes.** Identification of cultivable and currently not cultivable bacterial species. (Modified after Leys et al,[7] courtesy of the American Society for Microbiology.)

**a** Sampling of subgingival bacteria.
**b** Isolating and denaturing DNA.
**c** Amplification of 16S rRNA gene with polymerase chain reaction (PCR).
**d** Ligation of 16S rRNA gene fragments in plasmids (vectors) of *Escherichia coli* and transfection into competent *E. coli* cells.
**e** Colonies of successfully transformed *E. coli* cells can be identified on agar plates.
**f** Sequencing of DNA of transformed cells; identification of inserts. Species identification in gene data banks (BLAST).

➤ Some oral bacteria (e. g., streptococci, *Veillonella* spp.), can be found in virtually all humans and do colonize most mucous membranes of the oral cavity.
➤ The majority of oral species, however, are very selective[8] and may colonize either periodontal pockets, the dorsum of the tongue, or carious lesions, for example.

By amplifying conserved and highly variable regions of 16S rRNA genes using the polymerase chain reaction (PCR), transferring amplicons to competent cells of *Escherichia coli* (cloning), and subsequently sequencing the respective DNA strands (**Fig. 2.1**, **Box 2.1**),[7] bacteria of the oral cavity have been presently assigned to 14 phyla (**Fig. 2.2** and **Table 2.1**).[5] Of special importance are:
➤ **Bacteroidetes**: Gram-negative bacteria of the genera *Prevotella, Bacteroides, Porphyromonas, Tannerella,* and *Capnocytophaga.*

➤ **Proteobacteria**: *Neisseria, Eikenella, Kingella, Aggregatibacter, Campylobacter*; all gram-negative.
➤ **Firmicutes**: Gram-positive bacteria; three classes:
– Bacilli-class: *Streptococcus, Lactobacillus, Staphylococcus, Gemella.*
– Clostridia-class: *Eubacterium, Parvimonas, Veillonella, Dialister, Selenomonas.*
– Erysipelotrichia: *Bulleidia extructa, Solobacterium moorei, Erysipelothrix tonsollarum, Lactobacillus* [XVII] *catenaformis.*
➤ **Tenericutes** (formerly class Mollicutes within the phylum **Firmicutes**): *Mycoplasma.*
➤ **Actinobacteria**: *Actinomyces, Rothia, Corynebacterium, Propionibacterium*; all gram-positive.
➤ **Fusobacteria**: *Fusobacterium, Leptotrichia*; gram-negative.
➤ **Spirochaetes**: All treponemes; gram-negative.

---

**Box 2.1 Basic principles of bacterial phylogenetics**

In order to compare and determine the phylogenetic similarities of different bacteria, whether or not they are currently cultivable, certain characteristics of genes may be used which decode ribosomal RNA.

After transcription of the genome by messenger (m)RNA, the genetic code is translated into an amino acid sequence on the ribosomes. Prokaryotes (for instance, bacteria) have 70S ribosomes, which consist of rRNA and protein. Each ribosome is composed of a large (50S) and a small (30S) subunit. The latter contains the specific 16S rRNA.

Since accurate transcription of the genetic code and its translation into the amino acid sequence (and, ultimately, the protein) is of utmost importance, a few crucial regions of ribosomal DNA are highly conserved, while less critical regions are variable. The presence of both highly conserved and variable regions enables differentiation at species level, so it is possible to distinguish similar species phylogenetically.

Highly conserved and variable regions are amplified by PCR and transferred via plasmid vectors into competent cells of *E. coli*. Subsequently, the respective DNA strands may be sequenced (**Fig. 2.1**).

Currently, more than 125,000 sequences of bacterial 16S rDNA can be called up in gene data banks. Unknown bacteria can thus be identified and compared with the sequences of known species. Highly conserved regions of different species are used to align the sequences in question. The number of differences in variable regions is then determined, which can be used in cluster analyses to construct a phylogenetic tree (**Fig. 2.2**) which displays evolutionary relationships graphically.

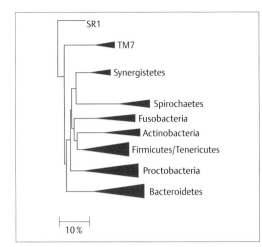

10 %

**Fig. 2.2 Phylogenetic tree of 10 of the 14 currently identified different bacterial phyla of the oral cavity.** (After Paster et al,[3] modified after Dewhirst et al[5]; courtesy of the American Society for Microbiology.) In phyla TM7 (Saccharibacteria) and SR1 so far no cultivable organisms were detected. Other phyla with very few phylotypes in the oral cavity (< 1%) are Chlamydia, Chloroflexi, GN02 and Euryarchaeota.

## The Oral Cavity as a Biotope

In order to describe a certain biotope, the following terms may be used:
➤ *Habitat*—a place where bacteria grow. Different bacteria form a bacterial community.
➤ *Ecosystem*—microbes in their environment.
➤ *Niche*—function of a bacterium in its habitat. Different bacteria compete for the same niche.
➤ *Resident flora*—microorganisms which are commonly found in a habitat. Equivalent terms are normal flora or commensals.
➤ *Opportunistic infection*—under certain circumstances, commensals can cause disease.

The oral cavity is a unique, complex *biotope* in the organism. Hard structures (teeth, dental implants) interrupt the mucosal lining. Teeth provide widely differing *ecosystems* which allow colonization by specific bacteria:
➤ Pits and fissures
➤ Smooth surfaces
➤ Cervical region of the teeth

**Table 2.1** Some bacteria in the predominant phyla (bold) and genera in the oral cavity (after Dewhirst et al[5]). Taxa in further phyla belong to Synergistetes, Chlamydiae, Chloroflexi, TM7 (Saccharibacteria), SR1, GN02, and (within Archaea) Euryarchaeota

| Firmicutes* | | Teneri-cutes** | Proteo-bacteria | Actino-bacteria | Fuso-bacteria | Bactero-idetes | Spiro-chaetes |
|---|---|---|---|---|---|---|---|
| **Bacilli** | **Chlostridia** | | | | | | |
| Strepto-coccus | Eubacterium | Myco-plasma | Neisseria | Actinomyces | Fusobac-terium | Prevotella | Treponema |
| Lacto-bacillus | Mogibac-terium | | Kingella | Rothia | Lepto-trichia | Bacteroides | |
| Entero-coccus | Peptostrepto-coccus | | Eikenella | Coryne-bacterium | | Porphyro-monas | |
| Abiotrophia | Parvimonas | | Haemo-philus | Propioni-bacterium | | Tannerella | |
| Granulica-tella | Peptococcus | | Aggregati-bacter | Bifido-bacterium | | Capnocyto-phaga | |
| Gemella | Catonella | | Entero-bacter | Atopobium | | | |
| | Veillonella | | Desul-fovibrio | | | | |
| | Dialister | | Desulfo-bacter | | | | |
| | Selenomonas | | Campylo-bacter | | | | |

* Phylum Firmicutes includes, apart from classes Bacilli and Clostridia, the class Erysipelotrichia with four species.
** Former class Mollicutes within the phylum Firmicutes.

➤ Root canal system
➤ Carious dentin

Further ecosystems, each with a special flora, include:
➤ Periodontal pockets
➤ Dorsum of the tongue
➤ Tonsils

The various habitats are colonized by very different bacterial communities[8,9]:
➤ Buccal mucosa: *Streptococcus mitis, Gemella haemolysans*
➤ Dorsum of the tongue: *S. mitis, Streptococcus parasanguinis, Streptococcus salivarius, Granulicatella adiacens, G. haemolysans*
➤ Masticatory mucosa of the hard palate: *S. mitis, Streptococcus infantis, Granulicella elegans, G. haemolysans, Neisseria subflava*
➤ Palatal tonsils: *S. mitis, Granulicalla adiacens, G. haemolysans*; in some cases also *Prevotella* spp., *Porphyromonas* spp.
➤ Crown of the tooth: *Streptococcus sanguinis, Streptococcus gordonii, Streptococcus mutans, Actinomyces oris, Rothia dentocariosa, G. haemolysans, Granulicella adiacens.*
➤ Carious lesions: *Lactobacillus* spp.
➤ Subgingival region: Predominantly obligately anaerobic, gram-negative bacteria including spirochetes and motile rods
➤ Root canal system: Obligately anaerobic, gram-negative bacteria

*Note*: Changes in the ecosystem may have a considerable influence on bacterial populations and thus a decisive therapeutic effect. For instance:
➤ Subgingival administration of oxygen (e. g., by applying 3 % $H_2O_2$) may kill anaerobic bacteria.
➤ Complete pocket elimination of periodontal pockets by excision (see Chapter 11) may impede recolonization with anaerobic pathogens.
➤ Sealing of fissure systems, which establishes anaerobic conditions and prevents further supply of substrates, may render streptococci and lactobacilli metabolically inactive.

### Colonization Mechanisms

The oral cavity provides, for many bacteria, very comfortable living conditions[10]:
➤ Warm (about 36°C) and humid environment

➤ Frequent nutritional supply
➤ Solid surfaces to adhere to

On the other hand, host defense mechanisms may interfere with colonization. Bacteria must have certain capabilities if they are to establish themselves in the oral cavity:
➤ Various mechanical obstacles put up by the host have to be overcome:
  – Saliva flow
  – Gingival crevicular fluid flow, which is directed outwards from the gingival sulcus or periodontal pocket (see Chapter 3)
  – Epithelial desquamation
  – Self-cleansing during mastication
  – Personal oral hygiene
➤ Both the bacteria and the surface to be colonized are electronegatively charged. Protons (in an acidic environment) and other cations may bridge electrostatic forces.
➤ The adhesion of bacteria to the surface is mostly quite specific:
  – Lectinlike (i.e., proteins that recognize carbohydrate structures of the pellicle, see below) and hydrophobic adhesins react with complementary receptor molecules of the host surface.
  – Adhesins are located in threadlike pili or fimbriae, which can also bridge electrostatic forces and enable contact to the surface of the substrate.
➤ Secretory immunoglobulin A (sIgA) of the host and so-called agglutinins may recognize antigenic properties in fimbriae and specifically block them.
➤ Colonization of many bacteria further depends on:
  – Redox potential
  – Oxygen tension
  – Antagonisms and synergisms between microorganisms

### Biofilm Dental Plaque

Among different bacteria, a multitude of interactions may exist, for instance complex food webs, metabolic cooperation, etc. (**Fig. 2.3**). This might be the main reason for the organization of microorganisms of the dental surface in a highly complex biofilm:
➤ Note that biofilms comprise the typical bacterial population colonizing solid surfaces in a humid environment,[11] which can be

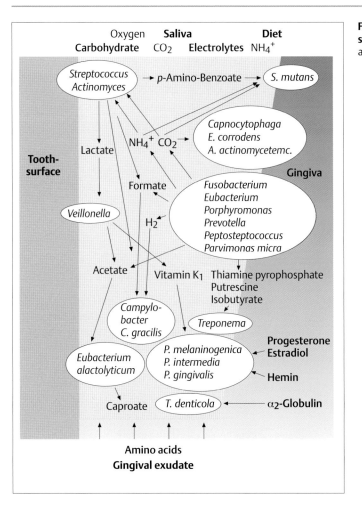

**Fig. 2.3 Bacterial interactions in subgingival biofilms.** (Modified after Carlsson.[10])

found, for example, on any object and on the ground beneath standing or flowing water or in any sewage installation.

➤ Extracellular structures of a multitude of very different bacteria, such as capsule polysaccharides or glycocalyx, surround the bacterial population as a *matrix*:

- It maintains the structure of the biofilm by formation of networked, cross-linked macromolecules. Biofilm bacteria are thus largely protected from external influences.
- Glycocalix facilitates survival and growth within the community.
- During periods of ceased nutrient supply, many bacteria can degrade exopolysaccharides.

➤ Another characteristic feature is defined microenvironments with different pH, oxygen tension, and redox potential.

➤ Bacteria may produce β-lactamase which cleaves the β-lactam ring of certain antibiotics; or catalase, or superoxide dismutases catalyzing dismutation of oxidizing ions released by phagocytes.

➤ A primitive *circulation system* supplies substrates and eliminates waste products and metabolites.

As compared to planktonic cultures where bacteria live individually in a fluid culture, bacterial communities in a biofilm (**Fig. 2.4**) exert remarkable properties,[12] which include:

➤ Close metabolic cooperation

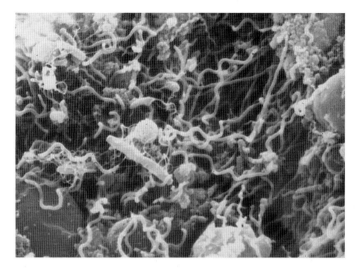

**Fig. 2.4 Scanning electron microscopic image of the dental biofilm.**

➤ A primitive communication system with exchange of genetic information[13]

➤ Resistance against phagocytosis and killing by neutrophil granulocytes, irrespective of presence of specific antibodies and complement.

➤ Resistance against antibiotics due to incorporation of bacteria in a matrix. *Note*: Minimum inhibitory concentrations (MICs) are determined for bacteria living in a planktonic environment. More realistic *minimum biofilm eradication concentrations* may be 100 or even up to 1,000 times higher.

➤ Accumulation of signaling compounds may mediate a sort of communication, so-called quorum sensing. For instance, gene expression for antibiotic resistance may be activated after reaching a certain threshold level of respective molecules (quorum cell density).

In general, as a community, the capacity for increased pathogenicity might be drastically increased. Examples of biofilm-associated body infections, which are often serious, are:

➤ Catheter infection

➤ Infectious endocarditis in patients with prosthetic heart valves

➤ Infection of artificial joints

➤ Conjunctivitis in patients wearing contact lenses

In particular, dental caries, periodontal disease, peri-implantitis and denture stomatitis are typical biofilm (i.e., plaque-induced) infections (see Chapter 13), which are characterized by delayed onset and a chronic course. Causative agents are endogenous microorganisms. *Note*: Localization of bacterial masses more or less outside of the host organism essentially determine the treatment:

➤ Mechanical disruption of the biofilm

➤ Adjunctive use of antiseptics

➤ Changes in the ecosystem

## Formation of Supragingival Plaque

With the commencement of plaque formation, that is, aggregation of bacteria on the tooth surface, microorganisms of the oral cavity may become pathogenic. Within minutes up to two hours of undisturbed plaque formation, an organic deposition of glycoproteins from the saliva is formed on the tooth surface and other hard structures of the oral cavity, the so-called *acquired pellicle*. On this pellicle, pioneer bacteria are seen after about four hours[10]:

➤ Streptococci, especially *Streptococcus mitis*, *S. sanguinis*, and *S. oralis*

➤ Small proportions of gram-positive rods such as *Actinomyces oris*. These plaque bacteria adhere loosely to start with but soon become firmly attached.

➤ Interestingly, most of the bacteria that adhere first to the pellicle are dead.

The primary adhesion of *Streptococcus mutans* onto the acquired pellicle is partly due to lectin-

like adhesins binding to α-galactoside receptors of salivary glycoproteins.
➤ Subsequent production of extracellular glucans promotes further accumulation of these bacteria.
➤ Dental plaque is stabilized by *extracellular polysaccharides*, in particular the extremely insoluble 1,3-α-glucan (mutan), which are synthesized by *S. mutans, S. sanguinis, S. oralis,* and *Streptococcus salivarius.*
➤ *Aggregations* between streptococci and *Actinomyces* spp. are particularly important for further plaque formation.
➤ Salivary bacteria colonize the plaque surface, while bacteria that are only loosely attached are washed away.
➤ Irregularities of the tooth surface are preferentially colonized and rapidly leveled.
➤ With a generation time of about 1 to 2 hours, the main reason for increase of plaque mass during the first 24 hours is bacterial proliferation.[14]

If plaque is allowed to further accumulate undisturbed, its composition becomes more complex[15]:
➤ The proportions of streptococci decrease while proportions of facultative or obligate anaerobic *Actinomyces* spp. increase.
➤ Among gram-negative bacteria, *Veillonella* spp. predominate.
➤ Gram-negative anaerobic rods of the genera *Fusobacterium, Prevotella,* and *Porphyromonas* appear in small proportions in supragingival flora. Note: *Fusobacterium nucleatum* plays a key role in dental biofilm formation because of its multigeneric coaggregation properties.[13]
➤ After about one week of undisturbed plaque growth, *spirochetes* and *motile rods* may be observed in plaque.

Thus, plaque formation and its maturation go through four phases:
➤ Minutes to two hours: Pellicle formation (specific adsorption of salivary glycoproteins).
➤ First day: Gram-positive (*Streptococcus mitis, S. sanguinis, S. oralis*) and gram-negative cocci (*Veillonella parvula, Neisseria mucosa*) and rods (*Actinomyces odontolyticus, A. viscosus, A. oris*). Extracellular polysaccharide production (e.g., mutan: 1,3-α-glu-

can) of *S. mutans.* Leveling of surface irregularities.
➤ Second to fourth day: Decrease of streptococci, increase of *Actinomyces* spp., gramnegative cocci and rods.
➤ After one week: Spirochetes and motile rods.

## Colonization of the Subgingival Region

Deepening of the sulcus as well as edematous swelling of the gingiva, as a response to supragingival plaque accumulation, ultimately leads to formation of a subgingival space. Later this space may further increase when junctional epithelium proliferates apically as the result of loss of connective tissue attachment.

As mentioned above, cloning in *Escherichia coli* and subsequent sequencing of 16S rDNA (**Box 2.1**) has revealed that the oral cavity is colonized by more than 700 different bacterial species, many of which are currently not yet cultivable. Most periodontal pathogens of the subgingival region are gram-negative and obligately anaerobic. Some exceptions are grampositive *Parvimonas micra* (formerly *Micromonas micra, Peptostreptococcus micros*), *Streptococcus intermedius* and *Eubacterium* spp. as well as facultative anaerobic *Aggregatibacter* (formerly *Actinobacillus*) *actinomycetemcomitans, Eikenella corrodens,* and *Capnocytophaga* spp. (**Table 2.1**).

The subgingival region provides comfortable conditions for many bacteria,[10] which are very different from those found in supragingival areas:
➤ Bacteria are protected from oral hygiene measures and saliva flow. This results in selective colonization of bacteria that are not able to adhere on solid surfaces— in particular, spirochetes and motile rods.
➤ Gingival exudate contains nutrients and essential growth factors for numerous periodontal pathogens:
 – Amino and fatty acids as energy source.
 – α₂-globulin is essential for *Treponema denticola.*
 – Hemin, iron, and vitamin K, which are all essential for the black-pigmenting, gramnegative anaerobes of the genera *Prevotella* and *Porphyromonas.*
 – *Prevotella intermedia, P. nigrescens* and members of the *P. melaninogenica* group

can substitute vitamin K for steroid hormones such as estradiol and progesterone. For that reason, an excessive increase of these microorganisms in gingival pockets is often observed during pregnancy, possibly leading to so-called *pregnancy gingivitis.*

➤ Favorable conditions for obligately anaerobic bacteria in deep periodontal pockets include a low redox potential and low oxygen tension.

➤ Specific relationships between periodontal pathogens and beneficial bacteria of the oral cavity (synergisms and antagonisms) may play an important role in the colonization of the subgingival space as well (see **Fig. 2.3**).

➤ *Note:* In contrast to colonization of supragingival tooth surfaces, an individual's diet (frequency and composition of meals) has no apparent influence on the colonization of the subgingival space.

## Dental Calculus

Dental calculus is mineralized bacterial plaque. It is not the primary cause of destructive periodontal disease. However, since it is always covered by vital plaque, its removal remains a cornerstone of all periodontal therapy (see Chapter 10).

➤ Mineralization of supragingival and subgingival plaque is brought about by minerals dissolved in saliva and gingival exudate, respectively[16]:

– After secretion from large sublingual, submandibular and parotid salivary glands, partial pressure of $CO_2$ in the saliva decreases rapidly in the oral cavity.

– As a result, pH rises and dissolved minerals precipitate. Therefore, *supragingival calculus* is mainly located adjacent to the excretion ducts of the large salivary glands, lingually at mandibular incisors, and buccally at the first and second molars in the maxilla. *Note:* the pH may also rise following production of ammonia and urea.

– *Subgingival calculus* covers the tooth/root surface within a gingival/periodontal pocket. Under the antibacterial influence of gingival exudate, a zone at the bottom of the pocket about 0.5 mm wide appears always to be plaque- and calculus-free.

➤ Various crystalline structures of calcium phosphate may be found in calculus (**Table 2.2**).

*Note:* The tendency to develop dental calculus and plaque differs greatly among individuals.

## ■ Periodontitis: an Infectious Disease

### Identification of Periodontal Pathogens

As most diseases of the oral cavity are caused by bacteria, traditional concepts of prevention have been based on the idea of largely reducing bacterial masses (see Chapter 7). However, both dental caries and inflammatory periodontal diseases are probably not caused by the total bacterial mass or plaque in general. Both have characteristics of *endogenous/opportunistic infections* (see below) which depend on certain preconditions:

➤ Presence of a specific habitat.

➤ Certain changes in the external conditions which promote the increase of particular segments of the complex flora.

➤ A change in the host's defense system which may lead to loss of control over the pathogenic flora in the habitat.

For most of the second part of the last century, periodontal diseases were assumed to be

**Table 2.2** Crystalline structures of calcium phosphate in dental calculus

| Name | Sum formula | Occurrence |
|------|-------------|------------|
| Brushite | $CaHPO_4 \times 2H_2O$ | Recent calculus |
| Octacalciumphosphate | $Ca_4H(PO_4)_3 \times 2H_2O$ | Mostly in outer layers of supragingival calculus |
| Hydroxyapatite | $Ca_{10}(OH)_2(PO_4)_6$ | Mostly in inner layers of supragingival plaque |
| Whitlockite | $Ca_3(PO_4)_2$ | Main component of subgingival calculus; contains small amounts of Mg |

caused by specific microorganisms (specific plaque hypothesis). In order to ultimately identify a specific pathogen as cause of a particular infectious disease, the traditional Koch-Henle's postulates have to be applied:

➤ The pathogen occurs without exception in every case of the disease and under circumstances which can account for the pathological changes and clinical course of the disease.

➤ It does not emerge in any other disease as a fortuitous and nonpathogenic entity.

➤ After being completely isolated from the body and repeatedly grown in pure culture, the pathogen can induce the disease anew and can be recovered from the experimentally infected host.

Lack of applicability of these postulates to oral infections prompted Socransky[17] to modify (and, in fact, considerably weaken) them as follows:

➤ An oral pathogen is *associated* with diseased sites. It should be absent in healthy sites or in different forms of the disease.

➤ *Elimination* of the pathogen should lead to healing of the lesion.

➤ Presence of abnormal cellular and/or humoral *immune responses* to the potential pathogen while responses to other microorganisms are normal.

➤ Further evidence for pathogenicity may arise from *animal* experimentation and identification of *virulence factors*.

Based on these criteria, in particular in the 1980s and 1990s, the following periodontal pathogens were identified[18,19]:

➤ Pathogens which are strongly associated with periodontal disease:
  – *Aggregatibacter actinomycetemcomitans*
  – *Porphyromonas gingivalis*
  – *Tannerella forsythia* (formerly *Bacteroides forsythus*)
  – *Eubacterium nodatum*
  – *Treponema denticola*

➤ Potential pathogens moderately associated with periodontal disease:
  – *Prevotella intermedia*
  – *Campylobacter rectus*
  – *Parvimonas micra* (formerly *Micromonas micra, Peptostreptococcus micra*)
  – *Eikenella corrodens*

  – *Fusobacterium nucleatum*
  – Other *Eubacterium* spp.
  – β-hemolytic streptococci

➤ Significant in certain cases:
  – *Staphylococcus* spp.
  – *Pseudomonas* spp.
  – Enterococci, enteric rods
  – *Candida* spp.

It should be critically emphasized that, in epidemiologic research of complex diseases, such as periodontitis, rather Sir Bradford Hill's criteria[20] of causal association are to be applied (see Chapter 5). Hill's criteria include:

➤ *Strength, consistency and specificity* of the association: What is the relative risk? Is there agreement among repeated observations in different places, at different times, using different methodology, by different researchers, under different circumstances? Is the outcome unique to the exposure?

➤ *Temporality*: Does exposure precede the outcome?

➤ *Experimental evidence*: Does controlled manipulation of the exposure change the outcome?

➤ *Biological gradient*: Is there evidence of a dose–response relationship?

A remaining set of criteria may support a hypothesis but is not regarded as evidence for causality:

➤ *Plausibility*: Does the causal relationship make biological sense?

➤ *Coherence*: Is the causal association compatible with present knowledge of the disease?

➤ *Analogy*: Does the causal relationship conform to a previously described relationship?

Further developments in molecular biology have even led to the formulation of molecular guidelines, namely the presence or absence of a specific nucleic acid sequence[21], for establishing microbial disease causation.

The breadth of bacterial diversity in the oral cavity, which became evident only after the application of novel, open-ended molecular methods, has led to critical revision of current concepts of the causative role of specific bacteria in the pathogenesis of periodontal diseases, which had been identified with traditional means such as cultivation of biofilm samples. Modern tools for a better characterization of the entire microbiota sampled at numerous periodontal sites in a given patient include:

➤ Checkerboard DNA-DNA hybridization of, say, 40 (or even 74) predominant species in subgingival biofilm[22]

➤ Microarrays with oligonucleotide probes for about 300 cultivable and yet not cultivable species in oral biofilm (Human Oral Microbe Identification Microarray, HOMIM).[23] *Note:* Possible cross-reactions and nonspecific target binding has been described with both methods, and this has currently not been settled satisfactorily.

➤ Next-generation sequencing[4] (e.g., HOM-INGS, species-level identification of nearly 600 oral bacteria taxa):
  - For further studies on microbial diversity in the oral cavity
  - To determine metabolic activities in dental biofilm
  - Sequencing of functional genes
  - Whole genomic analyses of certain species

After several decades of intensive research in periodontal microbiology it is presently unclear whether the flood of information from these novel techniques will ultimately lead to a paradigm shift of clinical concepts as regards diagnosis and treatment of inflammatory periodontal diseases.

## Types of Infection

It is possible that periodontal diseases comprise different kinds of infections which should then be differentiated (**Fig. 2.5**):

➤ *Endogenous/opportunistic infection* with bacteria that belong to the resident flora of the skin, nose, oral cavity, or intestinal and urogenital tracts. Opportunistic pathogens are usually not especially virulent. On the other hand, members of the resident flora at one site may cause life-threatening infections in other organ systems.
  - If oral hygiene is poor, or there are alterations within the habitat or drastic changes in the local or systemic host defense, some of these commensals—that is, potentially pathogenic bacteria found in every oral cavity—may increase disproportionately.
  - This may lead to periodontitis.

➤ *Exogenous infection* with microorganisms that are usually not members of the resident microflora:

  - Infections with enterobacteria, pseudomonads, or staphylococci are possible. These bacteria may negatively influence established periodontitis as *superinfection.*
  - Among periodontal pathogens, in particular a highly virulent clone of *Aggregatibacter actinomycetemcomitans*, JP2 (see below), may be considered an exogenous pathogen.

*A. actinomycetemcomitans, P. gingivalis, T. forsythia,* as well as *E. nodatum* and *T. denticola* are presently regarded as principal periodontal pathogens which are strongly associated with the disease. In most cases, however, bacteria alone cannot induce destructive periodontal disease. Whether periodontal infection actually occurs may depend on at least four factors[18]:

➤ A susceptible host
➤ Presence of pathogens
➤ Absence of beneficial bacteria
➤ A conducive environment in the periodontal/gingival pocket

## The Susceptible Host

Susceptibility for destructive periodontal disease is an old concept which is still not well understood. For some time, in particular in cases of aggressive periodontitis (see Chapter 4), impaired functions of neutrophil granulocytes had been suspected, in particular impaired chemotaxis and/or phagocytosis. Recent data have challenged this view (see Chapter 3).

In any case, a conspicuously increased susceptibility to periodontal infections may be regarded as a sequel of a systemically or locally excessive, impaired, or inappropriate response to the bacterial challenge:

➤ Excessive monocyte secretion of prostaglandin $E_2$ and interleukin-1β in reaction to outer membrane lipopolysaccharides of some gram-negative bacteria.

➤ A specific macrophage hyper-responsiveness trait which may expose the individual to an increased risk of various chronic inflammatory diseases and may actually comprise a general mechanism of a systemic component of periodontal disease.

In this context, some interesting associations between severe forms of periodontal disease

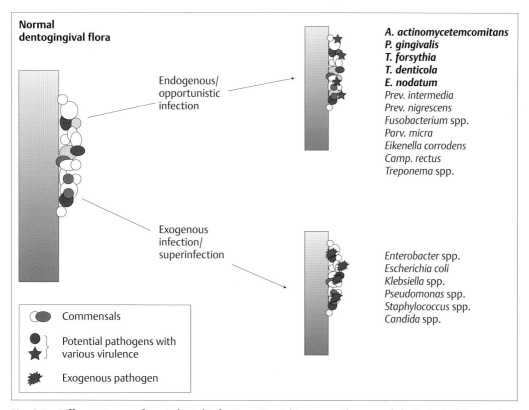

**Normal dentogingival flora**

Endogenous/ opportunistic infection

Exogenous infection/ superinfection

**A. actinomycetemcomitans**
**P. gingivalis**
**T. forsythia**
**T. denticola**
**E. nodatum**
*Prev. intermedia*
*Prev. nigrescens*
*Fusobacterium* spp.
*Parv. micra*
*Eikenella corrodens*
*Camp. rectus*
*Treponema* spp.

*Enterobacter* spp.
*Escherichia coli*
*Klebsiella* spp.
*Pseudomonas* spp.
*Staphylococcus* spp.
*Candida* spp.

Commensals

Potential pathogens with various virulence

Exogenous pathogen

**Fig. 2.5  Different types of periodontal infection.** *Top right:* Among the normal dentogingival flora, a few, mainly gram-negative, bacteria may increase disproportionately in numbers if local conditions in the habitat change, and this may lead to periodontal disease. In an especially susceptible host this is called "opportunistic infection." This applies in particular to virulent variants of some periodontal pathogens such as *Aggregatibacter actinomycetemcomitans*, *Porphyromonas gingivalis*, *Tannerella forsythia*, *Treponema denticola*, and *Eubacterium nodatum*. Note that many individuals harbor low numbers of these pathogens and are thus in a carrier status. *Bottom right:* Typical exogenous pathogens are commonly not found in the oral cavity. If they enter the oral cavity from outside, they may trigger periodontitis or accelerate its progression in the form of superinfection.

and chronic diseases and conditions may be considered (see Chapter 8):
➤ Coronary heart disease, coronary infarction
➤ Nonischemic stroke
➤ Adverse pregnancy outcome

Systemic diseases as, for instance, insufficiently controlled type I and type II diabetes mellitus (see Chapter 8), or infection with the human immunodeficiency virus (HIV), do increase the risk for periodontitis.

Hormonal effects of psychological stress have been shown to increase susceptibility to certain inflammatory periodontal diseases, such as necrotizing ulcerative gingivitis/periodontitis.

Note that both stress and inadequate coping with stress have been associated with chronic periodontitis. Among behavioral factors which are related to all kinds of inflammatory periodontal disease, smoking is by far the most dominant (see Chapter 8).

Ultimately, susceptibility for periodontal disease may largely be influenced by a combination of genetic factors, gene expression, and gene regulation (see Chapter 3).

**Presence of Pathogens**

Periodontal infection with bacteria such as *A. actinomycetemcomitans*, *P. gingivalis*, and *T. for-*

*sythia* frequently leads to the production of specific antibodies in the host. In response to antigens of gram-negative bacteria of the subgingival biofilm, especially specific antibodies of the IgG2 subclass are produced. It has long been assumed that increased serum levels of antibodies against *A. actinomycetemcomitans* protect the host from developing generalized aggressive periodontitis. This view has recently been challenged (see Chapter 3).

To become pathogenic, bacteria must possess certain *virulence factors* (**Table 2.3**)[24–27]:

➤ Adhesion to tissues of the host
➤ Growth and multiplication within the habitat

➤ Evasion from and/or perturbation of host-derived defense mechanisms
➤ Active destruction of colonized tissue

Since virulence factors are partly genetically determined and largely depend on growth conditions in the periodontal pockets, their expression varies considerably among strains of a given species.

An especially toxic variant of *A. actinomycetemcomitans* (JP2), which has a 530 base-pair deletion in the promoter region of the leukotoxin gene, produces considerable amounts of leukotoxin,[28] It has so far been identified mainly in individuals with a Northwest and Sub-Saharan African affiliation (Africans, Afro-Americans,

**Table 2.3** Some virulence factors of periodontal pathogens *Aggregatibacter actinomycetemcomitans*, *Porphyromonas gingivalis*, *Tannerella forsythia*, and *Treponema denticola*

| | Adhesion/colonization | Evasion/perturbation of host reponse | Tissue destruction |
|---|---|---|---|
| *A. actinomyce-temcomitans* | • Capsule antigen, pili, vesicles<br>• Antagonism to *S. sanguinis*, *Actinomyces oris* | • Leukotoxin, especially distinct in JP2 clone<br>• Inhibition of chemotaxis<br>• Fc-binding protein<br>• Suppression of lymphocyte functions<br>• Invasion of epithelial cells in vivo<br>• Degrades immunoglobulins | • Endotoxin<br>• Epithelotoxin<br>• Collagenase<br>• Inhibits fibroblast functions<br>• Cytolethal extending toxin, apoptosis<br>• Alkaline and acidic phosphatases |
| *P. gingivalis* | • Capsule antigen, pili, vesicles<br>• Synergism with *T. forsythia*, *Treponema denticola* | • Inhibition of chemotaxis<br>• Degrades complement and immunoglobulins<br>• Invasion of epithelial cells in vitro<br>• Does not trigger expression of E-selectin on inner endothelial surface<br>• Suppresses production and expression of IL-8 and ICAM-1 in junctional epithelium | • Endotoxin<br>• Collagenase<br>• Gingipain<br>• Fibrinolysin<br>• Phospholipase A<br>• Alkaline and acidic phosphatases |
| *T. forsythia* | • Synergism with *P. gingivalis*, *Treponema denticola* | • Invasion of epithelial cells in vivo | • Endotoxin<br>• Trypsinlike and other proteases<br>• Production of fatty acids<br>• Apoptosis induction |
| *Treponema denticola* | • Adhesion to fibronectin, laminin, plasminogen<br>• Synergism with *P. gingivalis*, *T. forsythia* | • Immune suppressive factor<br>• C3 activation<br>• Hydrolysis of numerous cytokines, IgG and IgA<br>• Induction of cytokines<br>• Activation of TLR2 & 4<br>• Resistence to β-defensins 1 & 2 | • Endotoxin<br>• Trypsinlike activity<br>• Active tissue invasion<br>• Cytoskeletal destruction of fibroblasts<br>• Degradation of host proteins |

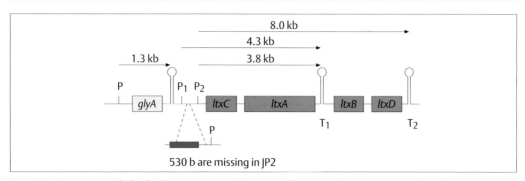

**Fig. 2.6  Gene map of the leukotoxin gene of *Aggregatibacter actinomycetemcomitans*.** The membrane-bound leukotoxin belongs, together with the hemolysin of *Escherichia coli* and the leukocidin of *Pasteurella haemolytica*, to the family of RTX toxins, which cause pore formation in the cell membrane of neutrophilic granulocytes and monocytes. The operon consists of four genes:
– *ltxC* is responsible for activation of the primary product of *ltxA*.
– *ltxA* decodes the toxin itself.
– *ltxB* and *ltxD* decode proteins for intracellular transport.
As compared to minimally leukotoxic strains, the highly toxic strain JP2 is characterized by a 530 base-pair deletion in the promoter region of the leukotoxin gene. These strains produce 10 to 20 times higher amounts of leukotoxin than minimally leukotoxic strains. An intraoral infection considerably increases the risk of development of aggressive periodontitis. (Adapted from Lally et al.[28])

Afro-native Americans).[29,30] Oral infection with this highly leukotoxic clone (**Fig. 2.6**) considerably raises the risk for aggressive periodontitis.[31]

Destructive effects of various virulence factors of different pathogens may add up within the environment of the periodontal pocket (**Table 2.3**):
➤ Leukotoxin and cytotoxin of *A. actinomycetemcomitans*
➤ Bacterial collagenase
➤ Endotoxin (lipopolysaccharide)
➤ Factors, which suppress growth and proliferation of fibroblasts or activate osteoclasts
➤ Trypsinlike peptidases of *P. gingivalis*, *T. forsythia*, and *Treponema denticola*
➤ Fibrinolysin and other proteolytic enzymes
➤ Acidic and alkaline phosphatases
➤ Toxic substances such as hydrogen sulfide (H$_2$S), ammonia (NH$_3$), or fatty acids

## Absence of Beneficial Microorganisms

Bacteria and their products are necessary and beneficial components of a healthy periodontium. In the course of evolution, gram-positive bacteria have adapted more closely to the conditions in the human oral cavity and can sometimes keep certain less-robust periodontal pathogens in check (**Fig. 2.7**). Antagonistic microorganisms may have an adverse effect on the ability of pathogenic bacteria to successfully establish themselves in the periodontal pocket. Presence of beneficial bacteria appears to interfere, in a concentration-dependent manner, with the establishment of typical periodontal pathogens.[32] For example, growth of *A. actinomycetemcomitans* is inhibited by *S. sanguinis* which by-produces H$_2$O$_2$. On the other hand, a bacteriocin produced by *A. actinomycetemcomitans* interferes with growth of a number of streptococci.[34]

Identification of beneficial, or host-compatible, bacteria was based on frequent demonstration of presence in healthy periodontium or following successful treatment of periodontitis, and their predominance during inactive phases of periodontitis. Important beneficial bacteria include:
➤ *Actinomyces* spp.
➤ *Capnocytophaga ochracea*
➤ *Streptococcus mitis*
➤ *S. sanguinis*
➤ *Veillonella parvula*

Introducing probiotic bacteria into the oral cavity, such as *Lactobacillus reuteri* or *L. casei*, has shown beneficial effects on caries incidence and chronic periodontitis (see Chapter 13).[35] Some promising observations and preliminary evidence has to be confirmed in controlled studies.

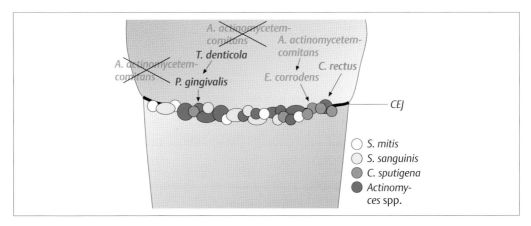

**Fig. 2.7  Colonization of periodontal pathogens is influenced by some beneficial bacteria** (*Streptococcus mitis, S. sanguinis, Capnocytophaga sputigena* and *Actinomyces* spp.) at the cementoenamel junction (CEJ). For instance, *Aggregatibacter actinomycetemcomitans* cannot colonize if *S. sanguinis* is already present (antagonism). If, on the other hand, *C. sputigena* has formed colonies, *A. actinomycetemcomitans, Campylobacter rectus* and *Eikenella corrodens* may establish (synergisms). *Treponema denticola* has no chance to thrive in the presence of *A. actinomycetemcomitans*. (Adapted from Socransky et al[32]; further observations by Müller et al.[33])

**Conducive Environment in the Periodontal Pocket**

Ecological conditions in the regions of the gingival sulcus and periodontal pocket may vary considerably. They partly determine the complex composition of the microflora, which mainly consists of obligately anaerobic, gram-negative, rather fastidious bacteria (**Fig. 2.8**). Many pathogenic microorganisms regulate expression of available virulence factors according to certain environmental signals:

➤ Specific responses to the present ecological condition make colonization and invasion of the host organism possible. Of importance are:
  – pH
  – Redox potential
  – Oxygen tension
  – Osmotic pressure
  – Temperature
  – Iron, magnesium and calcium concentrations
  – Antibody titers
➤ Absence of oxygen, for example, may increase leukotoxin production by especially virulent strains of *A. actinomycetemcomitans* more than three-fold.[36]
➤ The availability of iron does not seem to play an important role in the regulation of leu-

kotoxin expression by *A. actinomycetemcomitans*. On the other hand the amount of available iron does determine the expression of certain outer membrane proteins of *P. gingivalis*.[37]

The strong dependence of virulence of periodontal pathogens on conditions in their respective habitat may partly explain the long latency between first colonization and outbreak of disease as periodontal infection. Recent longitudinal studies on the incidence of aggressive periodontitis have suggested the role of an increasingly complex microflora (**Fig. 2.9**) which may contain, in addition to *A. actinomycetemcomitans, Filifactor alocis* and *Streptococcus parasanguinis*.[39]

**Transmission**

Major causes of caries and periodontal diseases —for instance, mutans streptococci, *A. actinomycetemcomitans*, and *Porphyromonas gingivalis*— can be transmitted between individuals. For instance, there seems to be a window of infectivity for mutans streptococci at the age of 24 months. The earlier the infection takes place, the more caries may be expected at the age of, say, 4 years. This may have important consequences for primary prevention of caries. If car-

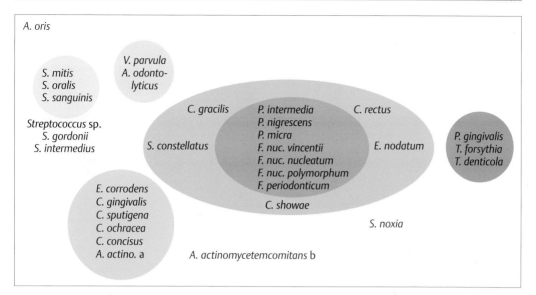

**Fig. 2.8  Bacteria of the periodontal pocket are organized in different complexes.** The figure also indicates a temporal sequence of colonization of the dental surface, from the left (primary colonizers *Actinomyces oris*, which occurs most frequently, and streptococci) to right. The large central complex in the middle contains potential periodontal pathogens (*Prevotella* spp., *Fusobacterium* spp., *Campylobacter* spp.), which are usually present at low concentrations in all oral cavities; only in response to changes in their ecosystem will they multiply excessively and cause pathological conditions. The red complex is comprised of periodontal pathogens (*Porphyromonas gingivalis*, *Tannerella forsythia*, and *Treponema denticola*), which are strongly associated with destructive periodontal disease. Serotype b of *Aggregatibacter actinomycetemcomitans* may be an outsider within the complex flora. Serotype a is associated with the complex containing *Eikenella corrodens*, *Capnocytophaga* spp., and *Campylobacter concisus*. (Adapted from Socransky et al,[22] courtesy of John Wiley and Sons.)

ious conditions in the maternal oral cavity can be resolved before tooth eruption in the child—such that the likelihood of infection of the neonatal child decreases because of low levels of mutans streptococci in the oral cavity of the mother—caries development in the deciduous and permanent dentitions may probably be delayed, reduced, or even prohibited (so-called primary primary prevention).[40]

It may be possible to change the oral flora of the expectant mother in a rather targeted way. Effective oral hygiene may be established and diet changed. Mutans streptococci may temporarily be eradicated by, for example, chlorhexidine-containing varnish. Any open carious lesions should be treated. It is important to provide consistent supportive care during pregnancy. Such a program would also be effective in the prevention of pregnancy gingivitis.

Early transmission of periodontal pathogens from the periodontally diseased mother or father to their child is very likely.

➤ *Aggregatibacter actinomycetemcomitans* may be acquired already in the mixed dentition. In contrast, stable colonization of *P. gingivalis* may occur only during adolescence.[38]

➤ These and other potential periodontal pathogens are found in numerous ecosystems outside the periodontal pocket, on the dorsum of the tongue and the tonsils, as well as in saliva.

➤ Transmission of *A. actinomycetemcomitans*, *P. gingivalis* and other periodontal pathogens is mainly accomplished through shared use of toothbrushes or cutlery, or exchange of saliva: vertically, from periodontally diseased parent to child; probably also horizontally, between adult partners.

*Note*: At least the highly leukotoxic clone of *A. actinomycetemcomitans* may be regarded an exogenous pathogen (see **Fig. 2.5**), which con-

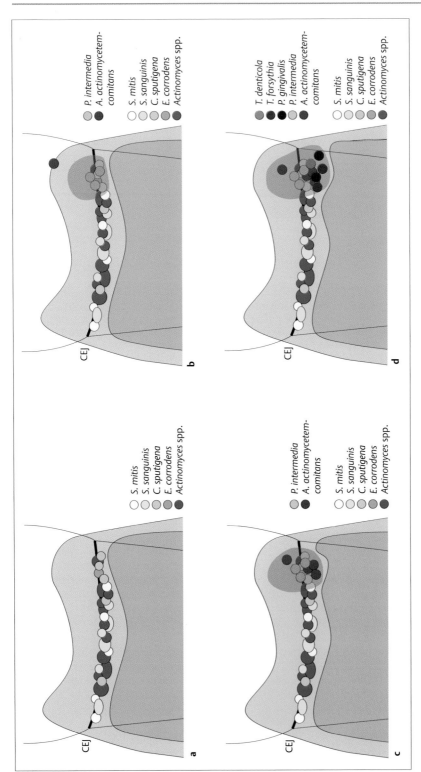

**Fig. 2.9 Development of pathogenic microbiota in aggressive periodontitis** (information retrieved by Könönen and Müller.[38])

**a** In healthy children, the flora mainly consists of the yellow- and green-complex bacteria (see **Fig. 2.8**) and *Actinomyces* spp.

**b** In case of gingivitis, *Prevotella intermedia* frequently colonizes the area at an early stage.

**c** *Aggregatibacter actinomycetemcomitans* may join the flora and cause, in susceptible patients, early alveolar bone loss in the deciduous and mixed dentitions.

**d** Once pocketing has occurred and lesions have spread, the flora becomes very diverse, soon resembling that of chronic periodontitis. In many cases, red-complex bacteria predominate while in others, *A. actinomycetemcomitans* is found in large numbers. Recent longitudinal studies have suggested, in addition to *A. actinomycetemcomitans*, an important role of (orange complex) *Filifactor alocis* and (yellow complex) *Streptococcus parasanguinis*.[39]

siderably enhances the risk of disease development if transmitted early in the lifetime.

### Peri-implantitis

At first sight, the flora which is associated with peri-implantitis does not differ significantly from that in periodontitis, where gram-negative anaerobes such as *P. gingivalis, T. forsythia*, and *Treponema denticola* predominate. There appears to be a certain risk for intraoral transmission of periodontal pathogens, which soon colonize implants after insertion. It is therefore strongly suggested that implants should be placed only after successful completion of periodontal therapy.

Recent in-depth analysis of the periodontal and peri-implant microbiomes revealed, however, significantly higher diversity in the former. Simple geographic proximity of teeth and implants seems not to be a sufficient determinant of colonizing topographically distinct niches.[41]

Whether exogenous *Staphylococcus aureus* and coagulase-negative staphylococci play a role in peri-implant diseases, similar as in orthopaedic infections, is currently controversially discussed.[42]

# 3 Pathogenesis of Biofilm-Induced Periodontal Diseases

## ■ Pathogenesis of Dental Biofilm-Induced Gingivitis

Complete lack of any inflammatory cells in gingival tissues—that is, *histologically healthy gingiva*—is achieved only after prolonged and total absence of any microbial plaque. This is only possible under experimental conditions.[1]

*Clinically normal* gingiva has several characteristic features. There is almost always an infiltrate composed of polymorphonuclear granulocytes and lymphocytes:

➤ In contrast to other tissues, the endothelium of the gingival vascular plexus expresses *adhesion molecules* such as E-selectin.
➤ Therefore, a continuous influx of polymorphonuclear (PMN) granulocytes occurs, leaving the plexus and migrating through the connective tissue and junctional epithelium into the sulcus.
➤ Leukocytes which reach the oral cavity are mostly vital, are able to phagocytose, and exert a high degree of enzymatic activity.[2]

Acute inflammatory reactions are associated with gingival redness, edematous swelling, and exudation. These lesions can be painful, especially if ulceration occurs. Main causes of *acute gingivitis*, besides bacterial plaque, are nonspecific trauma after thermal or chemical burn, and mechanical injury.

Histologically, different stages of dental biofilm-induced gingivitis have long been distinguished[3]:

➤ Initial gingivitis
➤ Early gingivitis
➤ Established gingivitis

Traditionally, any inflammatory process is divided into three phases:

➤ An *acute phase*, which is characterized by invasion of neutrophil granulocytes after tissue injury. Endogenous mediators influence the acute reaction:
  – Bradykinin and prostaglandins lead to *vasodilatation*.

  – Histamine and leukotrienes increase *vascular permeability*.
  – Complement and leukotrienes serve as *chemotactic factors*.
➤ The *immunologic phase* commences with the arrival of antigen-presenting cells.
➤ *Chronic lesions* are characterized by an increase of antibody-secreting plasma cells.

*Note*: The classical phases of acute and chronic inflammation cannot easily be distinguished in inflammatory periodontal diseases:

➤ Acute signs of inflammation (e.g., exudation) are found even in the case of clinically normal gingiva.
➤ Soon afterwards, acute and chronic (i.e., immunologic) inflammatory components coexist.

### Initial Gingivitis

Within 2 to 4 days after commencement of plaque accumulation, specific alterations in the junctional epithelium and the vascular plexus beneath may be observed. Clinically, the gingiva still appears to be absolutely healthy and normal (see **Fig. 1.3**).[1] Pathohistologically, characteristics of an *initial lesion* emerge (**Fig. 3.1**)[3]:

➤ Increase of vascular permeability occurs close beneath the junctional epithelium with loss of perivascular collagen.
➤ Exudation of plasma proteins. Polymorphonuclear granulocytes migrate through the junctional epithelium into the sulcus.
➤ As a consequence, intercellular spaces widen in the most coronal part of the junctional epithelium.
➤ Granulocyte migration leads to increased levels of leukotriene $B_4$—a product of degranulating neutrophils—in gingival exudate.

Endogenous mediators are responsible for triggering inflammation:

➤ Vasoactive amines such as histamine and serotonin
➤ Plasma proteases of the kinin-, complement- and plasmin-systems

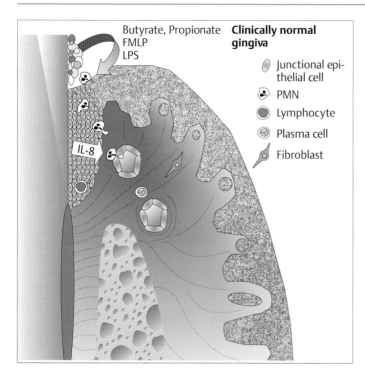

Butyrate, Propionate
FMLP
LPS

**Clinically normal gingiva**

- Junctional epithelial cell
- PMN
- Lymphocyte
- Plasma cell
- Fibroblast

IL-8

**Fig. 3.1 Components of clinically normal gingiva.** Histologically, an initial lesion is found. Bacteria of supragingival plaque produce metabolites such as butyrate and propionate, chemotactic peptides like *N*-formyl-methionyl-leucyl-phenylalanine (FMLP), and lipopolysaccharides (LPS). These trigger junctional epithelial cells to release the chemokine interleukin 8 (IL-8). A chemotactic gradient into the junctional epithelium and sulcus leads polymorphonuclear granulocytes to migrate from the vascular plexus. Scattered lymphocytes and plasma cells are seen. (Adapted from Page and Schroeder.[3])

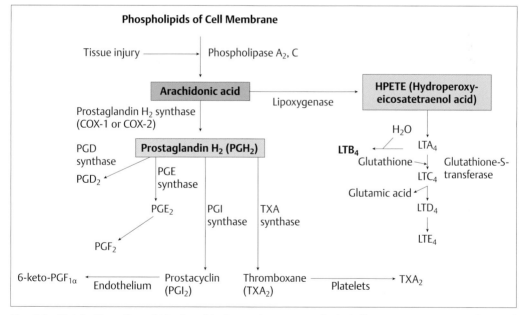

**Phospholipids of Cell Membrane**

Tissue injury ⟶ Phospholipase A$_2$, C

**Arachidonic acid**

Prostaglandin H$_2$ synthase (COX-1 or COX-2)

Lipoxygenase

**HPETE (Hydroperoxy-eicosatetraenol acid)**

PGD synthase

**Prostaglandin H$_2$ (PGH$_2$)**

PGD$_2$

PGE synthase

H$_2$O

LTB$_4$ ⟵ LTA$_4$

PGE$_2$

PGI synthase

TXA synthase

Glutathione ⟶ LTC$_4$ Glutathione-S-transferase

PGF$_2$

Glutamic acid ⟶ LTD$_4$

LTE$_4$

6-keto-PGF$_{1\alpha}$ ⟵ Endothelium ⟶ Prostacyclin (PGI$_2$)

Thromboxane (TXA$_2$) ⟶ Platelets ⟶ TXA$_2$

**Fig. 3.2 Metabolites of arachidonic acid play an important role in inflammatory reactions of several chronic diseases.** Arachidonic acid is usually esterified with phospholipids of the cell membrane. When tissue injury occurs, phospholipases are activated and arachidonic acid is released. Note that glucocorticosteroids prevent activation of phospholipases. Prostaglandins, prostacycline, and thromboxane originate after activation of cyclooxygenases COX1 and COX2 (inhibition by nonsteroidal anti-inflammatory drugs, NSAIDs), whereas lipoxygenase leads to formation of leukotrienes. Many metabolites of arachidonic acid exert important biological activities (**Table 3.1**).

**Table 3.1** Biological functions of metabolites of the arachidonic cascade

| Metabo-lite | Function |
|---|---|
| Prosta-glandins | • Vasodilation<br>• Pain<br>• Platelet aggregation<br>• Modulation of T lymphocytes, inhibition of cytokine production<br>• Stimulation of osteoclasts |
| Leuko-trienes | • Increase of vascular permeability<br>• Enable adhesion of polymorphonuclear granulocytes (PMNs) to endothelial cells<br>• Stimulate chemotaxis of PMNs and eosinophilic granulocytes<br>• Induce lysosomal degranulation of PMNs<br>• Enhance chemokinesis of T lymphocytes |

➤ Metabolites of arachidonic acid, prostaglandins, leukotrienes (**Fig. 3.2**), with numerous biologically important functions (**Table 3.1**)

**Complement.** The more than 20 proteins and protein fragments of the *complement system* comprise (like the clotting system, fibrinolysis, and kinin formation) a triggered plasma enzyme system. Such systems respond rapidly, in an amplifying reaction cascade, to a triggering factor. The product of each reaction is an enzymatic catalyst of the next.

Complement activation may take place via the *classical pathway*, which is triggered by antigen-bound antibodies.

➤ Serin proteases C1r and C1s, which are bound to C1q, are activated by IgG and IgM.
➤ C1s catalyzes cleavage of C2 into C2a and C2b, and C4 into C4a and C4b.
➤ The arising complex $\overline{C4bC2a}$ is able to catalyze the assembly of the C3 convertase (see below).

Activation of the complement cascade via the *alternative pathway* may be induced by microbial lipopolysaccharides (**Fig. 3.3**). Moreover, the so-called *lectin pathway* is a cascade reaction within the complement system, whereby mannose-binding lectin binds to certain sugars on the bacterial surface. Similar as in case of the classical pathway, initial reactions involve C2 and C4.

The central component of the complement system is C3, a protein with a molecular weight of 195 kDa and a plasma concentration of 1.2 mg/mL:

➤ Under normal circumstances and in the presence of $Mg^{2+}$, the larger fragment C3b, which is formed spontaneously at a very

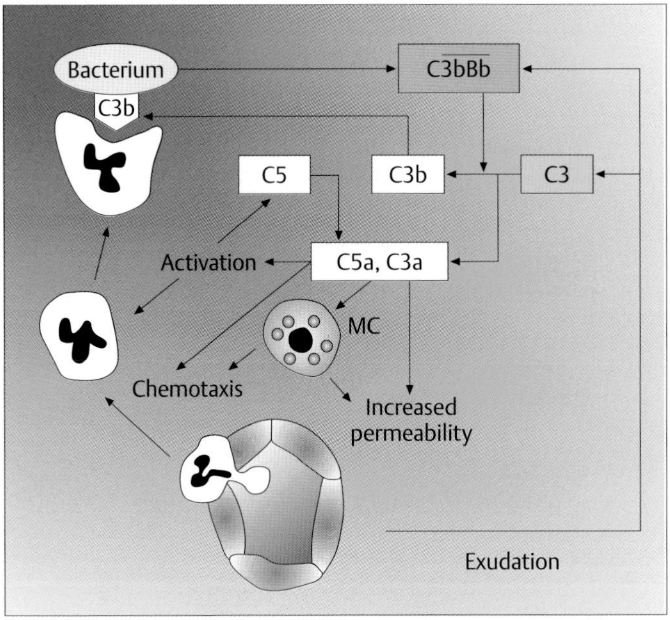

**Fig. 3.3  Acute inflammatory reaction by activation of the** *alternative pathway* **of the complement cascade.** First, C3 convertase is stabilized on the bacterial surface and cleaves large amounts of C3 into fragments C3a and C3b. Fragment C3b binds to the bacterium and serves as an opsonin. C3a activates C5. The cleavage product C5a is a chemotactic factor for polymorphonuclear granulocytes (PMNs), which leave the vessel and migrate directly to the bacterium. C3a and C5a are anaphylatoxins, which induce mast cells to release vasoactive mediators, resulting in a further influx of PMNs and complement into the tissue.

slow rate, may complex with complement component factor B. Following cleavage by plasma enzyme factor D, $\overline{C3bBb}$ is generated, which exerts enzymatic activity as C3 convertase.

➤ The C3 convertase $\overline{C3bBb}$ is stabilized on the bacterial surface by serum protein properdin and activated by microbial polysaccharides.
➤ C3 convertase cleaves large amounts of C3 into fragments C3a and C3b.
➤ C3b binds to the bacterium and thus serves as an opsonin for subsequent PMN phagocytosis.
➤ C3a activates C5, which is cleaved into C5a and C5b.

Complement components C3a and C5a exhibit several defense mechanisms:
➤ C5a is a strong chemotactic factor for PMN granulocytes.
➤ C3a and C5a are anaphylatoxins in that they are capable of triggering degranulation of mast cells and release of vasoactive mediators such as histamine, leukotriene $B_4$ (increase of vascular permeability) and prostaglandins (vasodilation).

Further activation of the complement cascade leads to pore formation in the bacterial cell membrane with subsequent lysis:
➤ C5b binds loosely to C3b.
➤ C6 and C7 bind successively to C5b.
➤ After formation of C8a and C9 the *membrane attack complex* (MAC) is formed.

**Leukocyte extravasation, chemotaxis, and phagocytosis.** For leukocytes to leave the vascular plexus of the gingiva, both leukocytes and endothelial cells must express adhesion molecules on their respective surfaces[4]:
➤ Bacterial products such as lipopolysaccharides (LPS) of gram-negative bacteria or proteins may react *directly*, in the form of split-off vesicles, with endothelial cells of capillaries and venules of the gingival connective tissue.
➤ *Indirect* activation by macrophages is also possible. After contact with LPS or bacterial proteins, these cells secrete proinflammatory cytokines as interleukin-1 (IL-1) and tumor necrosis factor alpha (TNF-α).
➤ In either case, the adhesion molecule E-selectin (or endothelial-leukocyte adhesion

molecule 1, ELAM-1) is expressed on the inner surface of the endothelial cell, which causes granulocytes to roll on the endothelium.
➤ After contact between the leukocyte adhesion receptor CD11/18 with the endothelial integrin ICAM-1 (intercellular adhesion molecule 1), the leukocyte can leave the vessel by amoeboid diapedesis (**Fig. 3.4**).

In order to be able to migrate, granulocytes need a sufficient number of functioning surface receptors. Migration follows a gradient of chemotactic factors, which include:
➤ Bacterial peptides such as N-formyl-methionyl-leucyl-phenylalanine (FMLP).
➤ Chemotactic cytokines (chemokines) such as IL-8, which is released in large amounts by cells of the junctional epithelium.
➤ Leukotriene $B_4$, which is released by other granulocytes.
➤ Complement component C5a.

Apart from its barrier function, junctional epithelium has also *sensory* and *signaling* functions[5]:
➤ Apart from secretion of the chemokine IL-8, junctional epithelial cells express ICAM-1. This allows neutrophils and certain lymphocytes to adhere by the leukocyte adhesion receptor CD11/18, signaling the presence of bacteria to the connective tissue below.
➤ Both junctional and pocket epithelia possess neural elements.

When PMN granulocytes reach the sulcus, complement and antibodies (both serve as opsonins) support phagocytosis of bacteria and their products. Leukocytes bind to opsonized bacteria by Fc receptors[6]:
➤ FcγRI binds with high affinity to immunoglobulins of the IgG1, IgG3, and IgG4 subclasses.
➤ FcγRII and FcγRIII bind with low affinity to antigen–antibody complexes or aggregations of IgG1 and IgG3.
➤ *Note*: FcγRII is the only Fc receptor that binds to IgG2, the IgG subclass formed mainly against polysaccharide capsule antigens of gram-negative bacteria.

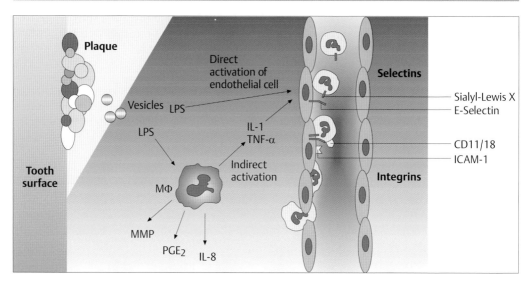

**Fig. 3.4   Activation of endothelial cells** may be triggered directly by split-off vesicles of lipopolysaccharide (LPS) of gram-negative bacteria residing on the tooth surface, or indirectly by proinflammatory cytokines interleukin-1 (IL-1) and tumor necrosis factor α (TNF-α), which are released by macrophages (MΦ) together with other cytokines, matrix metalloproteinases (MMP), prostaglandin $E_2$ (PGE$_2$), and chemokine IL-8. E-selectin is expressed on the inner surface of the vessel, where it binds loosely via Lewis blood group antigen to granulocytes. Their velocity in the blood stream is dramatically slowed down. As soon as granulocytes start to roll on the endothelium, stronger adhesion comes into effect by the leukocyte adhesion receptor CD11/18 and intercellular adhesion molecule ICAM-1. After this, the granulocyte migrates out of the vessel. (Adapted from Darveau et al.[4])

After phagocytosis, phagosomes fuse with cytoplasmic granules (**Table 3.2**) and become phagolysosomes. Bacteria are killed intracellularly:
➤ Oxygen-dependent killing:
  – Superoxide anion:
    $$NADPH + 2\,O_2 \xrightarrow{oxidase} NADP + H^+ + 2\,O_2^-$$
  – Hydroxyl radical:
    $$O_2^- + 2\,H_2O \longrightarrow 2\,H_2O_2 \longrightarrow {}^\bullet OH$$
  – Myeloperoxidase mediated: hypochloric acid, chloramines.
➤ Oxygen-independent killing:
  – Myeloperoxidase
  – Defensins: specific antibiotic peptides
  – Cathepsins
  – Lactoferrin
  – Lysozyme

Note that extracellular delivery of granular content for defense against invading bacteria may result in considerable host tissue destruction:
➤ Endopeptidases (proteases) are usually inhibited by $\alpha_2$-macroglobulin and $\alpha_1$-protease inhibitor.

➤ On the other hand, these inhibitors are easily cleaved by potent proteases of periodontal microorganisms, for example, gingipain by *Porphyromonas gingivalis*.

The concentrations of several plasma proteins, so called acute-phase reactants, increase under the influence of proinflammatory mediators such as IL-1:
➤ Acute-phase reactants that may increase enormously in concentration:
  – C-reactive protein (CRP): binds complement, opsonizes
  – Mannose-binding protein: binds complement, opsonizes
  – Serum amyloid P: initiates amyloid deposition
➤ Acute-phase proteins that may increase moderately in concentration (protease inhibitors):
  – $\alpha_2$-Macroglobulin
  – $\alpha_1$-Protease inhibitor

**Table 3.2** Cytoplasmic granules of polymorphonuclear granulocytes

| Enzymes | Primary (azurophilic) granules | Secondary (specific) granules |
|---|---|---|
| Microbiocidal enzymes | Myeloperoxidase<br>Lysozyme | Lysozyme |
| Neutral proteases | Elastase<br>Cathepsin G<br>Proteinase 3 | Collagenase |
| Acidic proteases | N-Acetyl-β-glucosamidase<br>Cathepsins B, D<br>β-Glucuronidase<br>β-Glycerophosphatase<br>β-Mannosidase | |
| Other | Defensins<br>Cationic proteins<br>Bactericidal/permeability increasing factor | Lactoferrin<br>Cobalophilin<br>CR3<br>Cytochrome |

## Early Gingivitis

After one or two weeks of undisturbed plaque accumulation some cardinal symptoms of inflammation, such as redness and swelling of the gingiva, become clinically visible. These alterations are due to increasing vascularity and an enhanced permeability of vessels with extravasation of plasma proteins leading to a strong increase in gingival crevicular fluid flow, which is clinically detectable.

The *early gingival lesion* represents the mounting of a competent immune reaction against plaque antigens.[3] It is the typical lesion found in healthy preschool children and has similarities with *lymphoid tissue.*

Any immune reaction is launched by cells residing in the junctional epithelium:
➤ Special mucosal T lymphocytes
➤ Antigen-presenting Langerhans cells
➤ Dendritic cells

In case of early gingivitis, the inflammatory infiltrate in the connective tissue consists mainly of *T lymphocytes.* It occupies about 10 to 15% of the volume of the free gingiva (**Fig. 3.5**). *B lymphocytes* are observed only in small numbers. They differentiate into antibody-secreting plasma cells. A systemic humoral immune reaction may be initiated[7]:
➤ Antigenic material from the bacteria is taken up by epithelial Langerhans cells and macrophages residing in the connective tissue of

the gingiva, and is transported to regional lymph nodes.
➤ Stimulated lymphocytes mount a specific immune response:
  – Plasma cells residing in lymph nodes produce specific antibodies.
  – They enter the circulation and arrive at the gingiva.
  – These specific antibodies can then be detected in the gingival crevicular fluid.

Whether a specific immune response can also be set up locally is not as clear:
➤ In this hypothetical case, *highly specific* for periodontal tissues, B and T cells would have to proliferate in regional lymph nodes and enter the circulation.
➤ These lymphocytes would then settle in the periodontium and start to execute their respective humoral and cellular functions.

*Plasma cells* produce, under the control of Th2 cells, antibodies. Th1 cells regulate cell-mediated immune responses (see below).

*Macrophages* always comprise only a small proportion of the cell population in the inflammatory infiltrate. They become effector cells after LPS exposure and secrete proinflammatory cytokines, prostaglandin $E_2$ ($PGE_2$), chemokines, and matrix metalloproteinases.[7] Thus, a continuous recruitment of lymphocytes and macrophages is facilitated.

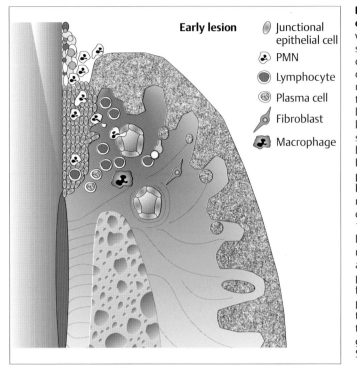

**Early lesion**

- Junctional epithelial cell
- PMN
- Lymphocyte
- Plasma cell
- Fibroblast
- Macrophage

**Fig. 3.5  Characteristics of the early lesion.** Further increase in vascular permeability leads to a strong influx of plasma proteins including acute-phase reactants, complement, and plasmin. Large numbers of PMNs pass the connective tissue and junctional epithelium, which expresses the chemokine IL-8. This is accompanied by structural alterations of the sulcus bottom, and lateral proliferation of basal cells. Activated macrophages produce proinflammatory cytokines IL-1, IL-6, IL-10, TNF-α, chemokines as IL-8, and the monocyte chemoattractant protein 1 (MCP-1), as well as $PGE_2$ and tissue collagenase, thus ensuring recruitment of additional T lymphocytes and monocytes from the venule plexus. T lymphocytes interact with fibroblasts, which exhibit cytopathic alterations. The infiltrate of the early lesion occupies about 10 to 15% of the volume of the free gingiva. (Adapted from Page and Schroeder.[3])

## Established Gingivitis

In adolescents and adults, further accumulation of bacterial plaque results, after an undetermined period of time, in the development of *established gingival lesions*.[3] A gingival pocket forms:

➤ An *intraepithelial tear* and subsequent degeneration of junctional epithelial cells lead to loss of the biological connection between the epithelium and the enamel surface.

➤ A pocket epithelium develops. Epithelial ridges proliferate, which extend into the infiltrated connective tissue. The epithelium between the ridges is frequently ulcerated. Some remains of junctional epithelium may be seen at the bottom of the gingival pocket.

Apical proliferation of bacteria ultimately results in the establishment of a *subgingival microflora*. Bacterial metabolites can now directly affect the connective tissue beneath.

Specific, very diverse populations of inflammatory cells migrate into the connective tissue lining the pocket[5]:

➤ Neutrophil granulocytes form a dense wall against microorganisms.

➤ Macrophages, lymphocytes, and plasma cells form the main cell populations in the connective tissue. There is selective immigration of:
  - antigen-specific memory cells,
  - activated lymphocytes,
  - mucosal, γδ receptor-positive T cells, and
  - CD1a-positive, antigen-presenting cells.

Selective expression of adhesion molecules plays a major role in regulation of specific migration. Chemotactic cytokines with a low molecular weight and potent, cell-type specific characteristics (chemokines) are especially important:

➤ IL-8 reacts specifically with neutrophil granulocytes and a small population of lymphocytes.

➤ MCP-1 (monocyte chemoattractant protein 1, CCL2) is responsible for migration of macrophages. Its production is regulated by IL-10.

➤ MIP-1α (macrophage inflammatory protein 1α, CCL3) enhances Th2 responses, contributes to recruitment of Th1 cells (see below), and facilitates migration of leukocytes through the junctional epithelium in early and late stages of inflammation.

➤ IP-10 (interferon γ-induced protein 10, CXCL10) is chemotactic for macrophages, monocytes, T lymphocytes, natural killer (NK) cells, and dentritic cells.

➤ RANTES (regulated on activation, normal T-cell expressed and secreted, CCL5) is selectively chemotactic for T cells, and eosinophilic and basophilic granulocytes.

Antibodies generated by plasma cells are not only directed towards specific antigens found in plaque. Rather, plaque bacteria may also induce a nonspecific, polyclonal B cell response.

Established gingivitis is an extremely frequent condition. Its lesions may be found virtually in every adolescent's and adult's mouth. It is not exactly known how long it takes for typical established lesions to develop if plaque is allowed to accumulate, but speculations range between a few weeks and several months.

Pathohistologically, established lesions are characterized as follows (**Fig. 3.6**):

➤ Persistent acute components of inflammation, in particular exudation and target-oriented migration of PMN granulocytes.

➤ Specific populations of inflammatory cells in the infiltrate.

➤ Immunoglobulins in extravascular connective tissue and junctional epithelium.

➤ Increasing proportion of plasma cells.

➤ Further loss of collagen.

➤ Lateral proliferation of junctional epithelium and gingival pocket formation.

Established gingivitis may remain quite stable for prolonged periods. Usually, there is a delicate balance between the bacterial challenge and the immune response of the host. After an indeterminate period of time, an *advanced lesion*—that is, destructive periodontitis—may develop. Thus, two forms of established gingivitis may exist concurrently:

➤ In most cases or sites, it is an independent, self-contained, stable lesion.

➤ Infrequently, it is a precursor of periodontitis.

These two forms cannot be distinguished clinically. Pathohistologically, active lesions (see below) may be characterized by a higher density (more than 50%) of plasma cells.[8]

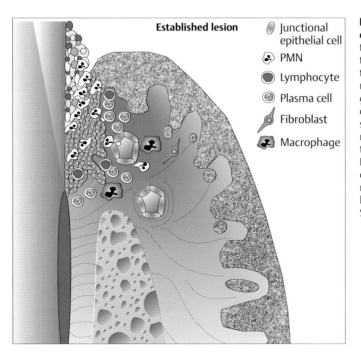

**Established lesion**

- Junctional epithelial cell
- PMN
- Lymphocyte
- Plasma cell
- Fibroblast
- Macrophage

**Fig. 3.6 Characteristics of the established lesion.** There is distinct lateral proliferation of junctional epithelium. An intraepithelial tear leads to gingival pocket formation and, subsequently, subgingival proliferation of bacteria. Acute components of inflammation persist. Specific populations of mononuclear cells dominate in the infiltrate. In addition to T lymphocytes, B lymphocytes and plasma cells occur, which produce γ-globulins, mainly nonspecific, polyclonal antibodies. (Adapted from Page and Schroeder.[3])

## Peri-implant Mucositis

If plaque is allowed to accumulate on oral implants, inflammatory lesions develop in peri-implant mucosa as well.

➤ Early responses resemble largely their respective lesions in the gingiva.

➤ In case of prolonged plaque accumulation these lesions tend to proliferate in an apical direction at a faster pace. As compared to inflammatory lesions in the gingiva, the proportion of fibroblasts, in particular, is largely reduced in peri-implant mucositis.[9]

## ■ Pathogenesis of Periodontitis

### Advanced Lesion

After an indeterminate period, continuous challenge by bacteria colonizing the subgingival space may result in the breakdown of specific and nonspecific defense mechanisms of the host. Further progression of the lesion (and, concomitantly, of the front line of plaque) beyond the cementoenamel junction leads to the stage of periodontitis, in which all structures of the periodontium are involved[3]:

➤ A *subgingival plaque microbiota* is ultimately established.

➤ Proliferation of the thin pocket epithelium with bizarre epithelial ridges is accompanied by apical proliferation of the remains of junctional epithelium on the cementum surface, covered by degenerated fibers of the supra-alveolar fiber apparatus.

➤ Root cementum is pathologically altered and might be penetrated by bacteria.

➤ Active phases with clinically apparent loss of periodontal attachment seem to occur infrequently and are probably of short duration (see below).

While inflammation becomes more severe, concentration of cytokines in the connective tissue of the gingiva decreases. Neutrophil migration gradually wanes. Granulocytes may even be activated in the connective tissue. If there is local shortage of $\alpha_2$-macroglobulin and $\alpha_1$-protease inhibitor in the tissues, this may lead to excessive periodontal destruction.

Immunoregulatory control of Th1/Th2 cytokine profiles appears to be crucial in the development of active periodontitis lesions.

**T lymphocytes.** T lymphocytes are differentiated according to their surface antigens[10]:

➤ *T helper cells* (Th: CD4+) bind major histocompatibility complex (MHC) class II molecules and recognize epitopes presented by dendritic cells, macrophages, and B-lymphocytes. Regulation of cell-mediated and humoral immune response is facilitated by different cytokines (**Table 3.3**):

– Th1 cells produce interferon-γ (INF-γ) and IL-2 with the following target cells and functions:

• Enhanced cell-mediated reactions against intracellular microbes and delayed hypersensitivity

• Enhanced phagocytosis of neutrophil granulocytes and activation of macrophages to contain the inflammatory lesion

• Enhanced production of proinflammatory cytokines including IL-1 and TNF-α.

• *Note:* The Th1 cytokine profile may be characteristic for rather stable periodontal lesions.

– Th2 cells produce IL-4, IL-5, IL-6, and IL-10 with the following target cells and functions:

• Suppression of cell-mediated reactions

• Effect on antibody-mediated and allergic reactions

• Differentiation of B cells to plasma cells

• Stimulation of mast cells and eosinophil granulocytes

• *Note:* The Th2 cytokine profile may be characteristic for progressive periodontal lesions.

– Th0 cells (immature CD4 + T lymphocytes) produce INF-γ, IL-2, IL-4, and IL-5.

– Th17 cells produce proinflammatory IL-17 [11]:

• IL-17 stimulates various cell types to secrete proinflammatory cytokines IL-1, IL-6, TNF-α, matrix metalloproteinases and chemokines.

• Increased serum concentrations of IL-17 have been found in particular in aggressive periodontitis.[12]

– Follicular B helper T cells (Tfh) prominently express IL-21. Upon B-cell exposi-

**Table 3.3** Origin and function of some cytokines

| Cytokine | Origin | Function during inflammation |
|---|---|---|
| **Interleukin (IL)-1** | Macrophages, fibroblasts | • Proliferation of activated B and T cells<br>• Induction of prostaglandin $PGE_2$ and cytokine production of macrophages<br>• Expression of endothelial adhesion molecules<br>• Induction of IL-6, INF-β1 and GM-CSF (granulocyte–macrophage colony-stimulating factor)<br>• Induction of fever, acute phase reactants, osteoclast activity |
| **Tumor necrosis factor (TNF)-α** | Macrophages, T cells | • Induction of acute phase reactants<br>• Activation of phagocytes<br>• Induction of IFN-γ, TNF-α, IL-1, GM-CSF, IL-6 |
| **Interferon (INF)-γ** | T cells, natural killer (NK) cells | • Induction of Th1 cells<br>• Inhibition of IL-4 activities<br>• Enhances production of IL-12<br>• Stimulates activities of macrophages, cytotoxic T cells, and NK cells |
| **IL-2** | T cells | • Stimulates growth of activated T and B cells, NK cells |
| **IL-4** | T cells, mast cells, basophilic granulocytes | • Induces differentiation of Th2 cells<br>• Inhibits IL-2 and INF-γ induced activities<br>• Inhibits production of IL-12<br>• Induces proliferation and differentiation of B cells<br>• Induces proliferation of T cells<br>• Downregulates monocyte production of IL-1, TNF-α, IL-6 |
| **IL-5** | T cells, mast cells | • Proliferation of activated B cells<br>• Production of IgM and IgA |
| **IL-6** | Th cells, macrophages, mast cells, fibroblasts | • Growth and differentiation of B and T cells<br>• Induction of acute phase reactants |
| **IL-10** | T and B cells, monocytes and macrophages | • Enhancement of Th2 reactions and concomitant suppression of Th1 reactions<br>• Suppression of proliferation and cytokine production of activated T cells<br>• Suppression of monocyte production of IL-1, IL-6, IL-8<br>• Enhances IL-1ra production<br>• Enhances proliferation and differentiation of B cells |
| **IL-12** | B cells, macrophages, dendritic cells, keratinocytes, neutrophilic granulocytes | • Key role in induction of Th1 reactions<br>• Stimulates growth and cytotoxic activity of NK and T cells<br>• Enhances receptor expression for IL-18 on Th1 cells |
| **IL-13** | T cells | • Downregulates IL-12-production<br>• Mounting of Th2 reaction<br>• Stimulation of B cells<br>• Inhibition of cytokine production of macrophages |
| **IL-17** | Th17 cells | • Stimulation of various cells to produce proinflammatory cytokines IL-1, IL-6, TNF-α, matrix metalloproteinases (MMP), and chemokines |
| **IL-18** | Monocytes, neutrophilic granulocytes | • Structurally homologous to IL-1β<br>• Induction of INF-γ<br>• Maturation of naive T cells to Th1 cells |
| **IL-21** | Activated CD4+ T cells, Th2, Th17 and Tfh cells | • Helps activate B cell function including Ig switch to IgG1 and IgG3 |

tion to a bacterial antigen, Tfh cells help in the differentiation of B cells to antigen-producing plasma cells, including an Ig class switch to IgG1 and IgG3, and memory B cells.

– Regulatory T cells (Tregs) are characterized as suppressor CD4+Th cells that prominently produce IL-10 and transforming growth factor beta (TGF-β) with immunosuppressive effects on Th1, Th2, Th17, and Tfh cells.

➤ *Cytotoxic/suppressor T cells* (Tc, Ts: CD8+) bind to class I antigens of the MHC complex:
  – Cytotoxic Tc cells produce IL-10 and INF-γ.
  – Ts suppressor cells produce IL-4.

T cells cooperate closely:

➤ A dendritic cell, which has engulfed virus particles or other microorganisms, presents the respective antigen to Th1 lymphocytes via MHC II molecules.

➤ Th1 lymphocytes condition the dendritic cell with INF-γ.

➤ The conditioned dendritic cell presents the respective antigen via the MHC I complex to immature Tc cells.

➤ Tc cells mature, proliferate, and kill all cells which present the respective MHC I antigens.

In (active) periodontitis, the ratio between CD4+ and CD8+ cells in the inflammatory infiltrate of the gingiva is increased. Among helper cells, Th2 cells seem to predominate:

➤ Their cytokines amplify the local humoral immune response.

➤ In particular, B-lymphocytes are stimulated by IL-4 to secrete IL-1.

➤ In contrast, IL-1 production by macrophages is suppressed.

The predominance of B cells and plasma cells in the inflammatory infiltrate underscores the important role of Th2 cells in the immune regulation of active, progressive lesions.[13] Under the influence of LPS and cytokines IL-1 and TNF-α, or other proinflammatory mediators such as PGE$_2$, junctional epithelial cells, fibroblasts, and vascular endothelia exert genetically programmed, destructive activities:

➤ In health, genes for the production of collagen and inhibitors of matrix metalloproteinases (MMP) are activated, while genes

for production of tissue collagenase are inactivated.

➤ Under pathologic conditions this relationship may be reversed: if stimulated by LPS, fibroblasts may secrete IL-1β themselves.

**Monocytes/macrophages.**    Monocytes/macrophages do play a central role as well.[7] The activity of macrophages is mainly genetically determined. It can be suppressed by INF-γ.

➤ LPS of gram-negative and lipoteichoic acid from gram-positive bacteria bind, via lipopolysaccharide binding protein (LBP), to the CD14 receptor of macrophages.

➤ Toll-like receptors (TLR, see below) transmit signals into the cell via their IL-1 receptor-like domain:
  – Nuclear transcription factor (NF)-κB, a key regulator of immune and inflammatory responses, is activated.
  – Production and secretion of prostaglandins, cytokines, and MMP is initiated.

➤ Alternatively, LBP or soluble CD14 (sCD14) may transfer LPS and lipoteichoic acid to nonactivating serum proteins (e.g., serum lipoprotein) for eventual removal of the offending bacterial components from the system without local activation of the innate host response.

➤ TNF-α and IL-1β bind to surface receptors of fibroblasts, inducing the production of MMP and PGE$_2$:
  – MMP leads to destruction of the extracellular matrix of gingiva and periodontal ligament.
  – PGE$_2$ activates osteoclasts and induces bone resorption.
  – IL-1β and TNF-α are also involved in bone destruction.

**Toll-like receptors.** Innate immunity provides not only a first line of antimicrobial host defense, but also has a profound impact on the establishment of adaptive immune responses.[14] Innate host responses, characterized by pattern-recognition receptor binding to microbial components, form a highly coordinated and dynamic process:

➤ Toll-like receptors (TLRs) link innate and acquired immunity.

➤ They may represent the most ancient host defense system, which is found, for example, in mammals, insects, and plants.

TLRs recognize pathogen-associated molecular patterns (PAMP) and, more significantly, discriminate between different classes of pathogens. The TLR expression repertoire varies on different cell types. Endothelial cells express more TLR4 (which responds to LPS from gram-negative bacteria) than TLR2 (ligand for lipoteichoic acid from gram-positive bacteria). Due to lack of TLR4 ligands, intestinal epithelia do normally not respond to LPS. Bacterial components and host signaling molecules may influence TLR expression.

**Osteoimmunology.** The interface between bone metabolism and immune pathology plays an important role in a number of diseases such as the development of bone cancer metastases, rheumatoid osteitis, osteoporosis and osteopetrosis, and periodontitis. The close relationship between the immune system and bone metabolism may ultimately lead to periodontal bone loss[15]:

➤ RANKL (receptor activator of NF-κB ligand), which belongs to the tumor necrosis factor ligand superfamily, is primarily expressed on osteoblasts and activated T lymphocytes under the influence of proinflammatory cytokines and mediators (IL-1, IL-6, IL-11, IL-17, TNF-α, PGE$_2$).

➤ RANKL signals respective progenitor cells to differentiate into mature osteoclasts.

➤ Among other cells, osteoblasts express osteoprotegerin (OPG) which acts as a scavenger receptor for RANKL.

**Virulence factors.** In turn, **virulence factors** of periodontal pathogens directly or indirectly interfere with defense mechanisms of the host (see Chapter 2, **Table 2.3**):

➤ Important virulence factors of *Aggregatibacter actinomycetemcomitans* include:
  – Leukotoxin, which kills neutrophil granulocytes, monocytes, and T-lymphocytes.
  – Cytolethal toxin, which causes apoptosis.
  – A low-molecular-weight protein, which suppresses chemotaxis of neutrophil granulocytes.
  – Immunosuppressive factors, which suppress production of IgG and IgM.
  – Fc-binding protein, which competes with specific receptors of neutrophil granulocytes and prohibits phagocytosis.

  – Moreover, RANKL is upregulated in the presence of *A. actinomycetemcomitans*.
➤ Virulence factors of *P. gingivalis*:
  – Expression of E-selectin on the endothelial inner surface is not triggered by the bacterium (see **Fig. 3.4**).
  – Its LPS only weakly activates IL-1 and TNF-α, being cytokines which would otherwise strongly induce expression of E-selectin.
  – The production, respectively expression, of IL-8 and ICAM-1 are suppressed.
  – Enzymes are produced that cleave most of the serum proteins, including immunoglobulins and complement.
  – Immunodominant molecules (gingipain, fimbrillin, heat-shock proteins, and other surface antigens), which are produced by *P. gingivalis* and other periodontal pathogens, may induce excessive immune reactions.

**Specific antibodies.** Serum titers of *specific antibodies*, especially IgG, against *A. actinomycetemcomitans* and/or *P. gingivalis*, may be considerably increased in patients with periodontitis and heavy subgingival infection with the respective bacteria. It has been suggested that periodontitis is frequently more generalized if antibody production does not occur. Recent studies, however, did not confirm this postulate.[16]

**Saliva.** Saliva plays an important role at the mucosal level in the maintenance of oral health. Saliva contains amongst others[17]:

➤ Lysozyme, a muramidase which can damage the bacterial cell wall
➤ β-defensins, cysteine-rich proteins with antibiotic activity
➤ Mucins, glycoproteins of small salivary glands
➤ *Note:* High serum antibody titers of IgA1 and large amounts of secretory IgA2 against oral pathogens such as *A. actinomycetemcomitans*, *P. gingivalis* or *Streptococcus mutans* may prevent the development of inflammatory conditions in the gingiva or dental caries, respectively. Some periodontal pathogens are able to cleave IgA1 and IgG.

Pathohistologically, the advanced periodontal lesion (periodontitis) has the following characteristics (**Fig. 3.7**)[3]:

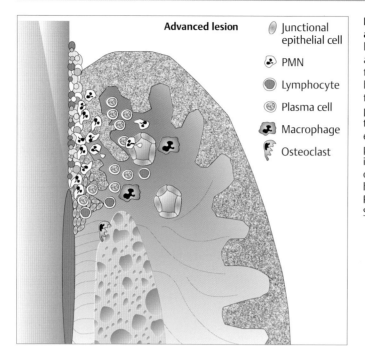

**Fig. 3.7 Characteristics of the advanced lesion.** Pocket epithelium with bizarre epithelial ridges and loss of connective tissue attachment to the tooth. The ratio between T helper cells and cytotoxic T cells is increased. Th2 cells produce cytokines which amplify the humoral immune response especially. Therefore, plasma cells predominate in the inflammatory infiltrate. Bone loss is induced by osteoclasts, which are activated by high concentrations of IL-1β and PGE$_2$. (Adapted from Page and Schroeder.[3])

Legend (within figure):
- Junctional epithelial cell
- PMN
- Lymphocyte
- Plasma cell
- Macrophage
- Osteoclast

Advanced lesion

➤ Persistence of all characteristics of the established lesion
➤ Involvement of alveolar bone and periodontal ligament
➤ Formation of a periodontal pocket
➤ Further loss of collagen in the area of the periodontal pocket, fibrosis in more distant areas
➤ Marked predominance of plasma cells, especially in active lesions
➤ Transformation of bone marrow into fibrous connective tissue

## Formal Pathogenesis—Progression

Destructive periodontal diseases may occur in an isolated fashion or at various sites and teeth in the oral cavity. If left untreated, the disease is characterized by progressive loss of parts of the tooth-supporting apparatus, which usually proceeds apically and is limited laterally:

➤ Loss of connective tissue attachment of supra-alveolar fibers
➤ Loss of supportive alveolar bone

Although periodontitis manifests itself locally, there is undoubtedly a systemic component as regards both its pathogenesis as well as its influence on the body's health (see Chapter 8).

Whether destructive periodontitis develops or not mainly depends on the ability of the host—in conjunction with neutrophil granulocytes, antibodies, and complement—to prevent exposure of the connective tissue to dentogingival plaque bacteria, their metabolites and, especially, LPS. In this case, only a mild, self-limited form of the disease will occur, namely gingivitis or mild periodontitis. Subsequent production of antibodies will in most cases keep the disease localized.

Destructive periodontal disease, on the other hand, may be the result of an activation of the *macrophage/lymphocyte axis* (**Fig. 3.8**).[18] Some individuals seem to respond to dentogingival plaque with an immediate activation of tissue macrophages and lymphocytes.

➤ In these cases a hyper-responsive macrophage trait has been postulated, which is probably genetically determined, may be influenced by smoking, stress, and some dietary factors, which may lead to high concentrations of IL-1 and PGE$_2$ in gingival connective tissue and crevicular fluid.

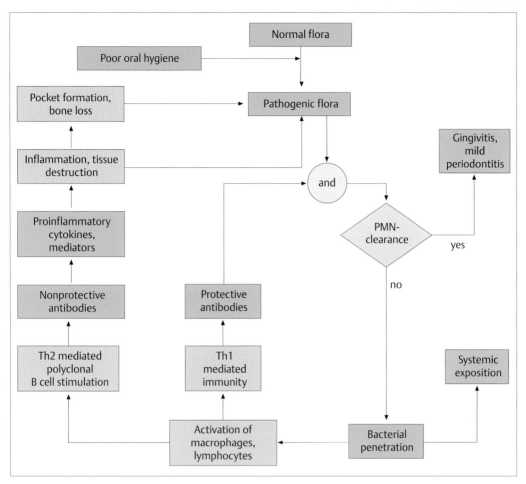

**Fig. 3.8  Pathogenesis pathway of periodontitis.** Pathogenic flora develops mainly due to neglect of oral hygiene. Usually, the first line of defense, namely the polymorphonuclear (PMN) granulocyte/complement axis, prevents penetration of bacteria or their metabolites into connective tissue. Gingivitis develops. If bacterial penetration or exposure to its metabolic products does occur, the macrophage/lymphocyte axis is activated. Under the influence of mainly Th1 reactions, specific antibodies are produced, which may be protective at later episodes of the disease. As a result, the advanced lesion is stable. In case of a predominant Th2 response polyclonal B cell activation is prominent. Proinflammatory cytokines and mediators such as IL-1 and PGE$_2$ lead to increased inflammation with tissue destruction and, consequently, pocket formation and bone loss. Pockets provide excellent conditions for the growth of most periodontal pathogens. (Adapted from Offenbacher.[18])

➤ It is assumed that in these individuals, during phases of undisturbed plaque accumulation, the gingivitis stage will rapidly develop further into destructive periodontitis.

An important characteristic of all chronic diseases, including periodontitis,[19] is alternating phases of progression and remission. Progression rates vary. Exacerbations with notable loss of attachment within a short time are relatively rare. After destructive phases, there may be prolonged periods of remission. Periodontitis may in some cases and/or at certain tooth surfaces also advance in a continuous manner.

## Characteristics of a Multifactorial Disease

As in all chronic diseases, there are initiating factors, factors which might impede development, and factors that influence clinical expression of periodontitis.

➤ *Note:* Although bacteria produce a great deal of substances that have deleterious effects on the host, almost all periodontal tissue destruction is due to inflammatory and immune reactions of the hosts themselves.

➤ Specific periodontal pathogens can explain only a minor part of the clinical variability of inflammatory periodontal disease. Tobacco consumption, for instance, appears to have a far greater impact (see Chapter 8).

➤ Inflammatory and immunological reactions, and connective tissue and bone metabolism are basically genetically controlled, but certainly influenced by acquired and behavioral risk factors as well.

In order to better understand complex diseases such as periodontitis, hierarchical *systems biology models* have recently been developed and subsequently applied (**Fig. 3.9**, **Box 3.1**).[20,21]

➤ While at the higher level clinically observable parameters such as smoking are considered, lower levels comprise tissues, cells, subcellular structures, and molecules.

➤ Biologic expression of the immune–inflammatory network as well as connective tissue and bone metabolism networks at the lower level may be determined by:
  – Bacterial profiles
  – Genetic make-up, gene expression, and gene-environment interaction[22]
  – Proteins and metabolites

For example, the predicted chemotaxis pathway and transepithelial leukocyte migration as well as immune responses have recently been confirmed in whole-transcriptome gene expression

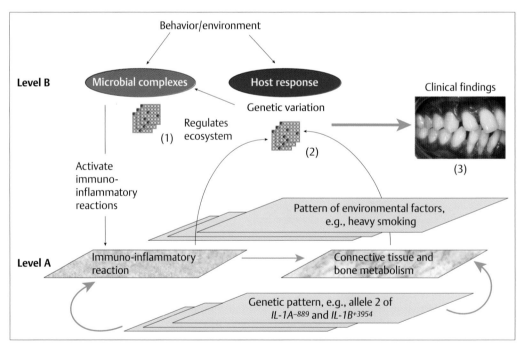

**Fig. 3.9   Systems biology based model of the pathogenesis of periodontitis.** Certain microbial complexes establish themselves on the tooth surface (cf. **Fig. 2.8**) in response to behavioral and environmental factors including host genetic factors. This leads to activation of immunoinflammatory reactions in the tissues and, in turn, influences connective tissue and bone metabolism which represent the lower level **A**. Observable components of the disease—for example, results of micro arrays of microbial complexes (1), inflammatory components as proteins and metabolites (2), and tissue alterations which are described by clinical parameters (3)—represent the higher level **B**. (Modified after Kornman[20]; courtesy of American Academy of Periodontology.)

during experimentally induced gingivitis and its subsequent resolution.[23]

➤ During gingivitis induction a significant, transient increase in the gene expression of inflammatory and oxidative stress mediators was observed, including *IL1A, IL1B, IL8, RANTES*, as well as genes encoding colony stimulating factor 3 (*CSF3*), and superoxide dismutase 2 (*SOD 2*).

➤ On the other hand, decreased expression of genes encoding INF-γ-induced protein 10 (*IP10*), interferon inducible T-cell alpha chemoattractant (*ITAC*), matrix metalloproteinase 10 (*MMP10*), and beta 4 defensin (*DEFB4*) were noted.

➤ These genes reversed expression patterns upon resolution, in parallel with the reversal of gingival inflammation.

As another example, gene transcriptomes in a large number of gingival biopsies from patients with chronic or aggressive periodontitis revealed, in fact, two distinct gene expression signatures, one primarily related to cell proliferation and the other to lymphocyte activation and unfolded protein responses, which may lead to novel classification of periodontitis.[24]

Among acquired and behavioral risk factors for destructive periodontal disease (see Chapter 8), the most important are:

➤ Type I and type II diabetes mellitus with a relative risk of 2 to 3, or even higher in patients with poorly controlled disease. There appears to be a bidirectional relationship since diabetic control is hampered in patients with periodontitis.

➤ Excessive tobacco consumption. The relative risk for periodontitis is estimated between 2.5 and 6, and may even be higher in smoking adolescents.

➤ Obesity, metabolic syndrome.

➤ HIV infection.

➤ Stress and inappropriate coping strategies.

➤ Osteoporosis.

All complex chronic diseases, such as cardiovascular disease, diabetes mellitus and periodontitis, have usually a *polygenetic* component which may lead to some typical characteristics:

➤ Comparably inconspicuous phenotype

➤ Rather slow progression

➤ Chronic course

➤ Delayed disease onset

---

**Box 3.1   Systems biology of the pathogenesis of inflammatory periodontal diseases**

The traditional, reductionist approach to demystify the pathogenesis of complex chronic diseases, including periodontitis, was helpful in the past for the identification of possible major players: bacteria in dental biofilm; acute and chronic components of local and systemic immune defense; connective tissue and bone metabolism (see **Figs. 3.1** and **3.5–3.7**).

A deeper understanding of previously rather blurred, largely nonlinear processes may be expected by applying systems biological, hierarchical models which analyze the interactive network of biological mechanisms locally, regionally, and systemically; and they may possibly allow coherent interpretations in the near future (see **Fig. 3.9**).

Systems biology tries to integrate huge amounts of complex data, which have been collected at different levels (genome, epigenome, transcriptome, proteome, metabolome), in an interdisciplinary approach and by use of appropriate mathematic models and computer simulations.

---

## Genetic Component

Previous heritability estimates of chronic periodontitis of about 50%, which were based on studies of twins and families,[25] have been called into question. In recent years, in particular, genetic polymorphisms (single nucleotide polymorphisms, SNPs) and combinations of SNPs (haploid genotypes, or haplotypes) in targeted genes, which are known to play a special role in immunological/inflammatory processes, have been identified:

➤ Taken individually, these SNPs, which have been observed in numerous genes, may contribute only minimally to the overall pathophysiology of periodontitis.

➤ In certain combinations and in sum they may determine the clinical picture or phenotype, in particular in combination with acquired diseases (e. g., diabetes mellitus) and/or behavioral factors such as smoking.

➤ The number and type of modifying genes, which had been associated with onset and course of periodontitis, may vary in different ethnicities.

➤ *Note:* Certain genetic patterns have been proposed for the observed association between several chronic diseases such as coronary heart disease, diabetes mellitus, obesity, and periodontitis.

It is long known that relatively rare, aggressive periodontitis actually cumulates in families (see Chapter 4):

➤ It is possible that a yet to be identified, single gene locus with autosomal dominant inheritance is responsible for increased susceptibility.

**Table 3.4** Certain single nucleotide polymorphisms (SNPs; common allele > rare allele), which have been related to increased susceptibility for chronic (CP) and/or aggressive periodontitis (AgP). (After Laine et al[27]; Vieira and Albandar[28])

| | Chromosome, gene locus | Polymorphism | Association with periodontitis |
|---|---|---|---|
| IL-1 family (IL-1α, IL-1β, IL-1RA) | 2q13-q21 | *IL1A* -889 (+4845): C > T<br>*IL1B* +3954: C > T<br>*IL1B* -511 (-31): C > T<br>*IL1RN* VNTR+2018: C > T | Moderate association of, in particular, haplotype *IL1A* (-889) / *IL1B* (+3954) with CP in Caucasian subjects |
| TNF-α | 6p21.3 | *TNFA* -1031: T > C; -863: C > A; -857: C > T; -367: G > A; -308: G > A; -238: G > A; +489: G > A | No association of any polymorphisms with CP or AgP |
| IL-4 | 5q31.1 | *IL4* -33: C > T; -590: C > T; 70 bp VNTR intron 2 | Haplotype of *IL4* -33, -590, 70 bp VNTR may be associated with CP |
| IL-6 | 7p21 | *IL6* -174: G > C | Possible association with CP |
| IL-10 | 1q31-q32 | *IL10* -592: C > A | Possible association with CP |
| Fcγ receptors FcγRIIa FcγRIIIb | 1q23-q24 | *FCGR2A* +131: H > R<br>*FCGR3B* +141: G > C (NA1 > NA2) | Limited evidence for association with CP and AgP |
| Vitamin D receptor (VDR) | 12q12-q14 | *VDR* Taq1: T > C | Possible association of rare variant of Taq1 (likely in combination with further VDR gene polymorphisms) with CP |
| CD14 | 5q21-q23 | *CD14* -260: C > T | Possible association with CP |
| Toll-like receptors TLR2, TLR4 | 4q32, 9q32-q33 | *TLR2, TLR4;* various SNPs | No association with CP |
| Prostaglandin endoperoxide-synthase 2 (COX-2) | 1q25.2-q25.3 | *COX2* rs6681231: C > G | Possible association with AgP |
| β-Defensin | 8p23.1 | *DEFB1* rs1047031: A | Possible association with CP and AgP |
| Glycosyltransferase | 9q34.3 | *GLT6D1* rs1537415: G | Possible association with AgP |
| Cathepsin C | 11q4 | *CTSC,* various SNPs | Causal in Papillon–Lefrévre syndrome; possible association with AgP |

➤ Alternatively, several modifying genes may control individual immune responses (e. g., IgG2 production in case of biofilm infections with gram-negative bacteria).

➤ A combination of both possibilities may hold true as well.

➤ For instance, in the very rare Papillon–Le-févre syndrome (PLS), which cumulates due to consanguinity of parents in certain families (see Chapter 4), numerous mutations in the cathepsin C gene have been identified which may lead to complete loss of respective enzyme activity. Whether and to what extent dermatological and periodontal symptoms of PLS and patients with prepubertal periodontitis with partial penetrant PLS are related to loss of cathepsin C activity is currently unclear.[26]

Various so far identified SNPs have been associated with increased susceptibility for periodontitis[27,28]:

➤ Polymorphisms in the IL-1 gene cluster on chromosome 2q13-q21 (see Chapter 6, **Box 6.1**):
  – In recent meta-analyses, a combination of allele 2*2 (C→T) of *IL1A*-889 and *IL1B* +3953/4 had been moderately associated in Northern European individuals with chronic (but not aggressive) periodontitis (odds ratio about 1.5) where it occurs with a prevalence of about 36%.

  – In these cases, certain cytokines have been found at greater concentrations in those with gingival exudate and/or tissue, respectively; for instance, as compared to homozygous carriers of allele 1 at locus *ILA1*-889, concentration of IL-1α in gingival exudate was up to four times increased.[29]

  – In particular, in Asian populations no association with this particular haplotype could be ascertained due to its low prevalence.

➤ Numerous polymorphisms in genes encoding other cytokines (e. g., IL-4, IL-6, IL-10), Fcγ receptors, the vitamin D receptor, COX-2, etc. have been associated with chronic and/or aggressive periodontitis as well (**Table 3.4**).

➤ Several further, possibly genetically determined, functional anomalies of the immune response have been suggested in aggressive periodontitis (**Table 3.5**).

Recently, *genome-wide association studies* with very large numbers (> 1,000) of well-defined cases and controls have been undertaken.[30] Their aim is a hypothesis-free collection of the entire genetic information. As a rule, identified gene loci are generally only weakly associated with disease (odds ratios of about 1.3). Respective results need to be (and in part have been) confirmed in even larger cohorts.[31]

**Table 3.5** Possible immune defense anomalies which have been discussed in aggressive periodontitis*

| Anomaly | Biological effects |
|---|---|
| Dysfunctions of neutrophil granulocytes | • Impaired chemotaxis<br>• Reduced number of receptors for FMLP, C5a, IL-8<br>• Mutation and defective FMLP-receptor<br>• Reduced phagocytosis, reduced bacteriocidal activity<br>• Reduced release of leukotriene B<br>• Enhanced release of superoxide anion |
| Protective antibodies of subclass IgG2 | May rarely be formed in generalized aggressive periodontitis (contradicting observations) |
| Monocytic response to bacterial lipopolysaccharides | Increased release of $PGE_2$ and IL-1 |
| Imbalance of activities of different T cell subpopulations | • Suppressed Th1 response (IL-2, INF-γ, TNF)<br>• Increased Th2 response (IL-4, IL-5, IL-6): polyclonal B cell stimulation |

* For key to abbreviations and symbols, see **Table 3.3** and main text.

**Peri-implantitis**

Pathohistologically, the composition of the inflammatory infiltrate does not differ in peri-implantitis from that in periodontitis:

➤ Predominance of plasma cells
➤ Lymphocytes
➤ Macrophages
➤ Polymorphonuclear granulocytes

However, the extension of the lesion in peri-implant tissues is distinctly different with grave consequences[32]:

➤ Frequently the infiltrate is in direct contact with the alveolar bone.
➤ In the apical part of the lesion there is no epithelial barrier between the infiltrate and the plaque-covered implant surface.

# 4 Classification of Periodontal Diseases

Plaque-induced periodontal diseases and a plenitude of common, infrequent or extremely rare nonplaque-induced disorders, more or less harmful or serious, may involve the mucous membranes of the oral cavity[1] and, in particular, the gingiva and other periodontal tissues.

## ■ Current Classification

Classification systems provide a framework within which the etiology, pathogenesis, diagnosis, and therapy of diseases can be scientifically studied. Furthermore, they enable the clinician to assess individual treatment needs. The current classification scheme of periodontal diseases is based on consensus reports of the 1999 International Workshop for a Classification of Periodontal Diseases and Conditions.[2] The most important results of this workshop were:
➤ Delineation of detailed criteria for classification of gingival diseases.
➤ A new classification of periodontitis. The previous classification which was largely based on age of onset and progression rate was dismissed:
  – The term "adult periodontitis" was dropped. Most of these cases are characterized by slow disease progression. Therefore, the term *chronic periodontitis* would be more appropriate. It was also noted that some cases of chronic periodontitis may also be found in children and adolescents.
  – The term "early-onset periodontitis" was dropped as well. This heterogeneous group previously brought prepubertal and juvenile periodontitis together. Many of these cases are characterized by rapid progression, and it was concluded that a more appropriate term would be aggressive periodontitis. Aggressive periodontitis may also develop at an older age. Many cases previously assigned to "refractory periodontitis" might be included in the category of aggressive periodontitis.

## ■ Plaque-Induced Gingival Diseases

Note that in all clinical aspects of periodontal diseases, dental plaque is mentioned—a typical biofilm (see Chapter 2), which commonly establishes itself on tooth and dental implant surfaces.

Dental plaque-induced gingivitis usually prevails on a periodontium without connective tissue attachment loss and bone loss. If it occurs on a periodontium with attachment and bone loss the situation should be considered stable or nonprogressive. Common characteristics of plaque-induced gingivitis are:
➤ Dental plaque in the region of the gingival margin.
➤ Well-defined histological alterations.
➤ Clinical signs and symptoms of inflammation which are confined to the (marginal) gingiva:
  – *Swelling* due to edema or fibrosis
  – Red or bluish-red *change in color*
  – *Gingival exudate.* Its flow rate (volume per time interval, see Chapter 6) increases with increasing severity of inflammation.
➤ Local factors may influence the clinical picture of gingivitis—for example, calculus, insufficient restorations, crowded teeth, etc.
➤ *Note:* Inflammatory alterations are completely reversible after removal of causative plaque.

### Systemically Modified Gingival Diseases

Inflammatory responses to dental plaque may be enhanced by *sex steroid hormones*:
➤ After the onset of puberty (Tanner stage 2 or higher).
➤ Immediately before ovulation during the menstrual cycle.
➤ During pregnancy, mostly during the second and third trimesters. Locally, a *pyogenic granuloma* may develop, that is, an exophytic granuloma of the gingiva, frequently involving an interdental papilla (so-called pregnancy tumor).

**Table 4.1** Current classification of periodontal diseases and conditions. (After Armitage [2])

| **I  Gingival diseases** |
| --- |

A  *Dental plaque-induced gingival diseases*

  1  Gingivitis associated with dental plaque only
    a  Without other local contributing factors
    b  With local contributing factors

  2  Gingival diseases modified by systemic factors
    a  Associated with the endocrine system
      1) Puberty-associated gingivitis
      2) Menstrual cycle-associated gingivitis
      3) Pregnancy-associated
        a) Gingivitis
        b) Pyogenic granuloma
      4) Diabetes mellitus-associated gingivitis
    b  Associated with blood dyscrasias
      1) Leukemia-associated gingivitis
      2) Other

  3  Gingival diseases modified by medications
    a  Drug-influenced gingival diseases
      1) Drug-influenced gingival enlargements
      2) Drug-influenced gingivitis
        a) Oral contraceptive-associated gingivitis
        b) Other

  4  Gingival diseases modified by malnutrition
    a  Ascorbic-acid-deficiency gingivitis
    b  Other

B  *Non-plaque-induced gingival lesions*

  1  Gingival diseases of specific bacterial origin
    a  *Neisseria gonorrhea*-associated lesions
    b  *Treponema pallidum*-associated lesions
    c  Streptococcal species-associated lesions
    d  Other

  2  Gingival diseases of viral origin
    a  Herpesvirus infections
      1) Primary herpetic gingivostomatitis
      2) Recurrent oral herpes
      3) Varicella-zoster infections
    b  Other

  3  Gingival diseases of fungal origin
    a  *Candida*-species infections
      1) Generalized gingival candidosis
      2) Linear gingival erythema
    b  Histoplasmosis
    c  Other

  4  Gingival lesions of genetic origin
    a  Hereditary gingival fibromatosis
    b  Other

  5  Gingival manifestations of systemic conditions
    a  Mucocutaneous disorders
      1) Lichen planus
      2) Pemphigoid
      3) Pemphigus vulgaris
      4) Erythema multiforme
      5) Lupus erythematosus
      6) Drug-induced
      7) Other
    b  Allergic reactions
      1) Dental restorative materials
        a) Mercury
        b) Nickel
        c) Acrylic
        d) Other
      2) Reactions attributable to
        a) Toothpastes/dentifrices
        b) Mouthrinses/mouthwashes
        c) Chewing gum additives
        d) Foods and additives
        e) Other

  6  Traumatic lesions (factitious, iatrogenic, accidental)
    a  Chemical injury
    b  Mechanical injury
    c  Thermal injury

  7  Foreign body reactions

  8  Not otherwise specified

| **II  Chronic periodontitis** |
| --- |

A  *Localized*
B  *Generalized*

| **III  Aggressive periodontitis** |
| --- |

A  Localized
B  Generalized

| **IV  Periodontitis as manifestation of systemic diseases** |
| --- |

A  *Associated with hematological disorders*

  1  Acquired neutropenia
  2  Leukemias
  3  Other

B  *Associated with genetic disorders*

  1  Familial and cyclic neutropenia
  2  Down syndrome
  3  Leukocyte adhesion deficiency syndromes
  4  Papillon–Lefévre syndrome
  5  Chediak–Higashi syndrome
  6  Histiocytosis syndromes
  7  Glycogen storage disease
  8  Infantile genetic agranulocytosis
  9  Cohen syndrome

continued ▶

**Table 4.1** Continued

| IV | **Periodontitis as manifestation of systemic diseases** |
|---|---|

*B Associated with genetic disorders*

    10 Ehlers–Danlos syndrome (types IV and VIII)
    11 Hypophosphatasia
    12 Other

*C Not otherwise specified*

| V | **Necrotizing periodontal diseases** |
|---|---|

*A Necrotizing ulcerative gingivitis*
*B Necrotizing ulcerative periodontitis*

| VI | **Abscesses of the periodontium** |
|---|---|

A Gingival abscess
B Periodontal abscess
C Pericoronal abscess

| VII | **Periodontitis associated with endodontic lesions** |
|---|---|

*A Combined periodontal–endodontic lesions*

| VIII | **Developmental or acquired deformities and conditions** |
|---|---|

*A Localized tooth-related factors that modify or predispose to plaque-induced gingival diseases/ periodontitis*

    1 Tooth anatomy
    2 Dental restorations/appliances
    3 Root fractures
    4 Cervical root resorption and cemental tear

*B Mucogingival deformities and conditions around teeth*

    1 Gingival/soft tissue recession
      a Facial or lingual surfaces
      b Interproximal (papillary)
    2 Lack of keratinized gingiva
    3 Decreased vestibular depth
    4 Aberrant frenum/muscle position
    5 Gingival excess
      a Pseudopocket
      b Inconsistent gingival margin
      c Excessive gingival display
      d Gingival enlargement (see I.A.3. and I.B.4.)
    6 Abnormal color

*C Mucogingival deformities and conditions on edentulous ridges*

    1 Vertical and/or horizontal ridge deficiency
    2 Lack of gingival/keratinized tissue
    3 Gingival/soft tissue enlargement
    4 Aberrant frenum/muscle position
    5 Decreased vestibular depth
    6 Abnormal color

*D Occlusal trauma*

    1 Primary occlusal trauma
    2 Secondary occlusal trauma

Increase of steroid hormones in gingival exudate during puberty and, much more pronounced, during pregnancy may result in:

➤ Distinct changes of ecological conditions in the dentogingival region (see Chapter 2), leading to possible advantage for colonization by *Prevotella intermedia*, *P. nigrescens* and members of the *P. melaninogenica* group.
➤ Enhanced inflammatory and immunological responses to microbial plaque due to presence of specific receptors for sex steroid hormones in the gingiva.

The inflammatory reaction to dental plaque is also enhanced in poorly controlled *diabetes mellitus*, particularly in children with type I diabetes mellitus.

In several forms of *acute leukemia* inflammatory reactions may lead to necrosis and/or gingival enlargement.

## Drug-Influenced Gingival Diseases

Drug-induced *gingival enlargements* have a genetic predisposition. Lesions are more prevalent at anterior teeth, especially interdental papillae. Drug-influenced enlargements are more frequently seen in young individuals. The following drugs may lead to gingival enlargement:

➤ *Anticonvulsants* (e. g., phenytoin):
  – Gingival enlargement in about 50% of patients.
  – Careful plaque-control cannot prevent gingival enlargement but may reduce extent and severity.
➤ *Calcium channel blockers* (e. g., nifedipine, varapamil, diltiazem):
  – Frequently prescribed in patients aged 50 years or older for hypertension, arrhythmia, and angina pectoris.
  – About 20% of patients develop gingival enlargement.
  – Oral hygiene possibly influences the development of lesions.
➤ *Immunosuppressants* (cyclosporin A [CsA], tacrolimus):
  – First choice prescription following organ transplantation or for the treatment of autoimmune diseases.
  – 60% of adult patients and more than 70% of children under CsA treatment may develop gingival enlargement. Under tacroli-

mus treatment, prevalence is less than 30%.[3]
- Meticulous plaque control cannot prevent development of lesions but may reduce their extent and severity.
- Combination therapy with calcium channel blockers has synergistic effects as regards gingival enlargement.
➤ *Note:* Neither low nor high dosages of estrogen and gestagen in *oral contraceptives* can enhance inflammatory reactions in gingiva. What has been described as "pill gingivitis" does no longer occur.[4]

### Gingival Diseases Modified by Malnutrition

As a result of *malnutrition*, immune defense mechanisms may be impaired, which may lead to an increased susceptibility to infections. In developed countries this is seen mostly in cases of:
➤ Anorexia nervosa
➤ Chronic alcohol abuse

Chronic *ascorbic acid* (vitamin C) *avitaminosis* (scurvy) may enhance inflammatory reactions to dental plaque.

### ■ Gingival Diseases Not Induced by Dental Plaque

### Gingival Diseases of Specific Bacterial Origin

Specific infections with bacteria, which are usually not residents in dental plaque, may involve the gingiva:
➤ *Neisseria gonorrhoeae.* Usually asymptomatic enanthema.
➤ *Treponema pallidum.* All three stages of syphilis may manifest in the oral cavity:
- Primary: asymptomatic chancre with regional lymphadenopathy
- Secondary: mucous patches
- Tertiary: gumma, especially of the hard and soft palate.
➤ Specific infections with β-hemolysing streptococci of Lancefield-group A, in particular *Streptococcus pyogenes* (scarlet fever).
➤ Specific infections with other bacteria (e.g., mycobacterial infections).

### Gingival Diseases of Viral Origin

Apart from measles and rubella, a number of viral diseases manifest in the oral cavity, some of them also at the gingiva:
➤ Herpesviruses:
- Herpes simplex virus (HSV-1 predominantly orally; HSV-2 predominantly anogenitally)
- Varicella zoster virus (human herpes virus 3, HHV-3)
- Epstein–Barr virus (HHV-4)
- Human cytomegalovirus (HHV-5)
➤ Human papillomavirus (HPV). Most HPV infections are subclinical and will not cause physical symptoms (warts, benign papillomas). *Note:* HPV-16 and -18 infections are a unique cause of oropharyngeal cancer.

Infections with herpesviruses usually induce acute symptoms:
➤ *Herpetic gingivostomatitis.* Primary infection with HSV-1 or HSV-2:
- Highest incidence at the age of 2 to 4 years; occurrence in young adults is also possible.
- Herpetic vesicles are found anywhere in the oral cavity, with no predilection: lips, cheek, tongue, gingiva, and pharynx.
- Vesicles have a high tendency of rupture leaving painful, fibrin-coated ulcers with diffuse erythema.
- Fever, malaise, regionary lymphadenitis.
- Halitosis.
➤ *Recurrent oral herpes infection.* Orolabial herpes, cold sores. After primary infection, HSV-1 or HSV-2 persists in sensory ganglia and may be activated. Local exacerbation may occur in cases of:
- Febrile common cold, UV-radiation, menstruation, local stimuli (e.g., during dental treatment, emotional stress).
- Suppression or dysfunction of the immune system, radiotherapy.
- In most cases local, highly contagious vesicles emerge, for instance on the lip or at the gingiva.
➤ *Infection with varicella-zoster virus* (HHV-3). Primary infection is chicken pox; the virus then persists in sensory dorsal root ganglia:
- When the virus is activated (e.g., after UV-radiation), lesions emerge within the

area of the main sensory branch: herpes zoster (shingles).
– *Note:* Virus activation may be a first indication of an unrelated, serious systemic disease.
➤ Infections with Epstein–Barr virus (HHV-4):
– Cause of infectious mononucleosis.
– Association with hairy leukoplakia on the lateral aspect of the tongue in HIV-seropositive patients.
– Epstein–Barr virus is also associated with Hodgkin's lymphoma, Burkitt's lymphoma, and nasopharyngeal carcinoma.
➤ *Infections with human cytomegalovirus* (HHV-5). Possible association with necrotizing ulcerative periodontal diseases.

## Gingival Diseases of Fungal Origin

Examples for oral manifestations are aspergillosis, blastomycosis, candidosis, and histoplasmosis. The most frequent oral fungal infections are due to *Candida* spp., mostly *C. albicans. Candida* spp. are usually nonvirulent commensals of the oral cavity. Opportunistic infection might occur in immunologically suppressed patients, during therapy with antibiotics, glucocorticosteroids, and antineoplastic drugs or in cases of poorly fitting dental prostheses, etc.
➤ Primary oral candidosis:
– Acute pseudomembranous candidosis—white patches which may leave a red, bleeding surface when removed
– Acute erythematous candidosis—diffuse erythematous areas
– Chronic candidosis—pseudomembranous, erythematous, hyperplastic, nodular, or plaque-like lesions
– *Candida*-associated denture stomatitis, angular cheilitis, or median rhomboid glossitis
– Superinfected lesions—leukoplakia, oral lichen planus, and lupus erythematosus
➤ *Secondary oral candidosis* as manifestation of systemic disease:
– in cases of diabetes mellitus.
– in patients under immune suppression. Refractory oral candidosis may be an early symptom of HIV infection. *Note:* Periodontal tissues may represent an entrance for systemic *Candida* infection in immune-suppressed patients.

– A therapy-resistant *linear erythema* of the gingiva in HIV-seropositive patients might also be a *Candida* infection.

## Gingival Lesions of Genetic Origin

Hereditary gingival fibromatosis (HGF-1)[5]:
➤ HGF-1 is an autosomal dominant disease with mutations on the *Son-of-Sevenless 1* (*SOS-1*) gene on chromosome 2p21-p22. The only clinical manifestation appears to be enlargement of the gingiva.
➤ An increased number of fibroblasts with high proliferation rate lead to collagen excess.
➤ Impaired tooth eruption with possible consequences as malocclusion, interference with food intake and speech, as well as esthetic handicap and psychological problems.
➤ Hereditary gingival fibromatosis may be part of other syndromes. Combinations with generalized aggressive periodontitis have been described.

Neurofibromatosis type 1:
➤ Autosomal dominant inheritance with complete penetration but variable expression. Numerous mutations of the complex q11.2 locus on the long arm of chromosome 17.
➤ Incidence: 1 per 3,000–4,000 people.
➤ Neurodermal dysplasia with multiple skin fibromas, focal melanosis (café-au-lait spots), bone malformation. Malformations develop during pubescent growth spurts and pregnancy.
➤ Oral manifestations in about 2 to 10% of cases.[6]

## Gingival Manifestations of Mucocutaneous Diseases

Some mucocutaneous diseases manifest in the oral cavity and in particular at the gingiva, for example:
➤ Lichen planus
➤ Pemphigoid
➤ Pemphigus vulgaris
➤ Erythema multiforme
➤ Lupus erythematosus

*Oral lichen planus* (OLP) is the most frequent mucocutaneous disorder involving the gingiva.

Lesions may occur in isolation in the oral cavity or in combination with cutaneous lichen:

➤ Prevalence is between 0.1% and 4%; 65% of cases are female.
➤ In contrast to cutaneous lichen ruber, oral lesions have a markedly chronic course.
➤ Malignant transformation occurs in 0.5 to 2.5% of cases.
➤ Bilateral involvement of cheek mucosa and/or lateral sides of the tongue is common.
➤ Polymorphic appearance:
   – Reticular and/or papular lesions are very characteristic.
   – Erosive lesions emerge after rupture of bullous lesions.
   – Atrophic lesions mainly develop following treatment with glucocorticosteroids.
   – Plaque-like lesions cannot be clinically differentiated from leukoplakia.
➤ Histopathology characteristically reveals:
   – A subepithelial, bandlike, mononuclear infiltrate mainly consisting of T-lymphocytes and macrophages, which resembles characteristics of a type IV (delayed hypersensitivity) immune reaction.
   – Degeneration of basal epithelial cells.
   – "Sawtooth" rete ridges of epithelium.
   – Hyperortho- or hyperparakeratinization of epithelium.
➤ The pathogenesis of OLP is still not well understood. It is presumed that OLP is either a T-cell-mediated immunological reaction to a presently unknown antigen at the border between the epithelium and the connective tissue; or an immune reaction to antigenically altered basal cells.
➤ So-called *lichenoid reactions* to dental materials (amalgam, gold, composite resin, see below) or certain drugs (gold salts, allopurinol, penicillamine, β-blockers, antimicrobial and antimalarial drugs, antihypertensives, sulfonylurea, etc.) may occur as well.[7]
➤ There appears also to be a connection with graft-versus-host disease (GVHD) and hepatitis C.

*Pemphigoid*—a group of autoimmune diseases. Autoantibodies are formed against components of the basal membrane, which leads to a split between epithelium and connective tissue:

➤ Bullous pemphigoid—predominately skin lesions, (oral) mucosal lesions are possible.

➤ Cicatricial pemphigoid—exclusively mucosal lesions, for example, of the conjunctiva (with tendency of scar formation and possible blindness), and oral or genital mucosa:
   – Subepithelial bullae
   – IgG deposits and C3 which are located at the basal membrane
   – Diagnosis may be confirmed serologically by detection of autoantibodies against keratinocytes.

*Pemphigus vulgaris*—a group of autoimmune disorders. Autoantibodies are formed against interepithelial adhesion molecules, resulting in destruction of desmosomes.

➤ Histopathology:
   – Acantholysis, intraepithelial vesicles
   – Free epithelial cells within the vesicle, so-called Tzank cells
   – Predominately mononuclear infiltrate with scattered neutrophil granulocytes
   – Intercellular IgG autoantibodies
➤ Poor general prognosis with rather high mortality.

*Erythema multiforme*—an acute, vesiculobullous disease, occurring particularly in young individuals in their teens and twenties. The disease is more frequently seen in males.

➤ There is a minor form with distinct, predominately skin lesions, and a major form (Steven–Jobson syndrome) with widespread skin and mucous membrane lesions.
➤ Skin lesions present as erythematous papules, which enlarge and form central vesicles or bullae and a characteristic "target" or "iris" lesion.
➤ Possibly allergic immune-complex reaction to various factors:
   – Herpesviruses, *Mycoplasma pneumoniae*, streptococcal infection of the upper respiratory tract
   – Drugs: sulfonamides, phenytoin, pyrazolones, barbiturates, phenyl butazone, penicillin, carbamazepine
➤ Self-limiting, infrequently recurrent disease.

*Lupus erythematosus* (LE)—autoimmune disease of the connective tissues. Formation of autoantibodies against various cell components (nucleus, cell membrane, etc.):

➤ Discoid lupus (DLE)—chronic form
➤ Systemic lupus erythematosus (SLE)—severe form with organ involvement
➤ In both forms oral mucosa may be involved:
  – In cases of discoid lupus, lesions are similar to leukoplakia or lichen planus.
  – Mucosal ulcerations occur in systemic lupus.

## Allergic Reactions

Allergic reactions which manifest themselves in the oral mucosa are very rare:
➤ Type I (anaphylactic) reaction. Massive release of IgE by mast cells; for example, in response to ingredients of toothpaste, mouthwash, or chewing gum. The reaction leads to acute inflammation of gingiva with ulceration.
➤ Type IV reaction (delayed hypersensitivity, T cell mediated). In cases of contact allergy to dental materials such as mercury, nickel, gold, chromium, palladium, or resin. It may manifest itself as a lichenoid reaction (see above). *Note*: Removal of material usually leads to resolution.

## Traumatic Lesions

Important elements in the differential diagnosis:
➤ In general: self-inflicted (factitious), iatrogenic, and accidental injuries.
➤ Mechanical injury of the gingiva by oral health remedies, dental instruments, or restorations.
➤ Chemical injury: local application of certain chemicals such as aspirin, cocaine, pyrophosphates, detergents, smokeless tobacco, or bleaching agents.
➤ Thermal injury: by hot food or drink, for example pizza, coffee.

## Foreign Body Reactions

Acute or chronic inflammation of the gingiva due to incorporated foreign material:
➤ Usually acute inflammation, gingival abscess (see below)
➤ Sometimes chronic foreign body reaction (e.g., amalgam tattoo)

# ■ Periodontitis

## Chronic Periodontitis

This is the most frequent form of periodontitis. Chronic periodontitis is an infectious, inflammatory disease of the tooth-supporting apparatus with progressive attachment loss and loss of alveolar bone.[8] Cardinal symptoms are pocket formation and/or recession and gingival inflammation.
➤ Chronic periodontitis frequently occurs after the age of 30 years. It may also be seen in children and adolescents.
➤ Periodontal destruction correlates well with the amount of local etiologic factors. Usually oral hygiene is suboptimal or poor and large amounts of supra- and subgingival calculus may be present.
➤ The associated subgingival microflora (see Chapter 2) contains various periodontal pathogens.
➤ Slow or moderate progression is typical, but periods of rapid progression may occur.

Further classification is based on extent and severity of the disease:
➤ *Localized* chronic periodontitis: ≤30% sites/teeth are affected.
➤ *Generalized* chronic periodontitis: >30% sites/teeth are affected.
➤ Severity of the disease may be described for a single site, a tooth, or the whole dentition, namely "slight": 1 to 2 mm attachment loss; "moderate": 3 to 4 mm attachment loss; "severe": ≥5 mm attachment loss.

Not all cases respond to therapy. This has been referred to as *refractory periodontitis*. The term does not designate a special disease category of chronic periodontitis (see below).

## Aggressive Periodontitis

Aggressive periodontitis is an infectious, inflammatory disease of the tooth-supporting apparatus with rapid attachment loss and loss of alveolar bone in otherwise healthy patients.[9] It cumulates in families, which may point to a genetic background. Secondary features which are generally, but not universally, present:

➤ The amount of microbial deposits is inconsistent with the severity of periodontal destruction.

➤ Numbers and proportions of *Aggregatibacter actinomycetemcomitans* (and/or *Porphyromonas gingivalis* in some populations) in subgingival plaque are elevated.

➤ Phagocyte abnormalities. *Note:* Whether neutrophil granulocyte dysfunction may be causative for aggressive periodontitis in nonsyndromic individuals (see below) has recently been questioned (see Chapter 3).

➤ Macrophage hyper-responsiveness leading to elevated tissue levels of $PGE_2$ and $IL-1\beta$.

In some cases aggressive periodontitis may be self-limiting (so-called burned-out lesions).

Diagnosis of aggressive periodontitis is usually based on history, and clinical and radiological data. Laboratory testing (see Chapter 6) may be helpful in certain cases but is not essential for diagnosis.[10] *Note:* In order to uncover possible differences in pathogenetic mechanisms in scientific studies of aggressive periodontitis and generalized severe chronic periodontitis, clear criteria have to be applied (**Box 4.1**).

---

**Box 4.1    Distinction between chronic and aggressive periodontitis**

Numerous suggestions for the classification of periodontal diseases have been made in the past half century, as detailed by van der Velden[11] (who proposes further classification); these include "official" amendments in 1989 (on the occasion of a World Workshop organized by the American Academy of Periodontology [AAP]), in 1994 (by the European Federation of Periodontology), and again in 1999 when an International Workshop on the Classification of Periodontal Diseases and Conditions was organized by the AAP and included delegations from Europe and Asia. The basic distinction between two major forms of periodontitis, chronic and aggressive, has sparked lots of controversy since it was formulated in 1999.

This distinction between chronic and aggressive periodontitis was largely based on different progression rates. The progression rate was and continues to be difficult if not impossible to reliably assess in individuals, let alone populations. Flemmig[12] pointed out that progression rates essentially have a normal distribution. Assigning one tail of the distribution to a different disease

entity would not make sense. Since periodontitis is manifested at different ages, and its extent and severity in relation to age correlate with future progression, prognosis in a particular case can probably best be assessed by considering both the extent and severity.[12]

Meanwhile, the search for different etiological factors, host response, genetic make-up, and more promising treatment modalities in patients with aggressive periodontitis have all revealed that there are surprisingly few differences when compared to chronic periodontitis (see recent issues of *Periodontology 2000* edited by Armitage et al,[13] and Albandar[14]). Moreover, review of the vast and burgeoning literature shows that the definitions are often ill-defined, with considerable overlap of phenotypes.

Apart from a downright awkward, essentialist, conception of "chronic" and "aggressive" periodontitis,[15] it is probably time to abandon the division and accept that periodontitis is a syndrome which comes at almost any age and in all sizes.

---

Aggressive periodontitis may be localized or generalized:

➤ Localized aggressive periodontitis:
  – Onset around puberty, but diagnosis is frequently made only when patients are in their early twenties.
  – First molars/incisors are affected. Interproximal attachment loss on at least two permanent teeth, one of which is a first

molar, and involving no more than two teeth other than first molars and incisors.

➤ Generalized aggressive periodontitis:
  – Onset is usually before the age of 30 years but the disease may be diagnosed later in life.
  – Generalized interproximal attachment loss affecting at least three permanent teeth other than first molars and incisors.

– If untreated, localized aggressive periodontitis often develops into generalized disease.

Whether strong and poor serum antibody responses to infecting agents may occur in localized and generalized aggressive periodontitis, respectively, has recently been questioned (see Chapter 3).

Localized periodontitis occurring before the onset of puberty may be either classified as localized chronic or localized aggressive periodontitis. Very rare, generalized forms of prepubertal periodontitis are usually a manifestation of systemic disease (see below).

## Periodontitis as Manifestation of Systemic Disease

### Hematological disorders.
➤ *Acquired neutropenia, agranulocytosis.* Mucosal necrosis and severe periodontal disease may develop during periods of markedly decreased numbers of neutrophil granulocytes.
➤ *Leukemia.* Periodontal lesions (gingival enlargement due to leukemic cell infiltrate or gingival necrosis) have been described in acute forms of leukemia, particularly in acute monocytic, or chronic lymphatic leukemia.

### Genetic diseases.
➤ *Familial benign, cyclic, and chronic neutropenia.* More protracted forms may lead to advanced periodontitis and generalized bone loss. Periodontal destruction may be limited by good oral hygiene and intensive dental care.
➤ *Down's syndrome (trisomy 21).* Generalized periodontitis develops before the age of 10 years and is characterized by rapid progression. Complete loss of teeth by the age of 30 years is possible.
➤ *Leukocyte adhesion deficiency syndromes (LADs).* These are rare, autosomal recessive diseases with poor overall prognosis. In LAD 1, expression of adhesion molecules CD11a/CD18, CD11b/CD18, and CD11c/CD18 (integrins) is suppressed (see **Fig. 3.4**). Patients with LAD 2 lack sialyl-Lewis$^X$ selectin (sLe$^X$, CD15s). Generalized periodontitis occurs already in the first dentition with considerable gingival inflammation, gingival proliferation, and development of clefts. LAD 2 has been observed in certain Arabic families due to consanguinity.
➤ *Papillon-Lefévre syndrome.* Very rare (1 case in 1–4 million), autosomal recessive disease characterized by hyperkeratotic skin lesions (palmoplantar hyperkeratosis) associated with severe generalized periodontitis. Several mutations in the cathepsin C gene (located in chromosome 11q14-q21) have been reported, which may lead to complete loss of enzymatic activity. Respective mutations may also be present in cases of prepubertal periodontitis independent of the syndrome. Periodontitis affects both dentitions.
➤ *Chediak-Higashi syndrome.* Very rare, autosomal recessive disease with poor overall prognosis. Patients display functional impairment of neutrophil granulocytes (chemotaxis, intracellular killing).
➤ *Glycogen storage disease.* Autosomal recessive disease. Patients have deficient carbohydrate metabolism associated with neutropenia and impaired function of neutrophil granulocytes.
➤ *Infantile genetic agranulocytosis.* Very rare, autosomal recessive disorder with severe neutropenia. There is generalized periodontitis of the first dentition.
➤ *Cohen's syndrome.* Autosomal recessive disease characterized by nonprogressive mental and motoric retardation, obesity, dysmorphia, and neutropenia. Patients have more periodontitis than matched controls.
➤ *Ehlers-Danlos syndrome.* Autosomal dominantly inherited group (10 types) of diseases characterized by impaired collagen synthesis involving mainly the skin and joints. Types IV and VIII are associated with severe periodontitis of the first dentition.
➤ *Hyperphosphatasia.* Autosomal recessive deficiency of alkaline phosphatase. There is severe periodontitis of the first dentition.

### Histiocytosis syndromes.
➤ *Abt–Letterer–Siwe syndrome.* Sepsislike disseminating (neoplastic) histiocytosis in infants and small children, with skin and organ affection. Fatal prognosis.
➤ *Hand–Schüller–Christian disease.* Chronic disseminating histiocytosis in children and

adolescents, with bone, skin, and organ lesions. Overall poor prognosis.
➤ *Langerhans cell tumor* (eosinophilic granuloma):
  – Solitary or multiple bony lesions without skin or organ involvement.
  – The mildest form of the disease may imitate localized aggressive periodontitis or necrotizing periodontal diseases (see below).
  – Biopsy is necessary to confirm suspected diagnosis. Thorough general examination is required to rule out further bony lesions.
  – Therapy: extraction of extremely mobile (floating) teeth, curettage of bony lesions; in certain cases low-dose radiation.

## ■ Necrotizing Periodontal Diseases

Various forms are distinguished depending on the extent of the disease and the topography of the lesions.
➤ Necrotizing ulcerative gingivitis:
  – Lesions are confined to the gingiva.
  – Epidemic-like dissemination was described in World War I in soldiers fighting in the trenches (hence "trench mouth").
➤ Necrotizing ulcerative periodontitis:
  – Rapid attachment loss, usually without pocket formation.
  – Bony sequestration may occur.
  – Close association with HIV infection.
➤ Necrotizing stomatitis:
  – Occurs independently or secondary to necrotizing ulcerative gingivitis/periodontitis.
  – In populations with very poor food supply and hygiene, noma (cancrum oris) may develop, characterized by severe soft and hard tissue destruction and high risk of facial mutilation.

*Note:* HIV test and differential blood count should be requested in any case of necrotizing periodontal disease.

## Necrotizing Ulcerative Gingivitis

Acute, painful disease confined to the gingiva. Symptoms are:
➤ abrupt onset of pain,
➤ necrosis of the tip of the interdental papilla,
➤ ulcer formation with white-yellowish or gray pseudomembranes, demarcated by linear erythema, and
➤ halitosis.
➤ Regional lymphadenitis and subfebrile condition may occur.
➤ Peak incidence is in patients in their early twenties.

**Etiology.**
➤ Invasive gram-negative, obligate anaerobes:
  – Spirochetes
  – *Selenomonas* spp.
  – Fusobacteria
  – *Prevotella intermedia*
➤ Presumed association with herpesviruses; for example, human cytomegalovirus (HCMV, HHV-5).

**Risk factors.**
➤ Poor oral hygiene
➤ Cigarette smoking
➤ Psychological stress, lack of sleep
➤ HIV infection

**Histopathology.**
➤ Nonspecific, acute necrotizing inflammation.
➤ Ulcerated areas are covered by pseudomembranes consisting of a network of fibrin, perished epithelial cells, leukocytes, erythrocytes, and bacteria.
➤ Connective tissue beneath lesions contains widened and proliferating vessels and a dense infiltrate of neutrophil granulocytes, plasma cells, and macrophages.
➤ Invasive fusobacteria and spirochetes.

## Necrotizing Ulcerative Periodontitis

Acute periodontal infection characterized by an expansion of necrotic lesions into the periodontal ligament and alveolar bone. Manifestation of severe impairment of the immune system (immune suppression, nutrition deficiency):

➤ Rapid attachment loss, often without formation of deep pockets, but with the possibility of bony sequestration.

➤ Closely associated with HIV infection/AIDS. *Note*: Necrotizing ulcerative periodontitis in HIV-seropositive patients may signal CD4+ cell depletion to less than 200/mm$^3$, which is a prognostic indication for AIDS development.

# ■ Abscesses of the Periodontium

## Gingival Abscess

Acute inflammatory condition of the gingiva characterized by purulent exudate without attachment loss:

➤ Following trauma—for example, injury caused by a fish bone, interdental brush, etc. Virulent bacteria may be implanted into gingival connective tissue and may cause an excessive inflammatory reaction.

➤ In hormonally exacerbated gingivitis—for example, pregnancy gingivitis and gingivitis associated with uncontrolled type I diabetes mellitus.

➤ In the context of drug-induced gingival enlargement (see above).

## Periodontal Abscess

A periodontal abscess is frequently observed in the final stages of periodontal disease. Acute exacerbation of already existing periodontitis may be due to:

➤ Increased numbers or proportions of virulent bacteria, such as *Porphyromonas gingivalis*, *P. intermedia*, *Fusobacterium nucleatum*, and *Tannerella forsythia* in the subgingival environment, which have penetrated the pocket wall.

➤ Local and general immune deficiency.

➤ Obstruction of the pocket entrance due to complicated morphology, for example, furcation or intrabony pocket (see Chapter 6).

Occasionally multiple periodontal abscesses may develop:

➤ Exacerbation of generalized severe periodontitis; for example, following administration of oral penicillins that are not β-lactamase stable.

➤ In patients with uncontrolled diabetes mellitus.

➤ In individuals with impaired immune system. *Note*: Differential blood count should be requested in any case of multiple periodontal abscesses.

## Pericoronal Abscess

A pericoronal abscess is a localized purulent infection within the tissues surrounding the crown of a partially erupted tooth, in particular a mandibular third molar. Peak incidence is between 18 and 24 years of age. Symptoms are:

➤ Red and swollen gingiva, purulent exudate.

➤ Mouth opening may be painful and is frequently limited.

➤ Lymphadenitis, fever.

➤ *Caution*: Inflammation may spread into the neighboring spaces, likely causing serious complications:
  – Posteriorly into the oropharyngeal space.
  – Medially to the base of the tongue: sublingual abscess, peritonsillar abscess, perimandibular abscess.

*Note*: Commensal periodontal pathogens may multiply excessively in the area of erupting third molars even without complaints and may spread to, and infect, other teeth.

## Combined Periodontal–Endodontic Lesions

Close periodontal–endodontic interrelationships exist via the apical foramen, lateral and furcal foramina, and dentinal tubuli after removal of root cementum.

Infections may spread from one area to the other:

➤ Retrograde pulpitis, if and when the plaque front within a periodontal pocket reaches the apex or accessory pulp channels.

➤ Spread of an endodontic (periapical) infection into the periodontal ligament.

*Note:* Differential diagnosis is of paramount importance, since treatment mainly depends on the origin of the lesion.

## ■ Developmental or Acquired Deformities and Conditions

### Localized, Tooth-Related Factors that Modify or Promote Plaque-Induced Gingival Diseases/Periodontitis

Anomalous positions of teeth in the dental arch as well as tooth anatomy, dental restorations and appliances, root fractures, cervical root resorption and cemental tear may all increase the risk for developing local periodontal disease. In particular in the latter cases, explorative surgery may be necessary for proper diagnosis.

### Mucogingival Deformities and Conditions around Teeth and on Edentulous Alveolar Ridges

Mucogingival deformities may occur around teeth and in edentulous areas of the alveolar ridge. In addition to the classification outlined in **Table 4.1**, severity and etiological characteristics may be used to describe the lesions and conditions. Recessions in particular may be localized or generalized.

### Occlusal Trauma

As a rule, excessive occlusal forces do not lead to periodontitis/attachment loss, but may accelerate the progression of already existing periodontitis. Primary occlusal trauma may be differentiated from secondary trauma.

➤ *Primary occlusal trauma*: periodontal injury due to excessive occlusal forces in a normal tooth-supporting apparatus (normal bone and attachment level).
➤ *Secondary occlusal trauma*: periodontal injury due to normal or excessive forces in a reduced periodontium (loss of bone and attachment).

*Note*: Increased tooth mobility (which is not synonymous with occlusal trauma) may have a negative impact on periodontal conditions and, especially, therapeutic results.

## ■ Peri-implant Mucositis, Peri-implantitis

Implant loss may occur early after implant insertion, or later. Early implant loss is often a result of surgical failures, lack of primary stability, postoperative complications, and untimely loading. Late implant failures are due to excessive loading and/or peri-implant infection. Inflammatory diseases at oral implants are plaque induced.
➤ *Peri-implant mucositis:* inflammatory reaction in the soft tissues surrounding the implant.
➤ *Peri-implantitis:* inflammatory response in the tissues surrounding osseointegrated parts of the implant, which leads to loss of the supporting bone.

# 5   Epidemiology of Periodontal Diseases

## ■ Epidemiological Terminology

Some definitions:
- *Incidence*: The number of new cases of disease within a certain time period in relation to the number of individuals in the population examined. In cariology, the term *caries increment* is used; that is, the number of new carious lesions within a given time period.
- *Prevalence*: The number of diseased individuals at a certain point of time in relation to the number of individuals in the population examined.
- *Lethality*: The number of fatalities of a given disease within a certain time period in relation to the number of diseased individuals.
- *Mortality*: The number of fatalities of a given disease in relation to the number of individuals in the population examined; mortality = incidence × lethality. Note that in dentistry, mortality may also relate to tooth loss.

Descriptive epidemiology deals with:
- the *distribution* of diseases in the population;
- possible *etiological factors* associated with health, disease, defects, handicaps, and fatalities.

Regularly conducted *surveys* may allow:
- trends and developments to be uncovered;
- new hypotheses to be formulated.

*Analytical epidemiology* attempts to verify certain hypotheses:
- Descriptive *cross-sectional studies* are generally unsuited for confirming potential risk factors. They may, however, allow assessment of a possible association between the disease and a particular (potential risk) factor.
- The same applies for retrospective *case–control studies*, in which cases of diseased individuals are matched with healthy controls.
- Particularly important are *prospective cohort studies*, which may actually allow identification of existing risk factors.

*Risk factors* are associated with the development and progression of the disease, but are not necessarily causative. In order to confirm a risk factor as part of the causal chain, criteria described by Bradford Hill (see Chapter 2) are usually considered:
- *Strength of association* between the risk factor and the disease:
  - One possible measure is the relative risk, which is given as the factor by which the likelihood of getting the disease on exposure to the agent is increased. A strong association is assumed if the relative risk is greater than 2.
  - Another measure of association is the odds ratio which approximates the relative risk when the disease incidence is rare, say less than 10%. It can (and needs to) be adjusted for confounders (variables that are associated with both an independent and the outcome variable) in a logistic regression model. Note that for more common outcomes (> 10%), the odds ratio always overstates the relative risk.
- *Consistency of association* in different populations:
  - Associations should be in the same direction (either positive or negative).
  - There should be no overt discrepancies in the strength of associations.
- *Temporal sequence*: A potential risk factor must precede development of the disease (principle of cause and effect).
- *Dose–response effect*.
- *Specificity of association*: Causative factors should generally be associated with only one disease. However, lack of specificity is not a reason to reject causality.
- *Biological plausibility*.
- *Experimental evidence*: A causal relationship can be confirmed only in intervention studies, that is, in randomized clinical trials. Note that elimination of the risk factor

does not inevitably lead to cure of the disease.

Findings from epidemiological investigations have a large impact on planning and conducting public health campaigns at the population level.

## Periodontal Epidemiology

Specific problems arise in periodontal epidemiology. For instance:
➤ Inflammatory periodontal diseases are almost ubiquitous.
➤ The progression of the disease is still not fully understood. Lesions usually develop very slowly. There is considerable evidence that progression is discontinuous, with short periods of disease activity followed by longer phases of remission (see Chapter 3).
➤ Since losses of the tooth-supporting apparatus are essentially irreversible, the disease or its sequels appear to be more severe at older age.
➤ Markedly polymorphous appearance. Although the current classification of periodontal diseases distinguishes different forms of periodontitis, it is still not entirely clear whether different expressions of the disease in fact represent different entities (see **Box 4.1**).
➤ Complex, multifactorial etiology of the disease.

In epidemiological studies on periodontal diseases in a given population, three different parameters have to be assessed simultaneously:
➤ *Prevalence*—the proportion of diseased individuals in the population.
➤ *Extent*—the number or proportion of affected subunits, teeth, tooth surfaces, or gingival units.
➤ *Severity*—the amount of attachment loss and/or the depth of periodontal pockets.

These fundamentals were not observed in investigations that had been conducted before about 1975. Therefore, data from older studies must not be compared with data from more recent surveys.

Recent evidence, in particular since the early 1990s, has profoundly modified our understanding of the natural history of periodontitis:

➤ Gingivitis does not inevitably lead to periodontitis.
➤ Aggressive forms of periodontitis, which in essence result in premature tooth loss, are quite rare.
➤ On the other hand, mild and moderate forms of periodontitis are widespread. Almost every adult shows some loss of attachment without experiencing any functional problems.
➤ Even after the age of 35 years, periodontitis may not be the main cause of tooth loss.

## ■ Examination Methods

Extent and severity of periodontal diseases and etiological factors such as plaque and dental calculus are often assessed as qualitative (ordinal) variables by means of index systems. Several problems inherent to this approach must be considered:
➤ A rather subjective element in data collection. For instance, researchers had disagreed on sulcus bleeding as an early sign of inflammation,[1] see below.
➤ Intermediate stages between scores are not defined.
➤ Opinions often differ about the best (or valid) method of statistical analysis.

### Assessment of Gingival Inflammation

Numerous indices for severity assessment of gingivitis have been developed. Many of those listed below have to be regarded now as historical while some are still in use, particularly in clinical studies:
➤ *PMA Index*: Papillae, as well as marginal and attached gingival units are assessed separately.[2] Grading of severity is done on an ordinal scale of up to six degrees (0 to 5 for papillae, 0 to 3 for attached gingiva).
➤ *Gingival Index* (GI)[3]: Assessment of the severity of gingival inflammation on an ordinal scale (0 to 3; **Table 5.1**). The GI is still used in many clinical studies.
➤ *Sulcus Bleeding Index* (SBI)[4]: Assessment of severity of gingival inflammation on a scale of six degrees (0 to 5). Authors had claimed that bleeding on probing the gingival sulcus (scores 1 to 5) preceeds color (scores 2 to 5) and tissue changes such as edema (scores 3 to 5).

**Table 5.1** Gingival Index (Löe and Silness[3])

| Degree | Description |
|--------|-------------|
| 0 | Normal gingiva |
| 1 | Slight inflammation <br> • Slight change in color <br> • Slight edema <br> • No bleeding after probing the sulcus |
| 2 | Moderate inflammation <br> • Redness <br> • Edematous swelling <br> • Glazy appearance, loss of stippling <br> • Bleeding after probing the sulcus |
| 3 | Severe inflammation <br> • Distinct redness <br> • Distinct edematous swelling <br> • Ulceration <br> • Tendency for spontaneous bleeding |

**Table 5.2** Papilla Bleeding Index (Saxer and Mühlemann[4])

| Degree | Description of bleeding after cautiously probing the sulcus |
|--------|-------------|
| 0 | No bleeding |
| 1 | Bleeding point |
| 2 | Several isolated bleeding points or small bleeding area |
| 3 | Interdental triangle fills with blood |
| 4 | Profuse bleeding |

**Table 5.3** Plaque Index (Silness and Löe[11])

| Degree | Description |
|--------|-------------|
| 0 | No plaque |
| 1 | Thin film of plaque, which is invisible to the naked eye and may be noticed only by running a probe along the tooth surface |
| 2 | Moderate accumulation of plaque which is clearly visible |
| 3 | Abundance of plaque |

➤ *Papilla Bleeding Index* (PBI)[5]: Assessment of bleeding upon probing the gingival sulcus on an ordinal scale (0 to 4; **Table 5.2**).
➤ In some index systems, the sulcus is cautiously probed and the proportion of bleeding gingival units calculated:
➤ *Gingival Bleeding Index* (GBI).[6]
➤ An especially simple diagnostic finding is absence or *presence of bleeding on probing* (BOP) to the base of the sulcus or pocket, which is preferably done by applying a standardized probing pressure (see Chapter 6).

## Bacterial Deposits

Index systems have been developed also for plaque and dental calculus, and many of them are still used in clinical studies:
➤ *Oral Hygiene Index* (OHI),[7] which may be subdivided into:
  – ODI: debris index (soft deposits)
  – OCI: calculus index
➤ *OHI-simplified* (OHI-S)[8]: This index system considers labial surfaces of teeth 16, 11, 26, and 31, as well as lingual surfaces of teeth 36 and 46. Grading: Deposits cover up to one-third of the tooth surface (grade 1), more than one-third (grade 2), or more than two-thirds (grade 3).
➤ *Quigley-Hein Index* (QHI)[9]: Assessment of plaque on labial surfaces of anterior teeth on a scale from 0 to 5.
➤ *Turesky modification of the QHI*: Assessment of facial and lingual surfaces of all teeth.[10]

➤ *Plaque Index* (PlI)[11]: Assessment of marginal plaque (**Table 5.3**).
➤ *Plaque Control Record* (PCR)[12]: Assessment of plaque on four surfaces of each tooth present. A simple system in which the presence of visible plaque is considered and the percentage of positive surfaces calculated.

## Combined Indices

Systems combining the assessment of gingivitis, periodontitis, and even etiological factors in just one index were popular in the middle of last century:
➤ *Periodontal Index* (PI)[13]. No special instruments are necessary. Four scores are defined:
  – 1 or 2: localized or circumferential gingivitis, respectively
  – 6: initial periodontitis without impairment of function
  – 8: advanced periodontitis with functional impairment

**Table 5.4** Community Periodontal Index for treatment needs (CPITN; Ainamo et al[15]), now known as the Community Periodontal Index (CPI; WHO[16]). It may also be used for individual periodontal screening and recording (PSR)

| Degree | Description |
|---|---|
| 0 | No bleeding after probing with a special WHO probe |
| 1 | Bleeding after probing |
| 2 | Supra- or subgingival calculus or insufficient restoration margins, probing depth less than 4 mm |
| 3 | Probing depth 4–5.5 mm |
| 4 | Probing depth of 6 mm or more |

➤ *Periodontal Disease Index* (PDI)[14]:
  – Scores 1 to 3: describe severity of gingivitis
  – Scores 4 to 6: indicate attachment loss of up to 3 mm, 4 to 6 mm, and 7 mm or more, respectively
➤ *Community Periodontal Index* (CPI)[15,16]: sextant-wise assessment (**Table 5.4**); measurements are conducted with the so-called WHO probe:
  – In order to standardize probing pressure and to identify subgingival calculus or insufficient restoration margins, the probe has a ball-shaped tip with a diameter of 0.5 mm.
  – Color coding demarcating 3.5 and 5.5 mm.
  – The probe may also be used for individual periodontal screening and recording (PSR, see Chapter 6).

**Attachment Loss**

The amount of supporting tissues that has actually been lost is measured with calibrated probes (see Chapter 6):
➤ Clinical attachment loss:
  – Vertical distance between the clinically probed bottom of the pocket or sulcus and the cementoenamel junction.
  – If the cementoenamel junction is located subgingivally, the periodontal probing depth may be determined first. Thereafter, the cementoenamel junction is identified with the tip of the probe and the distance to the gingival margin subtracted from the probing depth.

  – Horizontal attachment loss is usually related to furcation involvement and may be estimated as well.

An index that simultaneously assesses the extent and severity of periodontal destruction is the *Extent and Severity Index* (ESI),[17] giving a bivariate measure as follows:
➤ First value: extent of the disease; that is, the percentage of teeth or tooth surfaces involved for a defined threshold value, say, 3 mm.
➤ Second value: severity of the disease; that is, the average of attachment loss at sites above that threshold.
➤ Example: An ESI of 3: [60, 3.5] would mean that 60% of teeth or sites had attachment loss of 3 mm or more, and the average attachment loss of these teeth or sites was 3.5 mm, indicating widespread but rather mild periodontitis.

The entire information of full-mouth attachment level measurements, for instance at six sites per tooth, can largely be preserved in a multivariate representation of cumulative frequencies of probe parameters in the form of *percentile plots* (**Fig. 5.1**).[18]

**Case Definitions**

Based on joint recommendations of the US American Centers for Disease Control and Prevention (CDC) and the American Academy of Periodontology (AAP), the following case definitions have recently been applied in representative, population-based studies (**Table 5.5**)[19,20] in which full-mouth recording at six sites per tooth (see below) was done:
➤ *Advanced/severe periodontitis:* Two or more nonadjacent teeth with interproximal sites showing clinical attachment loss of 6 mm or more *and* pockets of 5 mm or more.
➤ *Moderate periodontitis:* Two or more nonadjacent teeth with interproximal sites showing clinical attachment loss of 4 mm or more *or* two or more interproximal sites with pockets of 5 mm or more.
➤ *Mild periodontitis:* Two or more interproximal sites showing clinical attachment loss of 3 mm or more and two or more interproximal sites with periodontal pockets of 4 mm or more (not on the same tooth), or one site with a periodontal pocket of 5 mm or more.

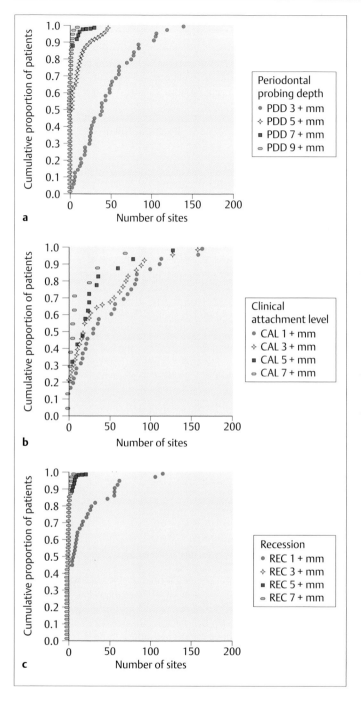

**Fig. 5.1 Percentile plots of cumulative frequencies** of (**a**) periodontal probing depth (PPD), (**b**) clinical attachment level (CAL) and (**c**) recession (REC) beyond certain thresholds (1 + ... 9 + mm) in a group of new patients who had visited a new university dental school between January and May 2003 (n = 46, 27 female; between 12 and 56 years of age; mean age 36, standard deviation 12 years). Periodontal probing was done at six sites for each tooth (between 96 and 192 sites per patient; mean 167, standard deviation 18). The gathered information as regards prevalence, extent, and severity of periodontal disease can be displayed in a multivariate way in which it is largely preserved (unpublished).
Example (cf. **Fig. 5.1b**): Attachment loss (at least one site with CAL ≥ 1 mm) was observed in 74 % of examined patients. At least one site with CAL of ≥ 5 mm was found in 43.5 % of patients. The proportion of patients with a considerable number of sites (e.g., ≥ 10) with severe attachment loss of ≥ 5 mm was 26 %.

Earlier, Tonetti and Claffey[21] had suggested case definitions which are widely used as well. Two threshold levels were proposed, one to identify, with high sensitivity, incipient cases, and a second to identify only cases with substantial extent and severity of disease:

➤ *Incipient and less extensive periodontitis*: Presence of proximal attachment loss of ≥ 3 mm in ≥ 2 nonadjacent teeth.

➤ *Widespread and severe periodontitis*: Presence of proximal attachment loss of ≥ 5 mm in ≥ 30 % of teeth present.

In order to differentiate, in epidemiological studies, aggressive from chronic periodontitis and to better interpret already collected data, age limits have recently been re-introduced (**Box 5.1**)[22]:

➤ In patients up to 25 years of age, moderate periodontitis according to the above-mentioned criteria would indicate aggressive periodontitis.
➤ Advanced/severe disease in patients between 26 and 35 years of age indicates aggressive periodontitis.

---

**Box 5.1    Worldwide distribution of chronic and aggressive periodontitis**

In a systematic review by Demmer and Papapanou[22] only studies of the previous decade were assessed, since it was assumed that the classification based on conclusions of the 1999 World Workshop (see Chapter 4) had been applied. It was expected that case definitions provided by the joint group of CDC and AAP (see **Table 5.5**) were increasingly being applied. Studies in which extent and severity of the disease based on certain thresholds were described—for example, the proportion of sites/teeth with clinical attachment loss of ≥ 3, ≥ 4, ≥ 5, and ≥ 6 mm—were also considered.

In order to reasonably interpret the 21 identified studies, the authors suggest that attachment loss of ≥ 4 mm at 2 or more nonadjacent proximal sites at different teeth in rather young subjects (≤ 25 years), which bleed after probing, would indicate aggressive periodontitis. In older subjects (26–35 years), attachment loss of ≥ 6 mm at ≥ 2 nonadjacent proximal sites of different teeth and bleeding on probing would indicate aggressive periodontitis.

At a global level, there are considerable differences in prevalence, extent, and severity of periodontitis. Definitive conclusions as regards the situation in different continents are hardly possible, since new data from Asia (60 % of the world population) have been published in just two studies from Thailand. There is no new information from Africa (15 % of the world population). Representative studies on a national level, in which usually lower prevalence than in preselected populations can be observed, are rare. Prevalence is also severely underestimated when partial recording (for instance, data in just two quadrants) is done. Furthermore, there is presently no information as regards incidence of periodontitis.

Relatively homogeneous estimates of prevalence of severe periodontitis in 40- to 50-year-olds, based on CDC/AAP criteria, are available for parts of Germany (SHIP study) and various populations in the United States (16–32 %). Representative national estimates for prevalence of severe periodontitis in all age groups have been reported for the United States (2 %) and Australia (4 %). However, in the recent US survey (2009–10 NHANES), which employed full-mouth recording for the first time, a much higher prevalence of severe periodontitis of 8.5 % was observed.[32]

In some nonrepresentative surveys from France, Canada, and Brazil, criteria of the 1999 World Workshop were applied. Severe generalized periodontitis was found in 50 % of subjects in Brazil, 19 % in France, and 6 % in Canada.

New epidemiological studies on aggressive periodontitis are difficult to conduct, since important criteria of the 1999 World Workshop such as occurrence in otherwise healthy subjects, rapid attachment loss, and accumulation in families may be difficult to observe in epidemiological studies. Just one study done on Israeli military personnel in the age range 18 to 30 years fulfilled workshop criteria for aggressive periodontitis.[23] Localized and generalized aggressive periodontitis was found in 4.4 % and 1.6 % of study participants, respectively. When taking the above-mentioned age criteria into account, prevalence among subjects up to 35 years old may be between 7 % and 15 %. In the German SHIP study, prevalence of moderate and severe periodontitis (CDC/AAP criteria) among subjects up to 29 years old was, in this instance, 13 %; among 30- to 39-year-olds, 7 % suffered from severe periodontitis.[24] There is no new information as regards prevalence of aggressive periodontitis in adolescents.

**Table 5.5** Joint recommendations of Centers for Disease Control and American Academy of Periodontology for case definitions in population-based surveys of periodontitis[19,20]

|  | **Definition** |
|---|---|
| Severe periodontitis | ≥2 interpromixal sites with clinical attachment loss (CAL) ≥6 mm (not on same tooth) and ≥1 interproximal site with periodontal probing depth (PPD) ≥5 mm |
| Moderate periodontitis | ≥2 interproximal sites with CAL ≥4 mm (not on same tooth); or ≥2 interproximal sites with PDD ≥5 mm (not on same tooth) |
| Mild periodontitis | ≥2 interproximal sites with ≥3 mm CAL and ≥2 interproximal sites with ≥4 mm pocket depth (not on same tooth) or 1 site with ≥5 mm PDD |
| No periodontitis | No evidence of mild, moderate, or severe periodontitis |

# ■ Epidemiology of Plaque-Induced Periodontal Diseases

Inflammatory periodontal diseases associated with dental plaque are among the most frequently occurring conditions, and one or more sites with clinical signs of gingival inflammation can most likely be found in each and every individual. There might be one notable exception: preschool children do not develop overt signs of gingival inflammation as a response to dental plaque.[25] Inflammatory alterations of the gingiva are not found in most children until a transitional dentition has developed.

The prevalence and extent of gingivitis reach their maximum at the onset of puberty, at about age 10 to 11 years in girls, and about two years later in boys (**Fig. 5.2**).[26] On the other hand, severity of gingivitis does not increase during puberty.

The epidemiology of periodontal disease has been studied since the early 1950s all over the world. Unfortunately, examination criteria have differed considerably. In the majority of older studies, only prevalence of the disease has been determined, and extent and severity not taken into account (**Fig. 5.3**). For instance, according to an early study by Marshall-Day et al,[27] prevalence of gingivitis seemed to decline rapidly after the age of 15 years. Concomitantly, the prevalence of periodontitis dramatically increased, reaching almost 100% after the age of 35 years, while tooth loss gradually affected more and more individuals.

## Natural History

The natural history of periodontitis was studied in a longitudinal investigation of Sri Lankan tea workers who had never received any dental care (**Fig. 5.4**)[28]:

➤ About 8% of the study population developed a rather severe form of the disease, possibly aggressive periodontitis. Average attach-

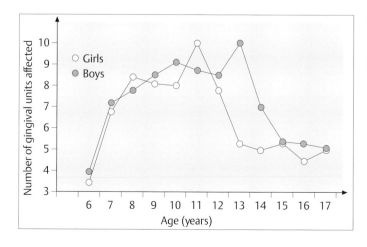

**Fig. 5.2 Extent of gingivitis in children according to an early study by Massler et al[26].** The PMA index[2] was applied, and inflammation of the papilla, marginal gingiva, and attached gingiva were assessed. Maximum gingivitis was observed at the onset of puberty: in girls at age 11 years and in boys at age 13 years.

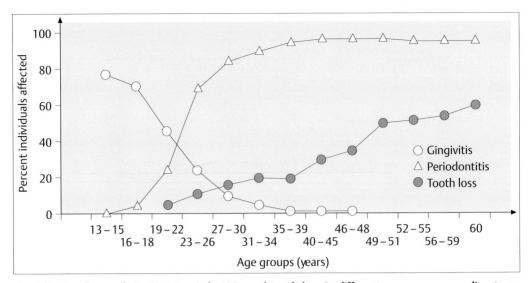

**Fig. 5.3 Prevalence of gingivitis, periodontitis, and tooth loss in different age groups according to an early study by Marshal-Day et al[27].** In adolescents, a very high prevalence of gingivitis was noted, which subsequently rapidly declined. Simultaneously, however, prevalence of periodontitis increased steeply, reaching almost 100% after the age of 35 years. The proportion of individuals with tooth loss increased linearly from the age of about 20 years onwards.

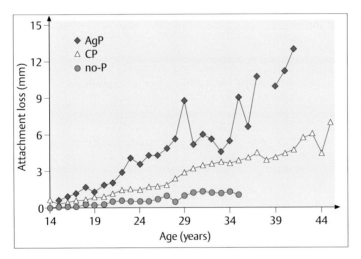

**Fig. 5.4 Natural history of periodontitis.** Average, age-dependent attachment loss in Sri Lankan tea workers, who were studied for 15 years. Eight percent developed a rather aggressive form of periodontitis (AgP), 81% a chronic form (CP), while in 11% no periodontitis was diagnosed (no-P). (Adapted from Löe et al.[28])

ment loss was more than 1 mm per year and virtually all teeth had been lost after the age of 40 years.

➤ The majority of tea workers (81%) developed a rather mild, chronic form of periodontitis. Annual attachment loss increased from an average of 0.3 mm by the age of 30 years to 0.5 mm at the age of about 45. Some tooth loss occurred, but generally this did not impair function of the dentition.

➤ In 11% of the study population, no relevant attachment loss was observed at all.

*Note*: This and other investigations have shown that about 7 to 15% of any given population may suffer from severe forms of periodontitis,[22] which actually leads to premature tooth loss. However, progression rates of periodontitis in general are normally distributed (see **Box 4.1**), one tail representing periodontally resistant individuals who hardly develop any periodontitis during their lifetime. The other tail may represent very susceptible persons prone to severe periodontitis which may develop early in life.

## Periodontitis in the United States

For decades, the Centers of Disease Control and Prevention have collected representative data for the US population in their National Health and Nutrition Examination Surveys (NHANES). Periodontal data of NHANES III (1988–94) has been extensively reported and could be summarized as follows[29]:

➤ At least 35% of the adult population (30 years and older) showed signs and symptoms of the disease, but most cases (22%) were mild.
➤ Moderate and advanced periodontitis was found in not more than 13%.
➤ Prevalence and extent of attachment loss increased with age, while in the oldest age group (80 years and older), prevalence of deep pockets decreased because of tooth loss and recession.
➤ Severe forms of the disease were more prevalent in males, and more so in Afro-Americans and Hispanics than in Whites.
➤ Furcation involvement was assessed as well (**Fig. 5.5**):
  – About 14% of individuals aged 30 years and older had at least one tooth with a furcation involvement.
  – On average, 7% of multi-rooted teeth were involved.

– A single furcation involvement was observed in 10% of individuals, whereas 4% had two or more furcation-involved teeth.

Since 1999, representative data have been collected on a continuous basis. NHANES examines a nationally representative sample of about 5,000 persons each year. These persons are located in counties across the country, 15 of which are visited each year. In general, minorities (adolescents, the elderly, Afro-Americans, Hispanics, pregnant women, low socioeconomic classes) are oversampled. Results are published biannually.

Comparing periodontal data of the 1988–94 NHANES III with those of the 1999–2004 continuous NHANES may allow assessment of possible improvements in oral health over the past 10 years (**Figs. 5.6–5.9**). A clear trend has been observed: prevalence, extent, and severity of periodontitis apparently declined over the 10-year period.[30] Both surveys do suffer from serious methodological flaws, though:

➤ In both surveys, only partial recording was done. Probing parameters, periodontal probing depth, recession, and clinical attachment loss, were assessed at two sites (mesiobuccal, midbuccal; since 1999 also distolingual) of each tooth only (except third molars) in two random quadrants, one in the maxilla and one in the mandible.
➤ It has been shown that partial recording considerably underestimates prevalence, extent, and severity of periodontitis.[31]

In the most recent NHANES of 2009–2010, full-mouth recording at six sites of each tooth was

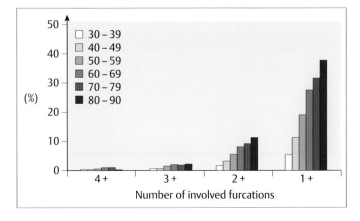

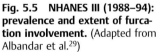

**Fig. 5.5 NHANES III (1988–94): prevalence and extent of furcation involvement.** (Adapted from Albandar et al.[29])

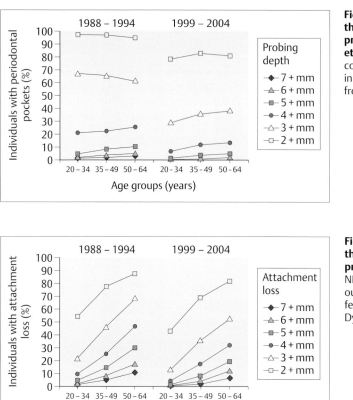

**Fig. 5.6   Periodontitis decline in the United States: comparison of prevalence of periodontal pockets** in NHANES III (1988–94) and continuous NHANES (1999–2004) in different age groups. (Adapted from Dye et al.[30])

**Fig. 5.7   Periodontitis decline in the United States: comparison of prevalence of attachment loss** in NHANES III (1988–94) and continuous NHANES (1999–2004) in different age groups. (Adapted from Dye et al.[30])

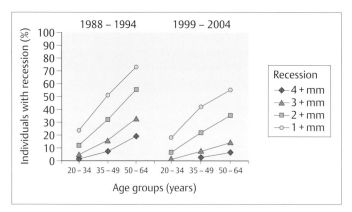

**Fig. 5.8   Periodontitis decline in the United States: comparison of prevalence of recession** in NHANES III (1988–94) and continuous NHANES (1999–2004) in different age groups. (Adapted from Dye et al.[30])

done.[32] Results have profoundly changed our current view of prevalence, extent, and severity of periodontitis:

➤ Periodontitis is much more prevalent than previously thought. More than 47% of the adult population 30 years and older have periodontitis (as compared to about 35% in NHANES III of 1988–94 and a decline in the continuous NHANES 1999–2004)

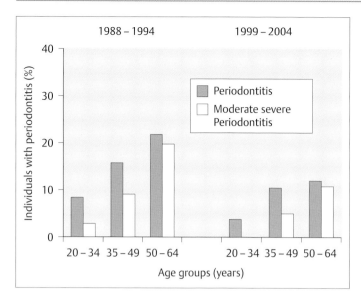

**Fig. 5.9  Periodontitis decline in the United States according to case definitions.** Comparison of prevalence of periodontitis in NHANES III (1988–94) and continuous NHANES (1999–2004) in different age groups. (Adapted from Dye et al.[30]) Note that the case definitions are not identical to those applied in the most recent NHANES of 2009–10 (**Table 5.5**).

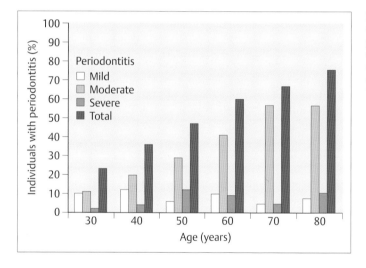

**Fig. 5.10  Application of the CDC–AAP case definitions for periodontitis.** Prevalence of periodontitis in most recent NHANES (2009–10). (Data from Eke et al.[32]) Case definitions are as listed in **Table 5.5**.

➤ By using the case definition presented in **Table 5.5**, mild periodontitis was diagnosed in 8.7%, while a majority of 30.0% presented already with moderate periodontitis. Severe periodontitis was found in 8.5% (**Fig. 5.10**).

➤ *Note:* Since different case definitions were applied in the 2009–2010 NHANES, the new data cannot be directly compared with NHANES III and the continuous NHANES of 1999–2004.

## Europe

A meta-analysis[33] of 47 studies from 24 countries in which the Community Periodontal Index (CPI; see **Table 5.4**) was employed and which had been conducted between 1982 and 1992 revealed the following:

➤ The weighted mean prevalence of shallow pockets (4–5 mm, maximum CPI score 3) was 36% in Western European countries and 45% in Eastern Europe.

➤ The weighted mean prevalence of deep pockets (≥6 mm, CPI score 4) was 9% in Western European countries and 23% in Eastern Europe.
➤ The average number of sextants with periodontitis (extent) was generally low, 0.2 to 2.4 for a maximum CPI score of 3, and 0 to 0.8 for a CPI score of 4.

## Global Trends

The World Health Organization's global database and other databases may provide information on recent trends in prevalence, extent, and severity of periodontal disease.[34] While in most studies the CPI (see **Table 5.4**) was used, periodontal probing depth and clinical attachment level measurements (see Chapter 6) were increasingly employed as well (see problems with partial recordings above).

In earlier surveys (similar as in the continuous NHANES 1999–2004) a decline of prevalence and severity could frequently be observed, for instance:

➤ In Australia, prevalence of increased periodontal probing depth of ≥4 mm in 35- to 44-year-olds was found to be 36.8% in the 1995–96 survey. In the survey of 2004–06, the respective figure was 23.9% in the age group of 35 to 54 years.
➤ Comparably high prevalence, in 1988, of CPI scores 3 and 4 in 35- to 44-year-olds in the United Kingdom of 62% and 13%, respectively, were lower in 1998, namely 54% and 5%, respectively. Comparably high prevalence of CPI scores 3 and 4 in 65-year-olds dropped from 60% and 17% to 52% and 15%, respectively, 10 years later.[34]
➤ Especially remarkable were data obtained in 35- to 44-year-olds in Oslo, Norway, where over a 20-year period the prevalence of CPI score of 4 decreased from 21.8% in 1984 to 8.1% in 2003.[35]

Recent surveys indicate a reversed trend, at least in some countries (**Fig. 5.11**), which might only in part be due to aging Western populations where most people tend to retain their natural teeth.

➤ In the most recent survey in Germany in 2005,[36] in both age groups (35–44, 65–77 years) prevalence of attachment loss of ≥3 mm had increased to 93% in men and 90% in women (48% and 42% in the 1997 survey, respectively) and almost 100% (72% and 67% in 1997), respectively.
➤ In 35- to 44-year-old persons, attachment loss of ≥3 mm affected 42% of tooth surfaces, while the respective figure for 65- to 74-year-olds was 73%.
➤ For the first time, 15-year-old adolescents were examined. A maximum CPI of 3 was found in 12.6% of the study population, while 0.8% had already a CPI of 4, which might indicate aggressive periodontitis (see below).
➤ Data from Hungary confirm an increase in prevalence of CPI scores 3 and 4 in 35- to 44-year-olds from 16% and 2%, respectively in 1991 to 21.9% and 5.5% in 2003–04 (**Fig. 5.11**).[37]

Concern has been raised regarding serious limitations of the CPI in epidemiological surveys. In future surveys, full-mouth recording of site-specific periodontal probing parameters, probing depth, clinical attachment level, and recession; as well as furcation involvement and plaque and bleeding on probing should be considered, even at the expense of not being able, at least for some time, to assess secular trends.

## Early-Onset (Aggressive) Periodontitis

Recent data on prevalence of aggressive periodontitis after the revision of its classification in 1999 (see Chapter 4) are still largely missing (see **Box 5.1**). In particular, no or few data are available from Asia and Australasia. The largest population-based study of 14- to 17-year-olds was conducted by the National Institute of Dental and Craniofacial Research (NIDCR) in years 1986–87 in the United States[38]:

➤ About 0.5% of individuals had localized aggressive periodontitis: 0.1% among Whites and 2% among Afro-Americans.
➤ 0.1% had generalized aggressive periodontitis: 0.03% Whites and 0.6% Afro-Americans. So, Afro-Americans had 20 times greater risk for aggressive periodontitis than Whites.
➤ A further 1.6% had incidental attachment loss which did not fulfill the criteria of aggressive periodontitis. While it was speculated that this might include both cases of periodontitis associated with restorative

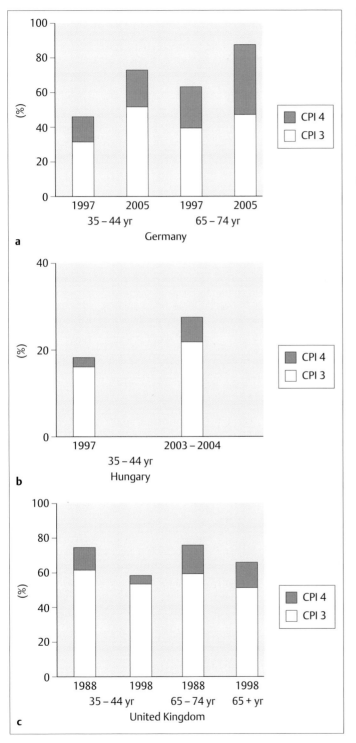

**Fig. 5.11  Global trends of periodontal key indicator CPI scores 3 and 4.**

**a** A recent study in Germany indicated a considerable increase in periodontitis prevalence (average percentage) and severity in both target age groups (35–44, 65–74 years) over an 8-year period.

**b** A similar trend could be observed for the age group of 35–44 years in Hungary.

**c** About a decade earlier, prevalence and severity had slightly improved in both age groups in the United Kingdom, albeit from a much higher level. (Data from Dye.[34])

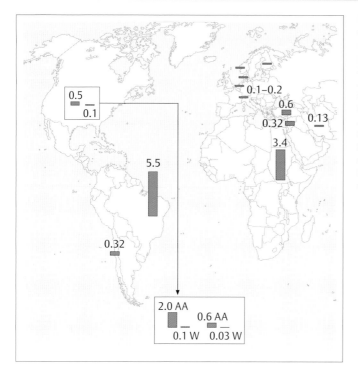

**Fig. 5.12 Worldwide distribution of aggressive periodontitis (%) in representative samples of target populations.** Data from the United States distinguish between localized aggressive periodontitis (about 0.5%: 2% in Afro-Americans [AA], 0.1% in Whites [W]) and generalized aggressive periodontitis (about 0.1%: 0.6% in Afro-Americans, 0.03% in Whites) in 14- to 17-year-olds. (Adapted from Löe and Brown,[38] supplemented with recent data compiled by Susin et al.[39])

treatment and incipient aggressive periodontitis, currently most of these cases would probably be characterized as chronic periodontitis.

Worldwide, prevalence of aggressive periodontitis seems to vary considerably (**Fig. 5.12**).[38,39] *Note*: While in European countries prevalence rates of 0.1 to 0.5% had been ascertained, the disease is apparently more prevalent in Africa (0.3% to >7%) and South America (0.3% to >5%).

### Prevalence, Extent, and Severity of Gingival Recession

Gingival recession basically occurs in two different forms (**Fig. 5.13**). One form is mainly induced by *injury*, especially due to inappropriate toothbrushing. In this form, gingiva is more or less free from inflammation. Most often, buccal surfaces of canines and premolars are affected. Less often, recession is seen at lingual or palatal surfaces—usually of the first maxillary molars. This kind of recession is mainly found in populations with high level of oral hygiene.

The other form is due to *longstanding chronic inflammation* in the course of periodontitis. Usually, all tooth surfaces may be involved. This form of recession occurs mainly in populations with poor oral hygiene.[40]

In the continuous NHANES of 1999–2004, the following observations were made[41]:

➤ 38% of 20- to 64-year-olds had at least one site with ≥1 mm recession (48% in NHANES III of 1988–94).

➤ Recession of at least 3 mm was found in 7.4% of individuals (16.7% in 1988–94).

➤ Recession of ≥1 mm and ≥3 mm were found in 60% and 21% of elderly, that is subjects ≥65 years old (87% and 32% in 1988–94, respectively).

### Peri-implant Diseases

For obvious reasons, population-based data are currently missing. A meta-analysis of nine prospective and retrospective cross-sectional and cohort studies with 5 years or longer functional loading time[42] yielded the following:

➤ Frequency of peri-implant mucositis was high, 63.4% (95% confidence interval [CI]:

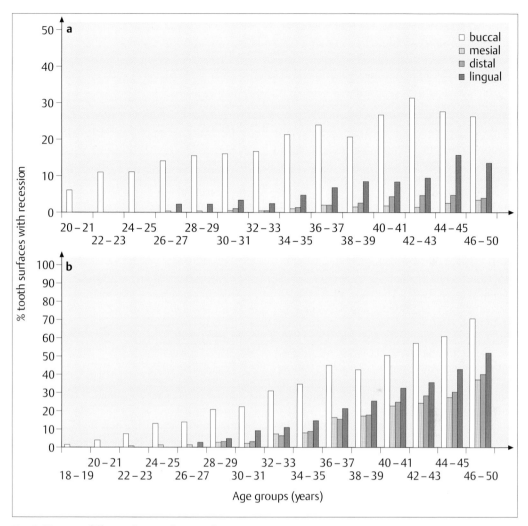

**Fig. 5.13 Two different forms of gingival recession.**
**a** Age-dependent increase of the proportion of tooth surfaces with recession in a Norwegian population with excellent dental service and a high level of oral hygiene. Recessions are mainly seen at buccal and, to a lesser extent, lingual surfaces.
**b** Age-dependent increase of the proportion of tooth surfaces with recession in workers in a tea plantation in Sri Lanka with no dental service and no special oral hygiene measures. In these individuals, extent of gingival recession increases also at proximal surfaces. (Adapted from Löe et al.[40])

59.8; 67.1). At the implant level, frequency was 30.7% (95% CI: 28.6; 32.8).

➤ Frequency of peri-implantitis was 18.8% (95% CI: 16.8; 20.8), while 9.6% (95% CI: 8.8; 10.4) of implants had peri-implantitis.

# 6   Diagnosis of Periodontal Diseases

The centerpiece of current dental treatment philosophy is comprehensive dental care. Careful examination of a patient usually yields numerous coexistent diseases and conditions in the oral cavity, typically:

➤ Dental caries and endodontic lesions
➤ Periodontal diseases
➤ Orthodontic and orthognathic disorders
➤ Temporomandibular disorders
➤ Diseases of the oral mucosa

While nowadays any treatment needs to be based on current evidence, the dentist should generally strive, within the context of comprehensive therapy, for esthetic and functional rehabilitation. The aim is to reach an optimum and stable situation under conditions of health that *meets the patient's needs* as regards esthetics and chewing comfort. An important aspect is planning treatment that is *appropriate* to each individual case, and which avoids both under- and overtreatment.

Major issues in treating periodontally diseased patients are:

➤ Anti-infective therapy
➤ Regenerative measures
➤ Risk modification

Before any therapy, detailed *diagnosis* is mandatory, which must be based on specific information in the patient's *history* and comprehensive clinical and, if required, radiological and/or laboratory *examination*. Relevant findings have to be properly recorded. *Note*: Appropriate diagnostic measures have to be carried out during all treatment phases.

## ■ Anamnesis

### Medical History

Information on the patient's *general history* can be gathered in the waiting room by means of a questionnaire, which the patient is asked to fill out. The patient's answers are checked and dis-

cussed in more detail during *dental consultation*.

The history is obtained in a systematic manner (**Fig. 6.1**). Right from the start of the first visit, any existing and possible risk factors for destructive periodontal diseases and conditions which might interfere with the treatment itself, patient management, or the expected therapeutic outcome should be taken into account. In particular the following has to be addressed in any case:

➤ Infectious diseases
➤ Increased risk of endocarditis
➤ Allergies and possible intolerance
➤ Cardiovascular diseases, high blood pressure
➤ Diabetes mellitus
➤ Pregnancy
➤ Osteopenia, osteoporosis
➤ Drugs, drug abuse
➤ Smoking habits
➤ Stress and coping behavior

During consultation, further important information will be acquired—often unconsciously—about the physical and psychological condition of the patient.

If necessary, the patient might be referred to a specialist. *Note*: Periodontally diseased patients present more frequently with systemic diseases, which can interfere with treatment planning.[1]

### Dental History

The first question is about the patient's chief complaint, the reason for consultation. Frequently patients mention:

➤ Pain or other alarming symptoms, such as tooth mobility, tooth migration, bad breath and/or bad taste
➤ Esthetic problems
➤ A desire for comprehensive treatment

Next, questions are asked about:

➤ Accidents, injuries, surgical operations of the head and neck
➤ Previous orthodontic treatment
➤ Previous periodontal treatment

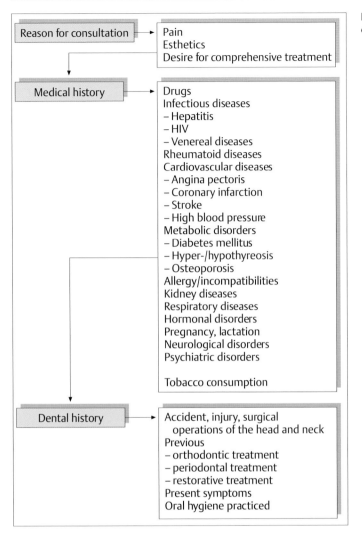

**Fig. 6.1   Systematic collection of medical and dental history.**

Reason for consultation → Pain
Esthetics
Desire for comprehensive treatment

Medical history → Drugs
Infectious diseases
– Hepatitis
– HIV
– Venereal diseases
Rheumatoid diseases
Cardiovascular diseases
– Angina pectoris
– Coronary infarction
– Stroke
– High blood pressure
Metabolic disorders
– Diabetes mellitus
– Hyper-/hypothyreosis
– Osteoporosis
Allergy/incompatibilities
Kidney diseases
Respiratory diseases
Hormonal disorders
Pregnancy, lactation
Neurological disorders
Psychiatric disorders

Tobacco consumption

Dental history → Accident, injury, surgical
   operations of the head and neck
Previous
– orthodontic treatment
– periodontal treatment
– restorative treatment
Present symptoms
Oral hygiene practiced

➤ Dental restorations
➤ Practice of oral hygiene

## ■ Clinical Examination

### Extraoral Examination

Clinical examination generally starts extraorally where the following are addressed:
➤ Color and perfusion of the skin, lip mucosa
➤ Asymmetries in the head and neck region
➤ Palpation of submandibular and sublingual lymph nodes

➤ Palpation of foramina of the trigeminal nerve
➤ Eyes: conjunctivae, possible nystagmus or exophthalmos
➤ Hands: tremor, clubbing of the last digits of fingers, sweat

### Intraoral Examination

First, mucous membranes are inspected. Using a dental mirror, the condition of masticatory, lining, and specialized mucosa (see Chapter 1) are assessed, typically beginning in the pharyngeal region. A systematic *stomatologic examination* is especially important for cancer screening and should be documented on a special form (**Fig. 6.2**).[2] This includes assessment of:

➤ Lips
➤ Tonsils, pharynx
➤ Mucosa of the soft and hard palate
➤ Cheek mucosa
➤ Dorsum and lateral sides of the tongue, floor of the mouth
➤ Gingiva: form, color, and consistency
➤ Flow rate and consistency of saliva

Next, the *dental examination* is done and the following recorded:
➤ Missing teeth
➤ Restored tooth surfaces, which are usually marked in blue
➤ Decayed tooth surfaces:
  – D 1, 2: Lesions to be monitored for caries after preventive measures have been initiated; they may be marked in green.
  – D 3, 4: Invasive therapy is required; lesions are marked in red.

➤ Other defects of enamel and/or dentin: erosion, attrition, abrasion
➤ Results of sensibility testing
➤ Dentin hypersensitivity
➤ Tenderness to percussion

For documentation of conditions before, during and after therapy, standardized intraoral photos should be taken:
➤ Focal distance of the objective between 60 and 110 mm
➤ Ring flash
➤ Anterior teeth: jaws closed, × 2/3
➤ Left and right lateral aspects: jaws closed, × 2/3
➤ Occlusal aspects of the upper and lower jaws with a mirror: × 1/2
➤ If necessary, close-ups at higher magnification

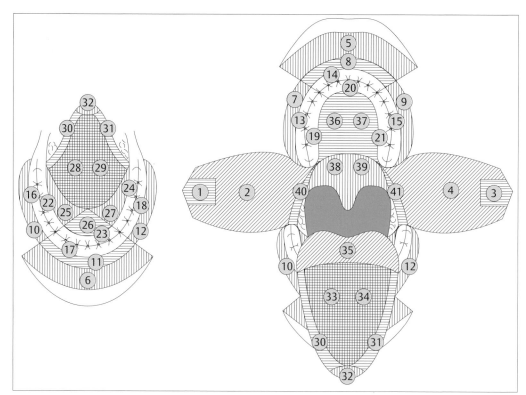

**Fig. 6.2  Form for the documentation of oral mucosal lesions.**[2] Teeth that are present are marked by circles (mandible left, maxilla right). White alterations are marked in black: (1) striae; (2) plaque-like lesions; (3) papular lesions. Red alterations are marked in red: (1) slight erythema; (2) overt erythema; (3) bulla; (4) desquamation/ulceration.

## Functional Examination

*Clinical functional analysis* during basic examination includes:
➤ Palpation of temporomandibular joints. Possible joint sounds (e. g., clicks or crepitation) are recorded.
➤ Palpation of jaw and face muscles for tenderness.
➤ Recording of the distance between incisal edges at maximum mouth opening and any deviation of the mandible during mouth opening.
➤ Assessment of any occlusal interference during retrusion, protrusion, and laterotrusion of the mandible; in particular, possible working side and balancing contacts.
➤ Wear facets, signs of bruxism.

Stone model casts for treatment planning:
➤ Alginate impressions are preferably taken with rim lock trays. They should completely reproduce occlusal conditions as well as the oral vestibule including lip and cheek frenula
➤ A maxillomandibular registration record is taken in maximum intercuspidation (e. g., wax bite registration)
➤ Stone model casts may be mounted in a semi-adjustable articulator.

## Periodontal Examination

**Table 6.1** lists standard instruments for periodontal examination. As an initial step, periodontal screening and recording by sextant (PSR, see **Table 5.4**) may be performed. PSR should ensure that periodontal lesions are not overlooked. It cannot replace, however, a detailed periodontal examination which is necessary in any patient scoring PSR 3 or higher.

Periodontal diseases usually exhibit cardinal symptoms of inflammation[3]:
➤ *Redness* of the gingival margin
➤ *Edematous swelling*
➤ *Pain*, especially in cases of ulceration and/or abscess formation
➤ *Impaired function*, for example, increasing tooth mobility and tooth migration

Important additional findings are:
➤ Tendency of the gingival tissues to *bleed* on being probed with a periodontal probe
➤ Inflammatory, sometimes purulent, gingival exudate

Findings are recorded on four or six gingival units/sites of all teeth:
➤ mesiobuccally
➤ midbuccally
➤ distobuccally
➤ distolingually/distopalatally
➤ midlingually/midpalatally
➤ mesiolingually/mesiopalatally

Basic periodontal examination inevitably employs various *periodontal probes* for very different purposes. Probes are used to assess the local destruction of the tooth-supporting apparatus

**Table 6.1** Standard instruments for periodontal examination

| Instruments | Description | Article no., manufacturer |
|---|---|---|
| Mouth mirror | Plane, front surface rhodium-coated, Ø 22 mm | M4C, Hu-Friedy |
| | Mirror handle | MHE6, Hu-Friedy |
| Dressing pliers | | DP18 or DP17, Hu-Friedy |
| Explorer | Double-ended For subgingival calculus detection For caries detection | EXD56, Hu-Friedy |
| WHO probe | For assessing PSI Ball-shaped tip WHO markings (3.5 mm, 5.5 mm) | PCP11.5B6, Hu-Friedy |
| Periodontal probe | Calibration in 1 mm steps Color-coded 3-3-2-3 mm | PCPUNC156, Hu-Friedy PCP116, Hu-Friedy |
| Furcation probe | Curved Nabers probe, calibration in 3-mm steps | PQ2N6, Hu-Friedy |

and the bleeding tendency of the gingiva, and to identify ecological niches for dental biofilm.

➤ Rigid, color-coded, not pressure-controlled periodontal probe:
  – 0.4–0.45 mm; examples: PUNC15, PCP11 (Hu-Friedy, Rotterdam, Netherlands)
  – The recommended probing force is about 0.2 N. Probing pressure may be estimated as about 1.6 MPa: $P=F/r^2\pi = 0.2/0.2^2\pi$ N/mm$^2$ =1.59 N/mm$^2$.
➤ Simple pressure-calibrated probes (1–1.5 MPa); examples: ClickProbe (KerrHawe, Bioggio, Switzerland, **Fig. 6.3**) and DB764 R (Aesculap, B Braun, Tuttlingen, Germany). These probes are particularly suitable for more objective assessment of gingival bleeding on probing. They should preferably be used in patients with plaque-induced gingivitis and those undergoing periodontal maintenance (see Chapter 12).
➤ Computer-assisted, automatic probes, such as the Florida probe, are only used for scientific research.

Since subgingival calculus and complicated root anatomy may obstruct the entrance of a periodontal pocket, pressure-controlled probes should not be used in untreated patients where rather forced probing with slightly high-er pressure may be useful in order to access the base of the pocket.

*Note:* Periodontal probing is generally unpleasant and may even be painful, in particular if the gingiva is inflamed. It is recommended to inform the patient about any discomfort before periodontal probing.

Several periodontal probing parameters have to be assessed during periodontal examination:

➤ *Periodontal probing depth*: The distance between the gingival margin and the clinically probe-able bottom of the pocket or sulcus.
➤ *Clinical attachment level*: The distance between the cementoenamel junction and the clinically probe-able bottom of the pocket or sulcus (**Fig. 6.4**). *Note:* The real bottom of the lesion or the sulcus bottom cannot be determined with periodontal probes:
  – If the gingiva is inflamed the probe will easily surpass the junctional epithelium. At 1.5 MPa the tip of the probe has then already reached the connective tissue.
  – On the other hand, the probe may not pass through a long junctional epithelium, which might have formed after periodontal treatment (see Chapter 11).
  – *Note:* The real attachment level, being the distance between the cementoenamel junction and first fibers of the supra-alveolar fiber apparatus, cannot be determined clinically.
➤ *Gingival recession*: The difference between the clinical attachment level and the periodontal probing depth. If this difference is found to be negative, recession is 0. See Miller's classification of recessions below.
➤ *Furcation diagnosis.* Periodontal lesions which reach the furcation area have a marked horizontal component.[4] The degree of furcation involvement has prognostic relevance:
  – Probing should be done with a curved, color-coded probe; example: the Nabers' probe (PQ2N, Hu-Friedy) with calibration in 3-mm steps.
  – In theory, measurements are done from an imaginary tangent to the prominences of both roots (**Fig. 6.5**)[5]:
    • Degree I: horizontal attachment loss of up to 3 mm
    • Degree II: horizontal attachment loss of more than 3 mm, but not encompassing the whole furcation area

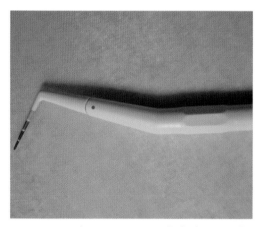

**Fig. 6.3  Simple pressure-controlled plastic probe** (ClickProbe) exerting a probing force of about 0.2 N when it bends (note the joint). Color-coded probe with 3 mm markings, probe tip diameter of about 0.5 mm. The probe is especially useful when assessing the number of gingival units bleeding after probing in patients with plaque-induced gingival disease or during periodontal maintenance.

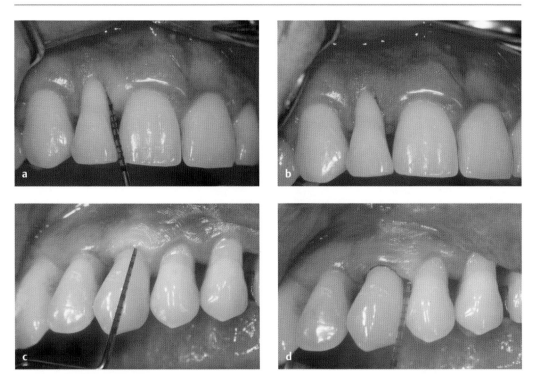

**Fig. 6.4   Periodontal probing.**

**a** The color-coded probe (UNC15) is calibrated in 1-mm steps. Periodontal probing depth at the mesiobuccal site of tooth 12 is about 3.5 mm. Clinical attachment level is 7.5 mm. Thus, gingival recession is 4 mm.

**b** After probing, the bleeding that follows should be recorded.

**c** Periodontal probing depth is 2 mm buccally at tooth 23, clinical attachment loss amounts to 3.5 mm while recession is 1.5 mm.

**d** Probing of the distobuccal surface of tooth 23 reveals 2.5 mm periodontal probing depth, 4 mm clinical attachment loss, and 1.5 mm recession. Profuse bleeding on probing should instantly be recorded.

- Degree III: through-and-through involvement
  - Detailed knowledge of the location of furcation entrances is necessary. Entrances need to be actively explored, so forced probing is recommended (see above):
    - In maxillary molars, the buccal, mesiopalatal, and distopalatal aspects are probed.
    - In maxillary first premolars, mesial and distal probing, from both buccal and palatal aspects, is required.
    - In mandibular molars, buccal and lingual furcation entrances are probed.
  - Furcation entrances are usually located subgingivally. Furcation involvement can therefore only be grossly estimated. More detailed assessment is performed intraoperatively (see below).

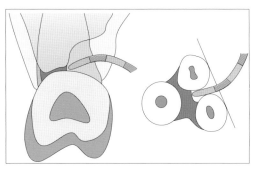

**Fig. 6.5   Probing the furcation area.** Measurements are performed with a curved probe (Nabers probe) to an imaginary tangent, which connects the prominences of both roots. Since the furcation entrance is usually in a subgingival location, the severity of furcation involvement can only be estimated. A more detailed assessment is recommended during surgery (see **Fig. 6.20**).

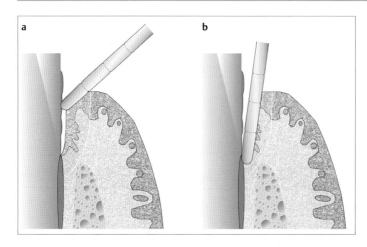

**Fig. 6.6  Bleeding on probing.**
**a** Bleeding tendency of the gingival margin (e.g., PBI, SBI, GBI, see Chapter 5). The probe is carefully inserted into the sulcus and run around the tooth at an angle of about 45°.
**b** Bleeding on probing to the (probe-able) bottom of the pocket or sulcus.

➤ Assessment of tooth mobility:
  – Manual assessment using two instrument handles:
    • Degree I: The crown can be tilted up to 1 mm horizontally.
    • Degree II: The crown can be tilted more than 1 mm horizontally.
    • Degree III: The tooth moves horizontally and vertically in response to cheek or tongue pressure; tooth function is severely compromised.
  – Electronic measurement (PerioTest, Medizintechnik Gulden, Modautal, Germany). The tooth's dampening characteristics are assessed.
  – *Note*: Tooth mobility is not in itself a prognostic factor.
➤ Bleeding on probing (**Fig. 6.6**):
  – Greater density of vessels and loss of collagen within the infiltrated connective tissue of the gingiva may lead to bleeding after minimal mechanical injury.
  – Various findings may be differentiated:
    • Bleeding after probing the marginal gingiva (sulcus bleeding): evidence for an inflammatory response in marginal tissues to supragingival plaque. It may be assessed with index systems (e.g., SBI, PBI, GBI; see Chapter 5) to document the course of periodontal therapy (**Fig. 6.6a**).
    • Bleeding on probing to the (probe-able) bottom of the pocket or sulcus indicates the presence of subgingival plaque. This finding should always be recorded in combination with the periodontal probing depth (**Fig. 6.6b**).

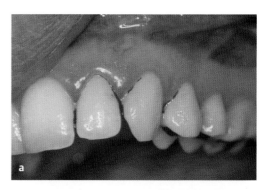

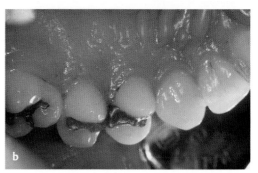

**Fig. 6.7  Different degrees of gingival bleeding on probing in plaque-induced gingival disease.**
**a** Profuse bleeding in a case of severe inflammation in particular of interdental papillae.
**b** Isolated bleeding spots distopalatally at tooth 14 and mesiopalatally at tooth 16.

    • Whether bleeding on probing occurs does not only depend on the degree of gingival inflammation (**Fig. 6.7**), but also on probing pressure (see above) or repeat probing.[6]

➤ *Purulent exudate.* Although this symptom was given a name a century ago ("pyorrhea alveolaris"), this sign of severe inflammation is nowadays infrequently observed.

All periodontal findings should be documented on a suitable chart (**Fig. 6.8**).

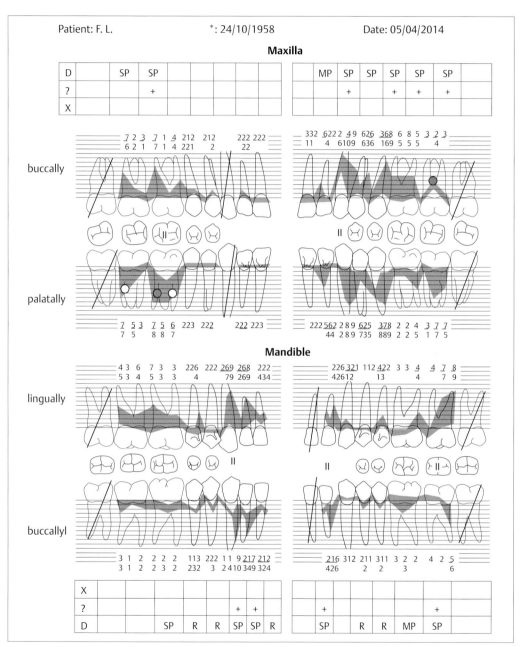

**Fig. 6.8 Filled-in periodontal chart.** Missing teeth ( / ), periodontal probing depths (*upper row* on each side), clinical attachment levels (*lower row* on each side, only attachment loss is recorded), bleeding on probing (underlined probing depth) and gingival margin (recession). Additional recordings (if applicable): caries and restorations, sensitivity, tooth mobility (*roman numerals*), furcation involvement: ○ incipient furcation involvement (degree I), ● advanced furcation involvement (degree II or through-and-through). Diagnosis (D): G: gingivitis, R: recession, MP: moderate periodontitis, SP: severe periodontitis. Preliminary prognosis (X: considered for extraction ?: guarded prognosis).

## Clinical Peri-implant Diagnosis

In order to assess peri-implant mucositis or peri-implantitis, similar clinical examination methods are applied as for natural teeth:

➤ *Bleeding on probing*: Absence indicates healthy and stable condition.
➤ *Purulent exudate*: In case of peri-implantitis, the inflammatory infiltrate may consist of large numbers of polymorphonuclear granulocytes. Pus may indicate an episode of active tissue destruction.
➤ *Peri-implant probing depth:*
   – When applying a probing force of 0.2 N, probing depths of 3 to 4 mm are considered normal, in particular if bleeding does not occur: The probe may then lie within long junctional epithelium (see Chapter 1).
   – Greater depth indicates an inflammatory infiltrate.
   – Note that variable probing pressure may influence measurements at implants to a greater extent than periodontal probing at natural teeth.
➤ *Degree of osseointegration:*
   – Resonance frequency analysis (RFA; Ostell ISQ, Neoss, Harrogate, UK). A transducer is connected to the implant and excited by means of a magnetic impulse. Resonance frequency values are highly correlated with the implant–bone contact surface.[7] The degree of osseointegration may be monitored and the moment when an implant can be loaded determined. Furthermore, at an ISQ value (implant stability quotient) of > 60, the implant may be immediately loaded with a fixed dental prosthesis.
   – In contrast, Periotest (see above) measurements are not suitable for assessment of successful osseointegration. *Note:* Clinically mobile implants have always to be explanted.

## Mucogingival Examination

When esthetics is compromised and/or gingival recessions are present, a detailed examination of the mucogingival situation is necessary. The following should be assessed:

➤ The depth of the vestibule, and aberrant lip and cheek frenula insertions.
➤ The *position* of the gingiva in relation to the cementoenamel junction.
➤ *Gingival width*:
   – Contrast may be enhanced by staining the glycogen-rich alveolar lining mucosa with an aqueous solution of 1% iodine with 2% potassium iodide.
   – The distance between the gingival margin and the mucogingival border may be measured with a periodontal probe or caliper. Subtracting the probing depth yields the width of the *attached gingiva*.
➤ *Gingival thickness*:
   – Sonometric measurement (e. g., Krupp SDM, Austenal, Cologne, Germany; the device is currently not available)[8]
   – If necessary, a precise measurement of gingival thickness can also be made by a caliper after piercing an endodontic reamer, which has been equipped by a rubber disc, to the bone surface.
   – Transgingival visibility of a periodontal probe which has been inserted in the sulcus may indicate rather thin gingiva.[9]
➤ Excessive gingival display, length of the upper lip.
➤ Assessment of the *periodontal phenotype* (**Fig. 6.9**)[10]:
   – Thin periodontal phenotype: combination of a narrow band of rather thin gingiva (< 1 mm) and scalloped contour of the alveolar bone. This fragile gingiva, with tendency for recession, is frequently associated with slender anterior teeth in the maxilla.
   – Thick phenotype: thick (about 1.5 mm) and wide gingiva (3–5 mm), wide interdental septa. Thickness and width are usually combined with rather square anterior teeth in the maxilla. This phenotype may have a low tendency for recession development.
   – *Note*: Gingival thickness is mainly tooth-related, and individual variation (the largely genetically determined "phenotype") may amount to just 4 to 5% of the total variability.[11]
➤ *Gingival recession*:
   – Depth and width of (buccal) recession as measured with a periodontal probe or caliper
   – Possible loss of papilla
   – Classification according to Miller[12] (**Fig. 6.10**):

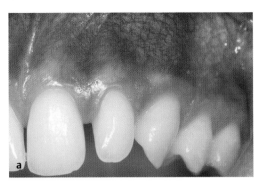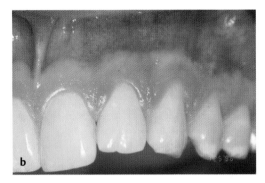

**Fig. 6.9   Periodontal phenotypes.**
**a** "Thin" periodontal phenotype. Slender form of anterior teeth and narrow band of apparently thin, only slightly keratinized, vulnerable gingiva.
**b** "Thick" periodontal phenotype. Rather wide, square anterior teeth and considerably wider and apparently thick and much keratinized gingiva.

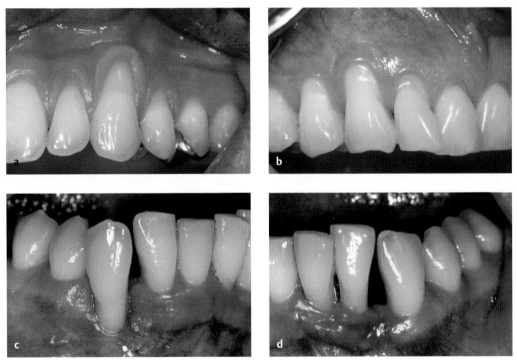

**Fig. 6.10   Classification of gingival recessions.[12]**
**a** *Class I:* Mucogingival border is not affected.
**b** *Class II:* A narrow band of free gingiva has been preserved but periodontal probing would extend beyond the mucogingival border. Note that class I and class II recessions may be surgically covered by up to 100%.
**c** *Class III:* Buccal recession extends beyond the mucogingival border. In addition, there is partial loss of the interdental papilla.
**d** *Class IV:* Interproximal attachment loss is more pronounced than buccal recession. Note that surgical root coverage of class III and class IV recessions may yield only suboptimal postsurgical results.

- *Class I.* Marginal tissue recession not extending to the mucogingival border; no loss of interdental bone or soft tissue.
- *Class II.* Marginal tissue recession extends to or beyond the mucogingival border; no loss of interdental bone or soft tissue.
- *Class III.* Marginal tissue recession extends to or beyond the mucogingival border. Loss of interdental bone; or soft tissue is apical to the cemento-enamel junction, but coronal to the apical extent of the marginal tissue recession. Malposition of the tooth may be present.
- *Class IV.* Marginal tissue recession extends beyond the mucogingival border. Loss of interdental bone extends to a level apical to the extent of the marginal tissue recession. Severe tooth malposition may be present.

*Stillman cleft* (**Fig. 6.11a**). Very narrow, comma-shaped recession within the marginal gingiva. It may be caused by trauma, usually during horizontal toothbrushing.

*McCall festoon* (**Fig. 6.11b**). Gingiva might be thickened around recession sites. Fibrous enlargement as a response to frequent toothbrush injury.

It is recommended to document all findings in a special recession chart (**Fig. 6.12**).

In edentulous parts of the jaw, alveolar ridge defects may occur which have also been classified[13]:
- ➤ Class I: *buccolingual loss* of bone, normal height of the alveolar process
- ➤ Class II: *loss of height* of the alveolar process, normal buccolingual width
- ➤ Class III: *combined loss* of width and height of the alveolar process

## Oral Hygiene

The level of oral hygiene has to be determined. Calculus and the topographical distribution of supragingival plaque and inflamed gingival units may be documented on special forms. As long as the therapist sees the need for further improvement of the patient's oral hygiene, the distribution of plaque should be assessed in each session:
- ➤ to motivate and inform the patient about progress in oral hygiene;
- ➤ to document any changes in oral hygiene level.

After disclosure with, for example, D&C Red #28 (Phloxine B) plaque-disclosing tablets (Disco-Tabs, Colgate-Palmolive, New York, USA), the presence of plaque on four surfaces of every tooth (mesial, buccal, distal, and lingual) is recorded using the Plaque Control Record (PCR, see Chapter 5).

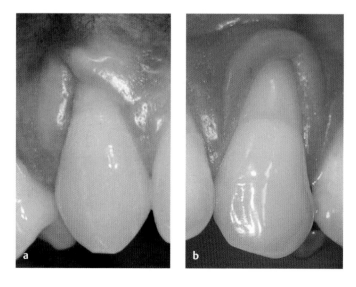

**Fig. 6.11 Special expressions of gingival recession.**
**a** Class I recession at tooth 13 with a Stillman cleft.
**b** Class I recession at tooth 23 with fibrous enlargement of the gingiva, so-called McCall festoon.

Patient: C. D.  *: 14/12/1975  Date: 08/06/2014

| 16 | 15 | 14 | 13 | 12 | 11 | | 21 | 22 | 23 | 24 | 25 | 26 |
|----|----|----|----|----|----|----|----|----|----|----|----|----|
| | | | 4.5 | 2 | 0 | Recession depth | 2.5 | 0 | 3.5 | | | |
| | | | 4 | 2 | 0 | Recession width | 3.5 | 0 | 4.5 | | | |
| | | | 1 | 1 | 2 | Probing depth | 2 | 1 | 2 | | | |
| | | | 0 | 2 | 3.5 | Gingival width | 2 | 3 | 0 | | | |
| | | | 0 | 1 | 1.5 | Attached gingiva | 0 | 2 | 0 | | | |
| | | | 1.2 | 0.9 | 1.3 | Gingival thickness | 1.2 | 1.0 | 1.2 | | | |
| | | II | II | I | 0 | Miller class | III | 0 | IV | | | |
| | | II | | | | Miller class | | | | | | |
| | | 0.8 | | | | Gingival thickness | | | | | | |
| | | 0 | | | | Attached Gingiva | | | | | | |
| | | 0.5 | | | | Gingival width | | | | | | |
| | | 1 | | | | Probing depth | | | | | | |
| | | 3 | | | | Recession width | | | | | | |
| | 2.0 | | | | | Recession depth | | | | | | |
| 46 | 45 | 44 | 43 | 42 | 41 | | 31 | 32 | 33 | 34 | 35 | 36 |

**Fig. 6.12   Filled-in recession chart.**

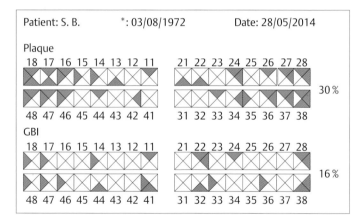

Patient: S. B.  *: 03/08/1972  Date: 28/05/2014

Plaque

18 17 16 15 14 13 12 11   21 22 23 24 25 26 27 28

48 47 46 45 44 43 42 41   31 32 33 34 35 36 37 38

30 %

GBI

18 17 16 15 14 13 12 11   21 22 23 24 25 26 27 28

48 47 46 45 44 43 42 41   31 32 33 34 35 36 37 38

16 %

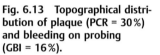

**Fig. 6.13   Topographical distribution of plaque (PCR = 30 %) and bleeding on probing (GBI = 16 %).**

➤ Similarly, presence of bleeding after probing of the sulcus (GBI, see Chapter 5) may be recorded on a regular basis as well (cf. **Fig. 6.6a**):
  – Starting distobuccally, for example, the probe is slightly inserted into the sulcus and run to the buccal and mesial surfaces of the tooth at an angle of about 45°. This is repeated at every tooth.
  – Probing is similarly carried out at palatal/ lingual sites.
  – Any gingival units that bleed are recorded.
➤ The percentage of tooth surfaces covered by plaque and the percentage of gingival units that bleed after probing of the marginal gin-giva are calculated. The patient is informed about the result, which is documented in the file (**Fig. 6.13**).

# ■ Radiologic Examination

To keep radiation exposure to a minimum, radiologic examinations should only be carried out if an appropriate indication is given, for example, to confirm or supplement uncertain clinical findings (**Table 6.2**). *Note*: In cases of generalized moderate and advanced periodontitis, a detailed radiographic survey is required. The following parameters are assessed:

➤ *Absolute bone loss*—the distance (in mm) between the cementoenamel junction and the alveolar bone crest or bottom of the bony lesion. Because of the supra-alveolar fiber apparatus, values within 1.5 to 2 mm are normal and do not represent bone loss. Note that on intraoral radiographs, bone loss may be underestimated by 1 to 2 mm.

➤ *Relative bone loss*—in relation to the root length (percent bone loss)
➤ Bone quality, presence of lamina dura (see Chapter 1)
➤ Presence of bony pockets. Furcation involvement
➤ Width of the periodontal ligament space
➤ Endodontic situation and periapical area

**Table 6.2** Recommendations for dental radiographic examinations (American Dental Association and US Department of Health and Human Services[14])

| Type of encounter | Patient age and dental development stage | | | | |
|---|---|---|---|---|---|
| | **Child with primary dentition** (prior to eruption of first permanent tooth) | **Child with transitional dentition** (after eruption of first permanent tooth) | **Adolescent with permanent dentition** (prior to eruption of third molars) | **Adult, dentate or partially edentulous** | **Adult, edentulous** |
| **New patient** being evaluated for oral diseases | Individualized radiographic exam consisting of selected periapical/occlusal views and/or posterior bitewing photos if proximal surfaces cannot be visualized or probed. Patients without evidence of disease and with open proximal contacts may not require a radiographic exam at this time | Individualized radiographic exam consisting of posterior bitewing photos with panoramic exam or posterior bitewings and selected periapical images | Individualized radiographic exam consisting of posterior bitewing photos with panoramic exam or posterior bitewings and selected periapical images. A full mouth intraoral radiographic exam is preferred when the patient has clinical evidence of generalized oral disease or a history of extensive dental treatment | | Individualized radiographic exam, based on clinical signs and symptoms |
| **Recall patient** with clinical caries or at increased risk for caries | Posterior bitewing exam at 6–12-month intervals if proximal surfaces cannot be examined visually or with a probe | | | Posterior bitewing exam at 6–18-month intervals | Not applicable |
| **Recall patient** with no clinical caries and not at increased risk for caries | Posterior bitewing exam at 12–24-month intervals if proximal surfaces cannot be examined visually or with a probe | | Posterior bitewing exam at 18–36-month intervals | Posterior bitewing exam at 24–36-month intervals | Not applicable |
| **Recall patient** with periodontal disease | Clinical judgment as to the need for and type of radiographic images for the evaluation of periodontal disease. Imaging may consist of, but is not limited to, selected bitewing and/or periapical images of areas where periodontal disease (other than nonspecific gingivitis) can be demonstrated clinically | | | | Not applicable |

**Table 6.2** Continued

| | Patient age and dental development stage | | |
|---|---|---|---|
| **Patient (new and recall)** for monitoring of dentofacial growth and development, and/or assessment of dental/skeletal relationships | Clinical judgment as to need for and type of radiographic images for evaluation and/or monitoring of dentofacial growth and development or assessment of dental and skeletal relationships | Clinical judgment as to need for and type of radiographic images for evaluation and/or monitoring of dentofacial growth and development, or assessment of dental and skeletal relationships. Panoramic or periapical exam to assess developing third molars | Usually not indicated for monitoring of growth and development. Clinical judgment as to the need for and type of radiographic image for evaluation of dental and skeletal relationships. |
| Patient with other circumstances including, but not limited to, proposed or existing implants, other dental and craniofacial pathoses, restorative/endodontic needs, treated periodontal disease and caries remineralization | Clinical judgment as to need for and type of radiographic images for evaluation and/or monitoring of these conditions | | |

- Number and shape of roots, topography of the root complex
- Adjacent areas: maxillary sinus, inferior alveolar nerve, mental foramen

Additional findings may include impacted teeth, remaining roots, cysts, root resorption, hypercementosis, etc.

Radiographs which are taken at regular intervals may allow comparisons between earlier and later exposures; for instance, before and after periodontal therapy.

## Panoramic Radiographs

An orthopantomogram (OPT) provides a general overview, which may be sufficient for periodontal diagnosis in mild or moderate cases.

- Advantages are:
  - Low effective radiation dose of 9 to 24 µSv.[15]
  - Neighboring structures such as temporomandibular joints, maxillary and nasal sinus, and impacted teeth can be assessed.
- Disadvantages, as compared to intraoral radiographs, include:
  - Images not in the plane of interest are blurred and distorted.
  - Uneven enlargement.
  - In anterior regions the cervical spine is superimposed.
- *Note*: Both periapical or periodontal lesions in the furcation area can sometimes more easily be detected on an OPT than on intraoral radiographs:

– A tomogram is preferably adjusted in a way that the central plane of the alveolar process is displayed.
– This is the layer that usually contains the respective pathological structures.

## Full-Mouth Radiographic Survey

A full-mouth radiographic survey is required in all patients with advanced periodontitis and in those undergoing comprehensive therapy:

➤ A standardized *paralleling technique* is implemented using special film holders with an adjustment device and a long cone (**Fig. 6.14a**). The central X-ray beam should be perpendicular to the film.
➤ D-speed and ultraspeed films yield a more detailed image because the grain size is smaller. Ektaspeed films need only half the exposure radiation because they have a larger grain size.
➤ Low kilovoltage (65–70 kV) is best to obtain more contrast, for example, to locate the tip of an endodontic instrument in a root canal.

➤ High kilovoltage (90 kV) yields films with lower contrast preserving more information regarding, for example, bone density and height of the bone crest.
➤ Nowadays, in most cases digital radiography (see below) is applied.

A full-mouth radiographic status usually consists of 14 periapical X-ray exposures (**Fig. 6.15**):

➤ Two exposures each for molars and premolars in upper and lower jaws (film size $3 \times 4\,cm^2$).
➤ Two exposures for maxillary canines (film size $2 \times 3\,cm^2$); the distal surface of the lateral incisor is usually imaged as well.
➤ One exposure for maxillary central incisors (film size $2 \times 3\,cm^2$); mesial surfaces of lateral incisors are also imaged.
➤ Two exposures for mandibular canines (film size $2 \times 3\,cm^2$).
➤ One exposure for mandibular incisors (film size $2 \times 3\,cm^2$).

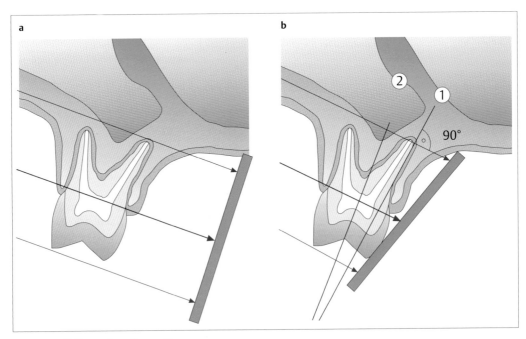

**Fig. 6.14 Full-mouth radiographic survey.**
**a** Paralleling technique. The film is positioned with a special film holder quite far from the tooth parallel to its long axis. The long cone of the X-ray machine is adjusted perpendicular to the film. The tooth image corresponds to the actual size of the tooth.
**b** Bisecting-angle technique. Similar results can be obtained, if the film is positioned close to the tooth and the long cone is positioned so that the central beam is perpendicular to the bisecting plane (1) of the angle between the film and the tooth axis (2), but this technique is not very reliable and is not recommended.

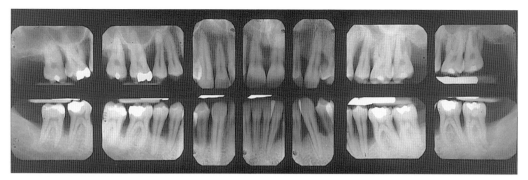

**Fig. 6.15** **Full-mouth radiographic survey:** 14 periapical X-ray photos.

Procedure:
➤ The patient sits upright in the chair.
➤ The film is positioned in its holder in the open mouth of the patient under visual control.
➤ A cotton roll is placed on the dental arch of the opposite jaw in order to fix the film holder when the mouth is closed.
➤ The long cone of the X-ray machine is adjusted, by reference to the adjustment device on the film holder, until it is perpendicular to the film.
➤ The film is exposed for a time that depends on film type and tooth group.

For bimaxillary assessment of bone loss of up to half of the root length of posterior teeth *vertical bitewing* exposures may be considered. This requires a special film holder (VIP-2, Dentsply Rinn, Illinois, USA). Several advantages include:
➤ The film is not or only minimally bent (related to the hard palate or floor of the mouth).
➤ The number of exposures is considerably reduced.
➤ Film holders can be individualized by occlusal impressions made with self-curing resin, which allows standardization of exposures to a large extent; e.g., for follow-up documentation in clinical studies.
➤ Note that anterior regions can usually not be assessed because of considerable overlap. Periapical regions are usually not imaged.

The *bisecting-angle technique* (**Fig. 6.14b**) is generally no longer recommended:
➤ Film positioning is uncertain. The film is held by the patient's index finger. Film distortion cannot be controlled.
➤ Cone adjustment is uncertain.
➤ *Note*: Nowadays, even for endodontic exposures complicated with rubber dam, rubber dam clamps, and inserted root canal instruments, special film holders are available for applying a paralleling technique.

A full-mouth periapical survey may be supplemented with *horizontal bitewing* radiographs to assess interproximal carious lesions. *Note*: In children and adolescents, bitewings may be sufficient to diagnose incipient bone loss at the alveolar crest.

Nowadays, indirect or direct *digital radiography* is usually applied to capture a radiographic image: intraoral detector (luminescence radiography with a scanner) or sensor chip (CCD). Numerous advantages include:
➤ Reduction in radiation dose, about 85 μSv as compared to 388 μSv when using D-speed films.[15]
➤ Digital image manipulation.
➤ Possibility of qualitative and quantitative subtraction radiography and computer-assisted digital image analysis (CADIA).

Subtraction radiography (**Figs. 6.16** and **6.17**) presupposes a high level of standardization with regard to radiation geometry, brightness, and contrast. The latter two can be adjusted by using appropriate software.

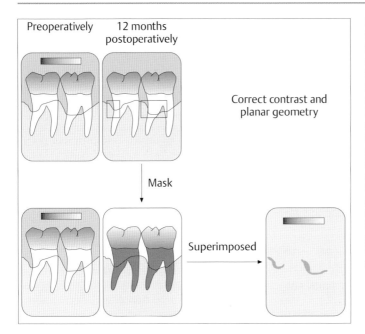

Preoperatively        12 months
                      postoperatively

Correct contrast and
planar geometry

Mask

Superimposed

**Fig. 6.16  Principles of subtraction radiography.** In this example there are two digital or digitized radiographs with acceptable radiation geometry, showing a particular region of interest and taken several months apart. Differences in contrast and brightness can be compensated for by appropriate software, as can small distortions of the planar geometry (some bending of the film). A mask (negative) is made of the postoperative radiograph and the two radiographs are superimposed. Leaving out the background noise, the bony alterations on the distal aspects of both molars and in the furcation area of the first molar now become visible.

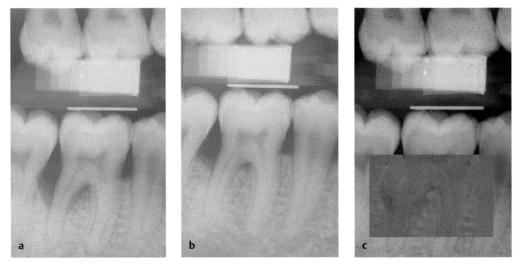

a      b      c

**Fig. 6.17  Subtraction radiography.**
**a** Intrabony lesion distally at tooth 46 with translucency in the furcation
**b** Situation 12 months after therapy
**c** Superimposition of regions of interest of mask (negative) exposure and original exposure. Bone gain is visible in particular in the distal bony pocket and furcation area.

## Computed Tomography

High-resolution computed tomography (CT) displays slices of the periodontium in two planes and allows a detailed assessment of furcation areas, intrabony pockets, and bony dehis-cences, for example. Several disadvantages have limited the use of CT including high costs and very high radiation dose (effective dose of up to about 2,000 µSv). Moreover, artifacts may arise from metallic restorations. Presently, CT is mainly employed in preimplantation diagnosis of height and width of available alveolar bone and neighboring anatomical structures, namely bone level and adequate thickness, course of the mandibular nerve channel, and topography of the sinus floor and the floor of the nasal cavity.

Nowadays, *cone beam computed tomography* (CBCT) has become increasingly important in treatment planning and diagnosis in implant dentistry:

➤ A cone-shaped X-ray bundle, with the X-ray source and the detector, rotates around a field of interest of the patient.
➤ As compared to conventional CT, advantages offered by CBCT are lower costs and less radiation exposure (effective dose of about 45–600 µSv).[15]
➤ Three-dimensional diagnosis of furcation areas, morphology of intrabony pockets, bony situation before placing implants, and possibly soft tissue dimensions are facilitated.

## ■ Intraoperative Diagnosis of Defect Morphology

When expensive and complicated regenerative measures are planned (see Chapter 11) a detailed examination of bony lesions together with careful documentation of the findings is highly recommended:

➤ Both the number of bony walls bordering the periodontal pocket and the morphology of a furcation lesion have prognostic significance:
 – The likelihood of bony regeneration increases considerably with the number of bony walls. *Note*: In an extraction socket (a "four-wall defect"), almost complete bony regeneration can be expected.
 – The treatment plan should be revised whenever the intraoperative situation leaves little hope for proper periodontal regeneration. *Note*: The final assessment of defect morphology can only be done intraoperatively.
➤ The dentist has furthermore an obligation to maintain proper documentation both for the patient and the insurance company or public health service that bears the treatment costs.

## Osseous Defects

Infrabony defects and furcation involvements (**Figs. 6.18–6.20**) may be preliminarily diagnosed on radiographs (OPT, periapical radiograph, CBCT). A definitive *classification* of bony defects (**Fig. 6.21**), however, can only be done during surgery:

➤ Three-wall bony defect: interproximal bony pocket where the buccal and lingual bony walls and proximal bone at the neighboring tooth are preserved. Also termed intrabony defect.
➤ Two-wall bony pocket: interproximal bony pocket with loss of either the buccal or lingual bony wall.
➤ One-wall bony pocket: Interproximal bony pocket with loss of both the buccal and lingual bony wall.
➤ Interdental crater: buccal and lingual bony walls are preserved while bony support at the neighboring tooth has been lost.

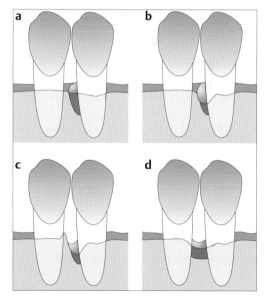

**Fig. 6.18 Infrabony defects.**
**a** Three-wall bony pocket.
**b** Two-wall bony pocket. The defect is bordered by either the buccal or lingual wall and the proximal bony wall.
**c** Mostly one-wall bony pocket, but note that apically there are several walls.
**d** Interdental crater with bony walls buccally and lingually.

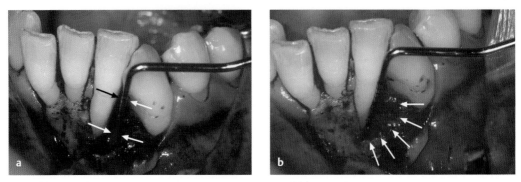

**Fig. 6.19   Intraoperative measurement of a circumferential bony pocket.**
**a** The entire defect, as measured from the cementoenamel junction to the bottom of the bony lesion, is about 15 mm deep. The depth of the two-wall bony pocket is 4 mm.
**b** Circumference of about 90°.

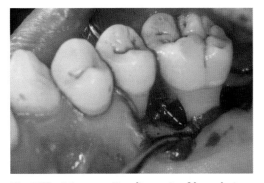

**Fig. 6.20   Intraoperative diagnosis of bony lesions in the furcation area.** The width of the furcation entrance at the level of the alveolar crest, the height and depth of the furcation, the height of the root trunk, and the distance between the cementoenamel junction and the bottom of the defect should be assessed.

Usually, combinations occur: A three-wall bony pocket at the bottom of the lesion, a two-wall component in the middle and a one-wall component more coronally. The circumference of the bony lesion is estimated, for example, in steps of 30°. Note that the number of walls of bony pockets can also be documented in lesions that are not located interproximally.

## Furcation Involvement

Since any clinical assessment of furcation involvement may be prone to considerable error (see above), a careful intrasurgical inspection of the situation at multirooted teeth (and possible revision of the treatment plan) is highly recommended (**Fig. 6.22**):

➤ The *depth* of the furcation, that is, the definite furcation degree (see above); and the *width* of its entrance
➤ The *height* as measured from the furcation roof to the alveolar bone has been subclassified[16]:
   – Class A: ≤ 3 mm
   – Class B: 4–6 mm
   – Class C: > 6 mm
➤ The height of the root trunk
➤ The height of interdental bone

Note that special circumferential bony pockets with indirect furcation involvement may occur, namely hemifurcal and crescent intrafurcal defects.

## ■ Advanced Diagnostic Techniques

In certain problematic cases such as aggressive periodontitis and periodontitis as a manifestation of systemic disease (see Chapter 4), or in refractory cases without acceptable therapeutic response, *special tests* may be useful. It should be self-evident that the amount of information gained must be proportionate to the costs in time and resources.

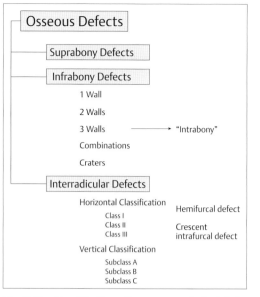

**Fig. 6.21   Classification of osseous periodontal defects.**

## Diagnostic Test Systems

Beyond clinical and radiographic findings, diagnostic tests should provide the doctor with further information. Clinicians are usually interested in:
➤ the nature of the infection;
➤ the prognosis;
➤ likely treatment outcomes.

Special diagnostic tests might answer typical questions:
➤ Is destructive periodontal disease likely to develop?
➤ Is the existing periodontal lesion active (i.e., progressive), or is it stable?
➤ Is the form of the disease aggressive (rapidly progressing), or rather, is it chronic (slowly progressing)?

Conventional diagnostic measures frequently lead to either over- or undertreatment. Ideally, diagnostic tests should enable the dentist to provide the appropriate therapy. The development of a diagnostic test requires a so-called *gold standard*, which ultimately signals the presence or absence of disease and which may be compared with the performance of the respective diagnostic test under scrutiny.
➤ The gold standard is usually very invasive—for example, histological evidence of attachment loss after the tooth has been extracted, probably together with its surrounding periodontal tissues.
➤ In clinical practice, the gold standard may be replaced by surrogates—that is, less invasive, previously validated (against the gold standard) test parameters. For example, a clinically determined attachment loss, or bone loss observed on radiographs that occurred in a relatively short period of time, may signal active ongoing destruction of the supporting apparatus of the tooth. Attention should be paid, however, to the following problems:
  – The real attachment level cannot be determined by clinical probing (see above).
  – The measurement error of periodontal probing is quite large, about 1 mm.
  – Qualitative or quantitative subtraction radiography (for observation of either bone loss or gain) requires a very high level of standardization of exposures.

By using inevitably inferior *surrogates* (as compared to the true, histological gold standard) numerous diagnostic tests have been developed which are based on completely different test systems. They include, for example:
➤ Presence or absence of specific periodontal pathogens or bacterial consortia
➤ Local or systemic mediators of the inflammatory and immunological host response
➤ Metabolic products of host and bacteria
➤ Deficiencies and peculiarities of the immune system
➤ Genetic polymorphisms

| Patient: N. L. | | *: 18/05/1946 | | Date: 20/05/2014 | | | | Tooth: 26 | |
|---|---|---|---|---|---|---|---|---|---|

Strategic importance:   high
Sensitivity:   +
Endodontic situation:   ./.
Mobility degree:   I
Restorative situation:   possible

| | mb | | b | | db | dl | | l | | ml |
|---|---|---|---|---|---|---|---|---|---|---|
| **Clinical findings** | | | | | | | | | | |
| PPD | 5 | 1 | 6 | 2 | 4 | 4 | | 2 | | 6 |
| vCAL | 3 | 3 | 7 | 2 | 2 | 2 | | 0 | | 4 |
| hCAL | | | Ø | | | 2 | | | | Ø |
| Furcation degree | | | FIII | | | FI | | | | FIII |
| **Radiographic findings** | | | | | | | | | | |
| Bone loss (% root length) | 40 | 0 | | | 0 | 30 | 15 | | | 40 |
| **Intraoperative findings** | | | | | | | | | | |
| *Bone height* | | | | | | | | | | |
| CEJ-BD | 3.5 | 3.5 | 5.5 | 2.5 | 2.5 | 2 | | 1.5 | | 5 |
| CEJ-AC | 3.5 | 3.5 | 7.5 | 2.5 | 2.5 | 2 | | 1.5 | | 5.5 |
| 3-wall comp. | | | 2 | | | | | | | 0.5 |
| 2-wall comp. | | | 0 | | | | | | | 0 |
| 1-wall comp. | | | 0 | | | | | | | 0 |
| *Furcation* | | | | | | | | | | |
| Depth | | | Ø | | | 2.5 | | | | Ø |
| Degree revised | | | FIII | | | FI | | | | FIII |
| Width | | | 2 | | | 2 | | | | 2.5 |
| Height | | | 2 | | | 1.5 | | | | 2.5 |
| Root trunk | | | 2 | | | 2.5 | | | | 2 |

**Fig. 6.22   Intrasurgical documentation of the morphology of bony lesions.** (After Müller and Eger.[4]).

mb:   mesiobuccal
b:   buccal
db:   distobuccal
dl:   distolingual
l:   lingual
ml:   mesiolingual
PPD:   periodontal probing depth

vCAL: vertical clinical attachment level
hCAL: horizontal clinical attachment level
FI-III:  furcation degrees I–III
CEJ-BD: distance from cementoenamel junction to bottom of defect
CEJ-AC: distance from cementoenamel junction to alveolar crest

Test parameters of a diagnostic test can be estimated in a screening experiment (**Fig. 6.23**):

➤ *Sensitivity* of the test is the conditional probability that a diseased individual is correctly identified by the test (true-positive result).

➤ *Specificity* is the conditional probability that an individual not affected by the disease is correctly identified by the test (true-negative result).

The usefulness of a diagnostic test in a clinical setting depends not just on these parameters but more essentially on three others:

➤ The *prevalence* of the disease in the population

➤ The *importance* of the disease for the single individual and for the population at large

➤ The *costs* of the test

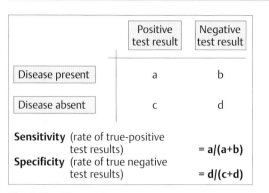

|  | Positive test result | Negative test result |
|---|---|---|
| Disease present | a | b |
| Disease absent | c | d |

**Sensitivity** (rate of true-positive
test results)        = a/(a+b)
**Specificity** (rate of true negative
test results)        = d/(c+d)

**Fig. 6.23   Diagnostic test parameters.**

Let's consider a *hypothetical example.* For a life-threatening disease with a high risk of transmission, very high sensitivity (e. g., 99%), and even higher specificity (e. g., 99.9%) is required for a useful diagnostic test. Consider the following:

➤ The prevalence, in a certain population, of individuals infected with a certain virus is, say, 0.1%.
➤ By applying a test with the above performance (99% sensitivity, 99.9% specificity), only $2 \times 10^{-6}$ per cent of negatively tested individuals are in fact infected by the virus. This *false-negative rate* may be ignored.
➤ On the other hand, about 50% of individuals who test positive are actually not infected— a rather high *false-positive rate*!
➤ Interpretation: The test is useful, since virtually all individuals infected with the virus are identified. Preventive and therapeutic measures can immediately be implemented and the population at large is protected.
➤ As a consequence of the high false-positive rate, persons who tested positive must be retested by a better, usually more expensive test, to reduce the false-positive rate.

For a non-life-threatening and common disease such as (active) periodontitis, which can be treated by simple measures like subgingival scaling (see Chapter 10), diagnostic test parameters are generally not so demanding. A moderate sensitivity of about 70% and a relatively high specificity of about 90% may result in a useful test if the costs of the test are not exorbitant. Consider, as another hypothetical example, the following:

➤ The prevalence of active periodontitis in a population may amount to 5%.

➤ Given the above test parameters (70% sensitivity, 90% specificity), 73% of positive test results would relate to periodontally stable individuals/tooth surfaces, a relatively high false-positive rate.
➤ 1.7% of negative test results would relate to periodontally active patients/tooth surfaces, a relatively low false-negative rate.
➤ Thus, the test would lead quite frequently to (over-)treatment of conditions that are actually stable. On the other hand, virtually every active lesion would be identified.
➤ The consequences of overtreatment (unnecessary costs) are outweighed by the risks of possible undertreatment (irreversible loss of tooth-supporting structures).

Traditional clinical parameters such as redness of the gingiva, bleeding on probing, purulent exudate, and probing pocket depth, are not very sensitive to identify active periodontal lesions and only moderately specific.[3] So, there has long been a great desire to develop test systems that have a potential to gain more information.

*Note:* Contrary to often-expressed recommendations by respective providers of chairside diagnostic tests, there is no necessity for expensive laboratory diagnostics which would just confirm clinical findings.

Test parameter sensitivity and specificity of a new diagnostic test are usually derived from a screening experiment. The sensitivity of the test is calculated as the proportion of true-positive results (as compared with the gold standard), while the specificity is the proportion of true-negative results. Note that so-called false-positive and false-negative rates of a test can only be determined if prevalence of the disease in the population of interest (for instance, patients who attend a clinic or private practice) is identical to the study population (which is rarely the case).

## Microbiological Tests

A microbiological approach to diagnosing periodontitis and, in particular, active disease has long appeared reasonable because of the infectious nature of both chronic and aggressive and an apparently limited number of potential pathogens being involved (see Chapter 2 and **Box 6.1**). Several commercial laboratories provide practitioners with fast and fairly cost-effective results for microbiological tests. This service includes usually semiquantitative detection of established periodontal pathogens such as *Aggregatibacter actinomycetemcomitans*, *Porphyromonas gingivalis*, *Prevotella intermedia*, *Treponema denticola*, and *Tannerella forsythia*. Often, therapeutic recommendations are given as well.

As a rule, subgingival plaque samples from the deepest pockets in each quadrant are collected and may be either pooled or analyzed separately. The following procedures should be observed:

➤ The teeth need to be isolated with cotton rolls.
➤ Any supragingival deposits have to be removed with a scaler.

➤ One or more absorbing endodontic paper points (ISO 30 or 35) are inserted to the bottom of the pocket (**Fig. 6.24**) and kept in place for about 10 seconds.
➤ The samples are then transferred to a suitable transport vial and mailed to the laboratory.

Nowadays **molecular biological methods** are used by almost all commercial laboratories which may use the following techniques:

➤ Species-specific, enzyme- or radiolabeled, oligonucleotide sequences (*DNA probes*) bind to complementary sequences of bacterial DNA:
  – Hypervariable sequences of 16S rDNA, which are known for a large number of species, are very suitable for constructing species-specific DNA probes (see Chapter 2 and **Box 2.1**).
  – Oligonucleotides consisting of 24 to 30 base pairs are either radioactively or enzymatically tagged, giving conjugates that emit fluorescence or chemiluminescence (digoxigenin-labeled). *Note:* In contrast to these oligonucleotide probes, whole genomic or cloned DNA probes more frequently show cross-reactions.

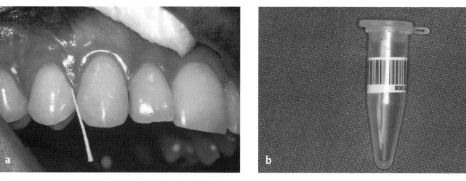

**Fig. 6.24   Collection of samples of subgingival plaque.**
**a** Subgingival bacteria are often sampled from periodontal pockets by use of an absorbing endodontic paper point (e.g., ISO 30), which is inserted down to the bottom of the periodontal pocket and left in place for about 10 seconds.
**b** As a rule, samples from the deepest pockets in each quadrant of the dentition are pooled in an appropriate vial and sent by mail for molecular biological analysis.

– Principle procedure (**Fig. 6.25**):
- The plaque sample is dispersed in a medium.
- Enzymes and detergents are added to lyse the cells.
- NaOH is added to denature bacterial DNA leading to single strands.
- DNA probes bind only to complementary fragments.

– Presently, commercial labs offer microbiological analyses based on species-specific DNA probes for up to 11 periodontal pathogens, namely *P. gingivalis*, *P. intermedia*, *A. actinomycetemcomitans*, *Eikenella corrodens*, *Fusobacterium nucleatum/periodonticum*, *Campylobacter rectus*, *T. forsythia*, *T. denticola*, *Eubacterium nodatum*, *Parvimonas micra*, and *Capnocytophaga* spp. (e.g., micro-Ident plus, Hain LifeScience, Nehren, Germany).

➤ *Polymerase chain reaction* (PCR). A pair of oligonucleotide primers is used to amplify a small sequence of genomic DNA several million times, thus making it detectable after gel eletrophoresis (**Fig. 6.26**). Primers usually consist of between 18 and 28 nucleotide bases.

– Various sequences of genomic DNA can be amplified, for example, species-specific 16S rDNA, sequences in the region of the leukotoxin gene of *A. actinomycetemcomitans* (**Fig. 6.27**), etc. PCR can identify target sequences with a very high sensitivity.
- DNA is denatured at 95°C in a thermocycler.
- At 55°C, species-specific sense and antisense primers, nucleotides and *Taq* polymerase (a thermostable DNA polymerase of the bacterium *Thermus aquaticus*) are added.

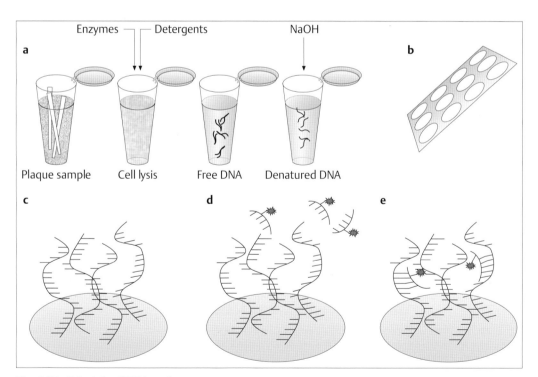

**Fig. 6.25 Principle of DNA probes.**
**a** Sampling and denaturation of bacterial DNA.
**b** Binding of denatured DNA to special filter material.
**c** High magnification of a spot showing floating, single-stranded DNA.
**d** Species-specific, labeled DNA probes are added.
**e** Probes bind only to target zones of homologous bacterial species. Labeling allows semiquantitative assessment. (Adapted from Murray and French.[17])

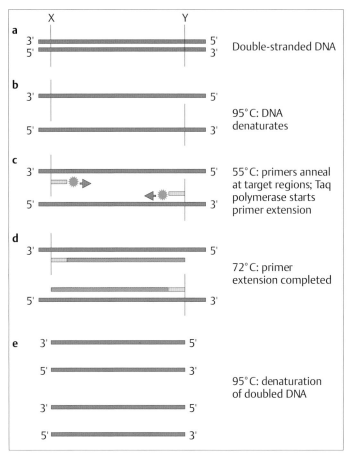

a 3' / 5'    X    Y    5' / 3'    Double-stranded DNA

b 3'    5'    95°C: DNA denaturates    5' / 3'

c 3'    5'    55°C: primers anneal at target regions; Taq polymerase starts primer extension    5' / 3'

d 3'    5'    72°C: primer extension completed    5' / 3'

e 3'    5'    95°C: denaturation of doubled DNA    5' / 3'

**Fig. 6.26  Principle of the polymerase chain reaction (PCR).**

a The genomic sequence between X and Y is to be identified by amplification.

b At 95°C the double-stranded DNA denatures; there are now two single strands of DNA available as template.

c After cooling to 55°C, a pair of specific oligonucleotide primers can anneal (hybridize) to the respective target regions. Heat-resistant *Taq* polymerase derived from *Thermophilus aquatus* starts primer extension. Nucleotides have to be added in excess.

d At 72°C, primer extension leads double-stranded DNA between the two primers.

e Two double-stranded pieces of DNA can now be further multiplied by repeating the cycle. The sequences are rapidly amplified a million times and can be identified by gel electrophoresis (**Fig. 6.27**).

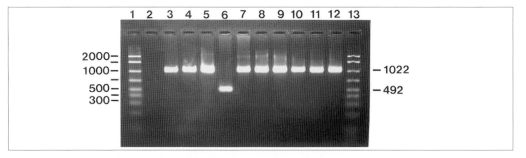

**Fig. 6.27   Gel electrophoresis of amplified sequences after PCR.**
A sequence within the promoter region of the leukotoxin gene of *Aggregatibacter actinomycetemcomitans* (cf. **Fig. 2.6**) has been amplified and visualized by ethidium bromide. Lanes 1 and 13 represent DNA size markers, lane 2 is a negative control (water). The analysis revealed two sequences with different sizes. In most species, 1,022 base pairs (bp) were amplified (Lanes 3–5, 7–12). One isolate (lane 6) had a deletion of 530 bp in the promoter region of the leukotoxin gene. (After Macheleidt et al.[18])

- Annealing of primers is accomplished at a temperature of 68° C.
- The temperature is raised to 72° C, and *Taq* polymerase starts primer extension.
- The process is stopped at 95° C when amplified DNA is again denatured.
  - Quantitative PCR (real-time PCR, e.g, Meridol Test, GABA, Basel, Switzerland):
    - A further, double fluorescence-labeled (fluorophore and quencher), species-specific, oligonucleotide probe (TaqMan probe) is added.
    - *Taq* polymerase reaches the TaqMan probe during primer extension and degrades it. Degradation of the TaqMan probe releases the fluorophore and, while breaking its close proximity to the quencher, allows its fluorescence.
    - The fluorescence signal relates to the amount of synthesized bacterial DNA in the sample and can be measured fluorometrically.
- ➤ RNA probes (e.g., IAI Pado Test 4·5, IAI, Zuchwil, Switzerland):
  - Direct hybridizing of specific oligonucleotide probes to bacterial rRNA without prior genetic amplification
  - Target bacteria: *A. actinomycetemcomitans, P. gingivalis, T. forsythia, T. denticola*
  - Universal oligonucleotide probe for estimating the total number of bacteria in the sample
  - Semiquantitative assessment of genetic material of living bacteria by chemiluminescence

**Direct observation** of bacteria in dental bioflm goes back to the late 17th century, when Antonie van Leeuwenhoek, with the aid of a microscope, described for the first time various bacterial morphotypes in dental plaque and their motility. In particular since the 1960s, microscopic assessment of dental biofilm has again become popular.

- ➤ *Direct microscopic techniques* (Gram preparation, dark field and phase contrast microscopy). Gram-negative bacteria increase drastically in number and proportion in pathologically deepened pockets. There is also a considerable increase in motile bacteria (motile rods and spirochetes). A major disadvantage of simple microscopic techniques is that bacteria cannot be differentiated at the species level.
- ➤ *Fluorescence in-situ hybridization* (FISH). As a research tool, target bacteria are labeled with oligonucleotide probes (see above), which carry a fluorescent dye. In thick biofilm, specific bacteria may be identified with confocal laser scanning microscopy. Direct assessment of the number and distribution of pathogens in biofilm is facilitated.
- ➤ *Vital fluorescence.* A dental biofilm sample is mounted on a glass slide. Fluorescein diacetate is added, which penetrates the bacterial cell membrane and is metabolized, in the living cell, to (green) fluorescein. The sample is counterstained with ethidium bromide (red), which binds to the nucleic acid of dead cells. The ratio of vital to dead bacteria in dental biofilm may be assessed, for instance in clinical studies on antibacterial mouthwash.
- ➤ *Indirect immune fluorescence.* Plaque samples are diluted and heat-fixed on a glass slide. Monoclonal mouse antibodies or species-specific polyclonal rabbit antisera are added, which bind to respective surface antigens of bacteria. Anti-mouse or, respectively, anti-rabbit IgG antibodies are added, which are labeled with fluorescein isothiocyanate. Fluorescent cells can be identified and counted in a dark field microscope. In older studies large numbers of samples had been assessed for the presence of a limited number of periodontal pathogens.

**"Chairside" tests.** Particularly in the 1980s and 1990s, numerous companies provided dentists with miniaturized test systems which were supposed to facilitate quick microbiological verification.

- ➤ Identification of *A. actinomycetemcomitans, P. gingivalis,* and *Prevotella intermedia* in dental biofilm by enzyme immune assay (EIA) or the latex agglutination test.
- ➤ Detection of trypsinlike peptidase in dental biofilm which may indicate the presence of *P. gingivalis, T. forsythia* and *Treponema denticola* (BANA test, OraTec, Manassas, Virginia, USA)

Due to high costs and questionable diagnostic value, hardly any chairside tests have prevailed in the market.

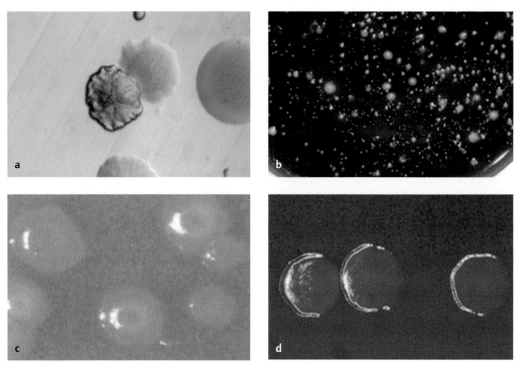

**Fig. 6.28   Typical colonies of periodontal microorganisms.**
**a** *Aggregatibacter actinomycetemcomitans* on selective TSBV medium. Note the starlike inner structure of the central colony.
**b** Numerous black-pigmented colonies of *Porphyromonas gingivalis* on an enriched blood agar plate.
**c** *Capnocytophaga* spp. on selective Thayer–Martin medium.
**d** *Eikenella corrodens* on clindamycin-containing selective medium.

**Bacterial culture.** Few laboratories still offer bacterial culture to dentists (e. g., LabOral, Amsterdam, Netherlands; **Fig. 6.28**). Several advantages of cultivating plaque samples include:

➤ Quantification of established periodontal pathogens can be done on enriched and selective media (**Fig. 6.29**).
➤ Unusual bacteria such as pseudomonads, enterococci, enteric rods, staphylococci, or *Candida* spp. may be identified
➤ Antibiotic susceptibility testing (e.g, agar diffusion [E-test] and agar dilution), is possible. *Note*: Minimum inhibitory concentrations of bacteria organized in a biofilm may be 100 to 1,000 times higher than those commonly determined in planktonic cultures.

Certain important pathogens such as *T. denticola* and *T. forsythia* are not easy to cultivate. Culture techniques are time-consuming and expensive. They were formerly important as tools for the identification of a number of periodontal pathogens, which meanwhile have become well established, but are nowadays no longer considered best practice in oral microbial diagnosis.

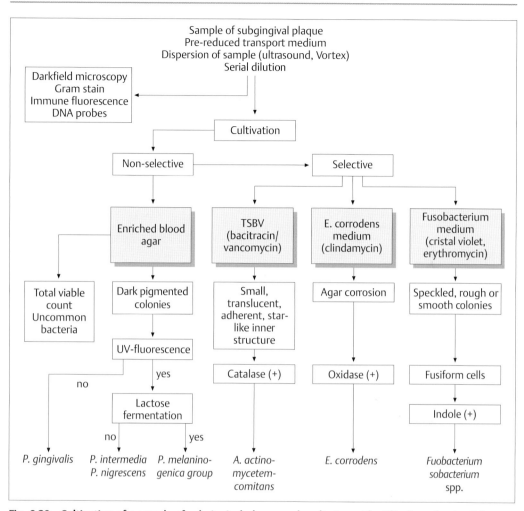

**Fig. 6.29 Cultivation of a sample of subgingival plaque and preliminary identification of potential gram-negative periodontal pathogens.** The total count of viable colony-forming units is determined on nonselective enriched blood agar taking account of the dilution factor. Some dark-pigmented colonies can be differentiated by their fluorescence capacity under long-wave ultraviolet light (*Porphyromonas gingivalis* or *Prevotella intermedia/ P. nigrescens*, *P. melaninogenica* group). Further differentiation is possible by lactose fermentation. Pink or opalescent, round, convex, colonies of fusiform bacteria are probably *Tannerella forsythia* (subcultivation and definitive differentiation on *N*-acetyl-muraminic-acid containing blood agar is necessary), while transparent, flat, spreading colonies may be *Campylobacter* spp. (subcultivation and definitive differentiation on formate-fumarate agar). Selective media for *Aggregatibacter actinomycetemcomitans*, *Eikenella corrodens*, and *Fusobacterium nucleatum* allow preliminary identification, enumeration, subcultivation, and definitive identification of these organisms. (Adapted from Slots.[19])

### Box 6.1    Advanced periodontal diagnosis

In two systematic reviews by Mombelli et al[20] and Listgarten and Loomer[21] the diagnostic value of microbiological diagnosis of periodontal disease was critically assessed. Concordantly, the presence or absence of periodontal pathogens *Aggregatibacter actinomycetemcomitans, Porphyromonas gingivalis, Prevotella intermedia, Tannerella forsythia* and *Campylobacter rectus* does not allow differentiation between the two major forms of disease, namely chronic or aggressive periodontitis. However, a clinical diagnosis of aggressive periodontitis is more likely in patients with than without detected *A. actinomycetemcomitans*.

A highly leukotoxic clone of *A. actinomycetemcomitans* has generally been found only in aggressive periodontitis but essentially in West African and Afro-American patients. Further variants of *A. actinomycetemcomitans* have been associated with aggressive periodontitis in young patients of Northern European/North American populations.

Microbiological monitoring may reasonably supplement treatment of certain periodontitis patients who do not properly respond to conventional therapy. In many cases, periodontal infections include *A. actinomycetemcomitans* and/or *P. gingivalis* which may require adjunct systemic antibiotic therapy (see Chapter 13).

Biochemical examination of gingival exudate for markers of the specific and nonspecific host response had been propagated notably in the 1990s in order to identify periodontal lesions at any risk of undergoing active destruction. Hardly any of the tests offered in the past are currently available.

For several years, a genetic test for the so-called IL-1 genotype had been propagated which might indicate an increased susceptibility for chronic periodontitis. A meta-analysis of 53 population-based case–control studies was done by Nikolopoulos et al,[22] in which various cytokine gene polymorphisms were addressed. Data from six studies limiting the analysis to Caucasians revealed quite a strong association of the above haplotype, that is, a combination of polymorphisms in the *IL1A* (-889) and *IL1B* genes (+3953/4), with chronic periodontitis (odds ratio [OR] 2.251, 95% confidence interval [CI] 1.207; 4.199). In a further five studies, a weak positive association with chronic periodontitis was ascertained for polymorphisms at *IL1B* (-511) (OR 1.481, 95% CI 0.941; 2.332). In a more recent systematic review,[23] 12 studies were considered in which combinations of polymorphisms in the *IL1A* (-889 or+4845, which are in more than 99% concordant) and *IL1B* (+3953/4) genes were associated with periodontitis in Whites. A moderate OR of 1.51 (95% CI 1.13; 2.02) was calculated. In both meta-analyses significant heterogeneity was observed.

A systematic review of 11 longitudinal studies[24] concluded that the presence of the respective haplotype did not allow inferences about further progression of periodontal disease after therapy. A commercial test based on this premise is no longer offered to dentists.

## Markers of Specific and Nonspecific Host Response

Results of **serological examinations** may be difficult to interpret. In cases of aggressive periodontitis, high antibody titers against periodontal pathogens such as *A. actinomycetemcomitans* always indicate presence of the microorganism. It has been suggested that insufficient production of antibodies may lead to a more generalized form of the disease. Recent studies did not confirm a respective postulate (see Chapter 3).

**Gingival exudate** contains numerous potential markers of the specific and nonspecific host responses.[25] It can be collected on special filter paper strips which may be placed in the sulcus or pocket entrance for, say, 10 or 30 seconds (**Fig. 6.30**).

➤ The area should be carefully isolated to avoid saliva contamination.
➤ The absorbed volume can be determined with a calibrated measuring device (Periotron 8000, Oraflow, Plainview, NewYork, USA).

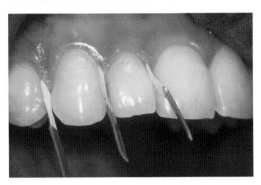

**Fig. 6.30 Sampling of inflammatory gingival exudate** at the mesial aspects of teeth using filter paper strips placed at the orifice of the sulcus/pocket.

➤ *Note:* The volume of the exudate depends largely on the degree of gingival inflammation. Therefore, the concentration of markers is of importance (mass per volume) rather than mass per unit of time.

Various biochemical markers have been identified in gingival exudate, which may have prognostic significance.
➤ Markers of the inflammatory reaction:
  – Monocytes of individuals susceptible to periodontitis respond to lipopolysaccharides (LPS) of gram-negative bacteria with increased secretion of prostaglandin $E_2$ (PGE$_2$):
    • PGE$_2$ may be found in gingival exudate and connective tissue and is strongly associated with local progression of periodontitis.
    • Similar observations have been made in relation to proinflammatory cytokines interleukin-1 alpha (IL-1$\alpha$), IL-1$\beta$, IL-6, and tumor necrosis factor alpha (TNF-$\alpha$), which can be detected by an enzyme immune assay in increased concentrations in gingival exudate of, in particular, refractory cases.
    • *Note*: A postulated *hyperreactive phenotype* of macrophages may essentially be controlled by genetic factors, but may be modulated by acquired and behavioral factors as well.
  – The *acute-phase reactants* C-reactive protein (CRP), $\alpha_1$-macroglobulin, $\alpha_2$-protease inhibitor, as well as transferrin and lactoferrin, each correlate with the degree of gingival inflammation but do not appear to be suitable for identification of active periodontal lesions.
➤ Host enzymes:
  – *Matrix metalloproteinases* (MMPs), such as collagenase and gelatinase, play an important role in periodontal tissue remodeling and turnover:
    • Neutral proteases may be nonspecifically detected in gingival exudate by a colorimetric assay.
    • A soluble, colored collagen fragment is cleaved enzymatically from a nonsoluble dye-and-collagen conjugate.
    • A chairside test for activated MMP-8 is currently available (Dentognostics, Jena, Germany).
  – Similar methods have been described for the detection in gingival exudate of *lysosomal enzymes* derived from polymorphonuclear granulocytes, for example:
    • Elastase
    • Cathepsins
    • $\beta$-Glucuronidase.
  – *Alkaline phosphatase* is released by osteoblasts, fibroblasts, and neutrophil granulocytes. This enzyme can be detected in gingival exudate by chemiluminescence.
  – *Aspartate aminotransferase* (AST) is released only after cell death. Increased concentrations of AST in gingival exudate (> 800 mIU) have been associated with active periodontal destruction. A test kit based on this reaction has been developed.
➤ Products of tissue metabolism:
  – Glycosaminoglycans are polysaccharide compounds which are bound to tissue proteoglycans. Especially the occurrence of *chondroitin-4-sulfate* and *chondroitin-6-sulfate* in gingival exudate has been correlated with gingival inflammation.
  – The amino acid *hydroxyproline* is a major component of collagen. Since it is detectable in gingival exudate, even in gingivitis, it appears not to be suitable as a marker of periodontal destruction.
  – The same holds for *fibronectins*, a heterogeneous group of glycoproteins in blood and connective tissue which play an important role during inflammation and wound healing.

– Further connective tissue proteins such as osteonectin, osteocalcin, or type-I-collagen peptides, carboxyterminal type-I propeptide, and aminoterminal type-III propeptide, and others can be detected in gingival exudate. Their diagnostic value seems to be limited.

**Critical remarks.** Some biochemical markers in gingival exudate appear to be associated with periodontal activity while others are highly correlated with clinical inflammation. *Note:* Expensive advanced diagnostics are only indicated if the results would actually modify therapy. At present, biochemical markers are not suitable for periodontal diagnosis:

➤ Possible tests yield little or no additional information.
➤ High costs are incurred if multiple sites are tested.
➤ As a consequence, most of the test systems developed to date have not been adopted in daily practice.

### Saliva Diagnostics

Most of the above-mentioned host-specific markers of periodontal inflammation in gingival exudate as well as microorganisms of the dental biofilm may also be detected in saliva[26]:

➤ The amount in relation to the saliva volume (i.e., concentration) generally correlates with the extent and severity of periodontal disease.
➤ Saliva samples can easily and noninvasively be obtained and analyzed at rather low costs.
➤ Promising candidates for periodontal saliva diagnostics are IL-1β, collagenase, in particular active MMP-8 (PerioMarker, Hager & Werken, Duisburg, Germany), and all established periodontal pathogens (**Fig. 6.31**).

### Human Genetic Tests

Among genetic markers (see Chapter 3), the diagnostic and prognostic value of, in particular, polymorphisms in the interleukin-1 gene complex have been studied in some detail (see **Box 6.1**):

➤ The haplotype of allele 2 (C→T) of *IL1A* (-889 or +4845) polymorphisms and allele 2 of *IL1B* (+3954) polymorphisms has been moderately associated with chronic periodontitis in Caucasians (**Box 6.1**), which may be related to an increased release of IL-1 by monocytes in contact with LPS of gram-negative bacteria (see Chapter 3).
➤ Gene–environment interaction: IL-1 genotype positive smokers have, in some populations, a higher risk for periodontitis as compared to IL-1 genotype negative smokers and nonsmokers.[28]

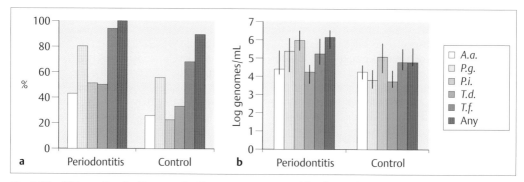

**Fig. 6.31   PCR results of saliva samples from 40- to 60-year-old individuals in the population-based Finnish Health 2000 study.** Eighty-four cases of moderate or severe periodontitis were compared with 81 controls without periodontal pockets. Note that differences in prevalence and load (numbers of bacteria in saliva) were surprisingly small. (After Hyvärinen et al.[27])
**a** Prevalence of *Aggregatibacter actinomycetemcomitans (A.a.), Porphyromonas gingivalis (P.g.), Prevotella intermedia (P.i.), Treponema denticola (T.d.)*, and *Tannerella forsythia (T.f.)*, or any of these pathogens.
**b** Results of quantitative PCR (log-transformed number of genomes per mL saliva, interquartile ranges).

➤ IL-1 genotype-positive patients with periodontal disease seem to lose more teeth despite proper supportive periodontal therapy (see Chapter 12).

*Note:* Human genetic tests for assessing the risk for a number of chronic diseases have been controversially discussed. A previously available commercial test for the IL-1 genotype (Genotype PST, Hain LifeScience) is no longer on offer due to conflicting results in various ethnicities.

## Halitosis

The chief complaint of many patients is actually present or assumed bad breath (halitosis). In most cases, halitosis is caused by oral bacteria releasing volatile sulfur compounds, for example, hydrogen sulfide, dimethyl sulfide, and methanethiol (methyl mercaptan).

As most probable sources, the following ecological niches should be considered:
➤ Periodontal pockets
➤ Open dental carious lesions
➤ Defective restoration margins
➤ In particular, the dorsum of the tongue, and tonsils.

Organoleptic (olfactory) assessment of expired air may be psychologically problematic and is certainly not very objective. On the other hand, *gas chromatography* is highly reproducible and an appropriate portable device is available for dentists (OralChroma, FIS, Kitazono, Japan).

## ■ Diagnosis

### General Diagnosis

The overall diagnosis relates to the following:
➤ The *form* of periodontitis (aggressive, chronic)
➤ Its *severity* (mild, moderate or severe)
➤ The *extent* of the disease (localized, generalized)
➤ Any modifying *systemic diseases* (e.g., generalized moderate chronic periodontitis, modified by type II diabetes mellitus, nonsmoker)

➤ If present, any mucocutaneous diseases (see Chapter 4).

### Tooth-Related Diagnosis

In addition, a diagnosis is made for *each tooth* (see **Fig. 6.8**):
➤ *Plaque-induced gingivitis:*
  – Periodontal probing depths of 3 mm or less.
  – Bleeding upon probing.
  – As a rule, no attachment loss has occurred. Note that gingivitis can also be present in case of recession or after proper periodontal treatment with no indication of progressive disease (see Chapter 4).
➤ *Periodontitis.* Severity may be classified by attachment loss: slight (1–2 mm), moderate (3–4 mm), and severe (≥ 5 mm).
  – Mild periodontitis:
    • Periodontal probing depth of about 4 mm and initial attachment loss, bleeding upon probing.
    • Loss of lamina dura of the alveolar bone (see Chapter 1), initial bone loss.
  – Moderate periodontitis:
    • Periodontal probing depth of about 5 mm and attachment loss up to 4 mm, bleeding upon probing.
    • Bone loss up to one-third of root length. Mild furcation involvement (degree I) may be present.
  – Severe periodontitis:
    • Periodontal probing depth of 6 mm or more and attachment loss ≥ 5 mm, bleeding upon probing.
    • Bone loss of more than one-third of root length, and/or advanced furcation involvement (degree II or III).
➤ *Recession* is present if the attachment loss is greater than the periodontal probing depth.
➤ If present, periodontal abscess, combined periodontal–endodontic lesion, etc.

### Prognosis

The individual diagnosis for each tooth is recorded together with its prognosis in the periodontal chart (**Fig. 6.8**). A preliminary statement should be made about:
➤ Which tooth can definitely be kept?

➤ Which tooth has a guarded prognosis but great strategic importance?
➤ Which tooth is hopelessly diseased and should be extracted?

## ■ Treatment Planning

Comprehensive treatment of periodontally diseased patients is conducted during well-defined phases (**Fig. 6.32**):
➤ Systemic diseases are registered and carefully considered.
➤ Emergency treatment and pain relief are provided.
➤ Phase I: Cause-related therapy, anti-infectious measures.
➤ Phase II: Corrective measures to regenerate lost tissue, restorative measures, etc.
➤ Phase III: Supportive care; risk assessment and risk management.

### Case Presentation

After medical and dental history, detailed examination and diagnosis, the treatment plan is developed and discussed with the patient:
➤ The patient is informed about all recorded findings.
➤ The dentist asks about the patient's main reason(s) for consultation.
➤ The patient's treatment-needs in regard to esthetics and chewing comfort as well as preferences and values are assessed.
➤ An optimum treatment proposal is developed based on medical evidence and the patient's preferences.

In addition, at least one medically acceptable minimum solution should be discussed:
➤ After briefing the patient about the pros and cons in relation to the time and resources at his/her disposal, it is the patient who ultimately decides which therapy is to be embarked upon.

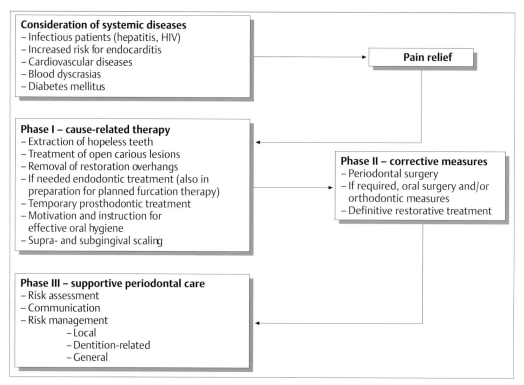

**Consideration of systemic diseases**
– Infectious patients (hepatitis, HIV)
– Increased risk for endocarditis
– Cardiovascular diseases
– Blood dyscrasias
– Diabetes mellitus

**Pain relief**

**Phase I – cause-related therapy**
– Extraction of hopeless teeth
– Treatment of open carious lesions
– Removal of restoration overhangs
– If needed endodontic treatment (also in preparation for planned furcation therapy)
– Temporary prosthodontic treatment
– Motivation and instruction for effective oral hygiene
– Supra- and subgingival scaling

**Phase II – corrective measures**
– Periodontal surgery
– If required, oral surgery and/or orthodontic measures
– Definitive restorative treatment

**Phase III – supportive periodontal care**
– Risk assessment
– Communication
– Risk management
    – Local
    – Dentition-related
    – General

**Fig. 6.32   Phases of comprehensive therapy of a patient with complex periodontal disease.**

**Table 6.3** Time schedule for comprehensive dental treatment of a patient with periodontal disease.[*]

| Treatment phase | Measures | Time schedule |
|---|---|---|
| **Phase I** | Detailed history, clinical examination, preliminary treatment plan | 1st session |
| | Preventive measures<br>• Oral hygiene assessment<br>• If needed, extraction of hopeless teeth<br>• If needed, provisional restorations for open carious lesions; removal of overhangs interfering with oral hygiene<br>• Instructions for improving oral hygiene<br>• Scaling/root planing | 2nd session |
| | • Oral hygiene assessment<br>• Scaling/root planing, polishing<br>• If needed, temporary prothesis<br>• Small definitive restorations | 3rd up to (if needed) 5th session |
| | Caries risk assessment<br>Periodontal reevaluation<br>Definitive treatment plan | • After 2 weeks (in cases of gingivitis/mild periodontitis)<br>• After 4–6 weeks (in cases of moderate/advanced periodontitis) |
| **Phase IIa** | If needed, periodontal surgery, oral surgery including inserting implants | |
| | Periodontal re-evaluation | After 6–8 weeks |
| **Phase IIb** | If needed, fixed and removable partial prostheses<br>If needed, orthodontic treatment, etc. | |
| **Phase III** | Supportive care | Depending on complexity of restorative supply and periodontal risk assessment |

[*] Phase I: cause-related therapy (see Chapter 10). Phase II: corrective measures. Phase IIa: surgical treatment of bony and furcation lesions, recession; IIb: restoration of function and esthetics (see Chapter 11). Phase III: supportive care (see Chapter 12).

➤ *Note*: Continuous monitoring of advanced periodontal or carious lesions should be avoided during comprehensive therapy.

Finally, a definitive schedule of the different treatment phases (**Table 6.3**) and emerging costs is provided. Written informed consent is obtained.

# 7 Prevention of Periodontal Diseases

## ■ Prevention-Oriented Dentistry

For many diseases, a primary objective is *prevention*. For dental caries and periodontal diseases, prevention is possible for the following reasons:

➤ Both are *infectious diseases*. Suppression and control of the oral pathogens responsible for the disease processes appears possible to a large extent.
➤ *Health awareness* among the general public is increasing.
➤ *Oral hygiene measures* are well established.
➤ As regards dental caries, *fluoridation* in one form or another is widely available to most parts of the population.

Preventive measures are traditionally divided into primary, secondary, and tertiary (**Fig. 7.1**). To prevent dental caries and periodontal disease, the following should be considered:

➤ *Primary prevention* usually consists of:
  – Improving individual oral hygiene
  – Appropriate diet which should not harm dental health
  – Local fluoridation
  – Regular check-ups
➤ *Secondary prevention*:
  – Early assessment and treatment of any diseases in the oral cavity
  – Professional tooth cleaning
➤ *Tertiary prevention:*
  – Systematic therapy
  – Prevention of complications

## Karlstad Study

The paramount importance of a consistently carried out preventive program for the establishment of oral health was ultimately suggested in the Karlstad study[1]:

➤ *Test group*: 375 adult patients were enrolled and received the following:
  – Oral hygiene training, professional tooth-cleaning and conventional dental caries therapy.
  – During the first 2 years patients were recalled every 2nd month, thereafter every 3rd month. Oral hygiene was reinforced and topical fluoride applied.
➤ *Control group*: 180 patients who were offered standard dental care:
  – Oral hygiene training, professional tooth-cleaning and conventional dental caries therapy.

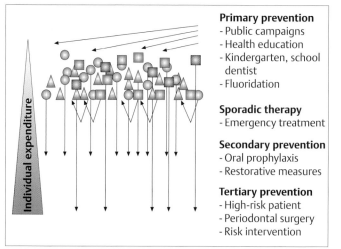

**Primary prevention**
- Public campaigns
- Health education
- Kindergarten, school dentist
- Fluoridation

**Sporadic therapy**
- Emergency treatment

**Secondary prevention**
- Oral prophylaxis
- Restorative measures

**Tertiary prevention**
- High-risk patient
- Periodontal surgery
- Risk intervention

Individual expenditure

**Fig. 7.1 Primary, secondary and tertiary prevention as related to risk groups.** Note that red boxes represent high-risk patients with need for tertiary prevention.

– Thereafter, patients were referred back to their original dentist with check-ups once a year.

➤ The controlled arm of the study had to be terminated after 6 years due to serious ethical concerns:
   – On average, a further 12 to 15 tooth surfaces decayed in patients of the control group as compared to only 0 to 1 surface in patients of the test group.
   – Additional periodontal attachment loss in the control group amounted to 0.7 to 1.5 mm on average. On the other hand, subjects in the test group even showed some clinical attachment gain (**Fig. 7.2**).
   – Based on these findings, control patients were offered the same care as the test group of patients.

An individual schedule for maintenance visits was established after 6 years: 95 % of the study participants then needed only 1 to 2 prophylaxis sessions per year. The study went on for decades, and in 257 patients, who could be reexamined after 30 years, altogether only 173 teeth had been lost.[2]

➤ Most teeth (62 %) were lost due to root fracture.

➤ 7 % teeth were lost due to dental caries, and 5 % due to periodontal problems.

➤ It was suggested that the main reason for generally stable conditions was a permanently low average proportion of 20 % or less of tooth surfaces covered with dental plaque.

The long propagated messages of the Karlstad study were:

➤ The two most important diseases of the oral cavity, dental caries and periodontal disease, can be totally prevented.

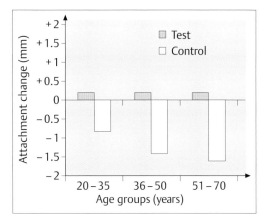

**Fig. 7.2   Karlstad study. During the first 6 years, attachment losses occurred only in the control group (yearly visits to the dentist).** (Adapted from Axelsson et al.[1])

➤ However, at the population level, this can only be achieved by an enormous and probably disproportionate effort.

**Critical assessment.** The Karlstad study does not meet the contemporary stringent standards of a double-blind, randomized clinical trial:

➤ During the first 6 years, treatment goals in the test group did differ significantly from those in the control group.

➤ After 6 years, participants were followed up in a longitudinal cohort study.

➤ Far-reaching conclusions as regards sound evidence for the possibility of complete prevention of both dental caries and periodontitis by appropriate measures may therefore not be justified. Quality of evidence (**Box 7.1**): moderate.

**Box 7.1   Is there any evidence?**

Apparently, periodontists are in the comfortable situation that they may base their everyday decisions on a large and further emerging body of evidence from randomized controlled trials, numerous systematic reviews and meta-analyses which are on top of the evidence pyramid. There may be serious quality issues with the available evidence, though. This concerns basically the study design and execution, inconsistency of study results, indirectness, imprecision of estimates, and possible reporting bias. Low-grade evidence from observational studies, on the other hand, may be upgraded due to strong association, a dose–response gradient, and proper confounder adjustment. There is obviously a need for grading the evidence. In accordance with, for example, the Cochrane Collaboration, the quality of evidence is assigned based on Grading of Recommendations Assessment, Development and Evaluation, or GRADE[3]:

**High quality**—Further research is very unlikely to change our confidence in the estimate of effect.

**Moderate quality**—Further research is likely to have an important impact on our confidence in the estimate of effect and may change the estimate.

**Low quality**—Further research is very likely to have an important impact on our confidence in the estimate of effect and is likely to change the estimate.

**Very low quality**—Any estimate of effect is very uncertain.

Recommendations, either strong or weak, in favor of or against certain therapeutic measures, may be given based on quality of evidence, but also on uncertainty about the balance between desired and undesired effects, uncertainty or variability in patient's values and preferences, or uncertainty about whether the intervention represents a wise use of resources. Note that both lowering and moving up quality of evidence as well as recommendations are certainly a matter of judgment.

Patient-oriented evidence outcomes are usually morbidity, mortality, symptom improvement, cost reduction, and quality of life. Preventing tooth loss and improving esthetics are major patient-oriented outcomes in clinical oral research.[4] Others may be side-effects, treatment costs and the time to complete treatment. Disease-oriented evidence measures are immediate, physiologic, or surrogate end points that may or may not reflect improvements in patient outcomes (e.g., blood pressure, blood chemistry, physiologic function, pathologic findings). As regards periodontal disease, measures of periodontal probing parameters, host response characteristics and microbiological findings are typically considered surrogate outcomes.[4]

Real evidence-based medicine does include a strong interpersonal relationship between the patient with chronic disease and the therapist. Thus, continuity of care and emphatic listening is of paramount importance for conjoint decision-making which does not entirely rely on the available scientific evidence but, to a large extent, also on individual circumstances.

## Possibilities of Prevention

For the past three decades our general view of periodontitis in the population at large has been thoroughly revised:

➤ Susceptibility to the disease seems to differ considerably among individuals. Not every case of gingivitis inevitably develops into destructive periodontitis.

➤ Although the prevalence of generalized severe chronic periodontitis and aggressive forms of the disease is rather low, it is not

expected that it will further decrease in coming years.

➤ Whether the risk group of periodontally susceptible individuals will benefit from further improvement of oral health in general is doubtful.

➤ In particular in aging Western populations, many people will keep their full dentitions despite having moderate and even severe forms of periodontitis.

This reassessment has important consequences for dental public health:

➤ Prevention of early stages of gingivitis at the population level may be an unrealistic aim and most probably not necessary.

➤ Although the dogma of a causal chain, viz. plaque→gingivitis→periodontitis, can still be found in many contemporary textbooks, the concept of pre-eminent importance of dental plaque for pathological conditions in the oral cavity has been questioned.

➤ In many countries, the decline of smoking prevalence and smoking being banned in public places nicely relates with an observed decline of periodontitis prevalence.

➤ While the periodontitis epidemic during the 20th century, which was to a great extent fueled by smoking, may in fact cease in the near future, the socioeconomic polarization of the disease will inevitably dictate new approaches to periodontal care.[5]

Instead of suggesting periodontal surgery for the masses, one of the more important tasks in coming years may be intensive diagnostic, preventive, and therapeutic care for a small group of highly susceptible patients. Periodontal conditions in large parts of the population may be managed without periodontal surgery by taking a more conservative approach to periodontal therapy (secondary prevention). With few exceptions (e.g., emergencies, traumatic injury, handicapped patients), *no definitive treatment* should be provided unless relevant preventive measures have achieved some measurable success:

➤ Detailed information on the etiology of periodontal diseases and how to prevent them (patient motivation) should be provided in any case. Oral hygiene instruction and oral prophylaxis, including restoring the patient's ability to practice proper oral hygiene, can usually be accomplished in about two to three sessions.

➤ A conscious distinction should be made between patients who visit a dentist only sporadically when they have an acute complaint and the relatively small group of patients who desire systematic therapy, that is, comprehensive care.

➤ In most patients, professional tooth-cleaning needs to be repeated only at relatively long intervals, say, every 6 or 12 months.

*Note*: It has been shown that continuous non-surgical periodontal therapy may reduce the rate of tooth loss by more than 50 %.[6]

Prevention of certain, in particular acute, infectious diseases with well-known causal agents is usually accomplished by vaccination, avoiding contact, improving overall hygienic standards, and/or protection from food contamination. Exposure avoidance and risk factor modification are theoretically also applicable in complex chronic diseases such as diabetes mellitus, cardiovascular diseases, and cancer. On the other hand, best protection is still provided by regular follow-up examinations and early diagnosis, despite rather moderate achievements. Without any doubt, periodontitis does belong to these complex chronic diseases.

Apart from poor oral hygiene, future strategies for prevention must take further important risk factors into account (see Chapter 8):

➤ Tobacco consumption
➤ Diabetes mellitus
➤ Socioeconomic factors

By considering the *relative risk* (*RR*, the ratio of disease incidence among exposed individuals divided by the ratio of disease incidence among nonexposed) and the *prevalence* of a particular risk factor (*Prev$_{RF}$*), the *attributable risk* (*AR*) may be calculated as $AR = Prev_{RF}(RR-1) / [(1+Prev_{RF}(RR-1)]$:

➤ The attributable risk relates to that particular portion of diseased individuals which can directly be attributed to the risk factor. In other words, if it would be possible to eliminate the risk factor, incidence of the disease would decrease by the proportion given by the attributable risk.

➤ Thus, in view of still-high prevalence of smoking in Western populations and strong association between smoking and periodontal disease it can reasonably be assumed that periodontitis may be more effectively prevented by smoking cessation[7,8] than by oral hygiene improvement alone (**Table 7.1**).

➤ It is noteworthy that in many countries in which smoking has been banned in public, the decline of smoking in the population seems to correlate with decreased prevalence of, in particular, moderate periodontitis.

**Table 7.1** Poor oral hygiene as a risk factor for periodontitis in relation to other risk factors

| Risk factor | Preventable? | Relative risk | Prevalence (%) | Attributable risk (%) |
|---|---|---|---|---|
| Poor oral hygiene | yes | 1.9[a] | 25[a] | 18 |
| Smoking | yes | 2.5–6[b] | 18[d] | 21–47 |
| Diabetes mellitus | no (controllable) | 2.8–3.4[c] | 8[e] | 13–16 |

[a] Haffajee et al.[9]
[b] American Academy of Periodontology.[10]
[c] American Academy of Periodontology.[11]
[d] World Health Organization,[12] United States.
[e] Centers for Disease Control and Prevention,[13] United States.

## Measures at the Population Level

*Strategies that affect the whole population* (**Fig. 7.1** and **Box 7.2**). At the population level, even small improvements in oral hygiene can have a dramatic impact on periodontal health in general. To achieve success at this level, more information about factors that interfere with improvement of oral hygiene is needed. Educational measures and public campaigns for oral health improvement should be implemented within the context of *established general health education*[16]:

➤ This education should be based on individual need rather than an objective deficiency.
➤ Basic information about plaque, mechanisms of prevention, the possibility of treatment, the efficacy of commercial products, etc.
➤ Facilitate rather than prescribe.
➤ Less professional intervention, more self-support.
➤ Make healthier alternatives easier to accomplish.

Health education has to be implemented at various levels. Kindergarten nurses, teachers, pediatricians, and the whole dental team should promote oral hygiene within the framework of general education programs:

➤ General cleanliness and body care
➤ Disease prevention
➤ Improving self-esteem

All health care workers participating in these programs should receive training in the professional teaching of effective oral hygiene. Oral hygiene measures should be possible in schools and in the workplace, and are regarded as a matter of course:

➤ Sanitary installations should be accessible to all.
➤ Supply proper and low cost oral hygiene aids.
➤ Differing age groups and levels of education should be taken into account.

---

**Box 7.2    Preventive impact of individual oral hygiene and oral health promotion on gingival health and incidence or progression of periodontitis**

A systematic search for randomized controlled studies on the importance of individual oral hygiene measures for prevention of incidence or progression of chronic periodontitis[14] revealed only three studies. Although no single study provided evidence for a statistically significant advantage of certain individual oral hygiene measures for the prevention of chronic periodontitis after 3 to 4 years, it is, according to the authors, unclear whether new randomized studies should be initiated, since the whole concept of a pivotal role of insufficient oral hygiene (the nonspecific plaque hypothesis) has been questioned in recent epidemiological studies. Quality of evidence: low

A systematic search for current data on the effect of oral health promotion revealed 5 systematic reviews and another 13 randomized controlled studies in which the impact of oral health promotion on gingival health could be assessed.[15] Most studies aimed at interventions in schools and at the workplace. Up to 6 months after intervention, considerable reduction of dental plaque was reported. Long-term and sustainable effects were, according to the authors, unlikely. Quality of evidence: low

## Secondary and Tertiary Prevention

Secondary and tertiary prevention has to be implemented in the context of *comprehensive dental care*. Secondary preventive measures are indicated whenever comprehensive treatment of all pathologic conditions in the oral cavity and oral rehabilitation are planned. For most patients with periodontal diseases, simple measures are sufficient for long-term maintenance of the dentition:
- ➤ Training for effective oral hygiene measures
- ➤ Regular supra- and subgingival scaling
- ➤ Periodontal surgery, which is indicated in only a few cases and situations

A central aspect of treatment planning is to consider the *strategic importance* of individual teeth:
- ➤ Extraction of any periodontally diseased tooth from an intact dental arch is a matter of great responsibility. Considerable costs and risks may be associated with prosthetic rehabilitation.
- ➤ Greater therapeutic efforts should be made in case of strategically important teeth. An early referral to a periodontal specialist is desirable.
- ➤ On the other hand, early extraction of diseased, strategically irrelevant teeth may be indicated in order to prevent costly and risky prosthetic constructions (e. g., periodontally diseased wisdom teeth and second molars).

## Preferential Treatment of High-Risk Groups

Patients in high-risk groups should be identified and given priority. Note that a fairly small group of patients (not more than 15% of the population) is responsible for virtually all tooth loss due to periodontitis:
- ➤ General risk factors such as smoking, diabetes mellitus, genetic factors etc. are now well established.
- ➤ Presence of a number of periodontal pathogens such as *A. actinomycetemcomitans*, *P. gingivalis* and *T. forsythia* seems to increase the risk of active periodontitis in certain individuals.

As a matter of fact, high-risk patients may incur considerable diagnostic and therapeutic costs:
- ➤ Microbiological and, in some cases, genetic tests
- ➤ Periodontal surgery, including regenerative measures
- ➤ Adjunctive antibiotic therapy
- ➤ Expensive epithetic and/or prosthetic constructions, including oral implants

*Note*: Patients with periodontal disease who are in a high-risk group should preferably be treated by periodontal specialists.

# 8 General Medical Considerations

## ■ Systemic Phase

Before comprehensive therapy commences, all medical and dental history information is checked for clinical relevance (see Chapter 6). Any *systemic diseases* must be taken into account for proper treatment planning. The dental team should be protected from infections (infectious hepatitis due to HBV, HCV, infection with HIV, etc.). In patients known to be at increased risk as regards possible treatment restrictions, allergy or drug interactions have to be considered in order to achieve an optimum therapeutic result.

### Infectious Patients

Relevant clues in the medical history should be followed up. In high-risk groups, specific antibody titers should be assessed.

For example, HIV-seropositive patients often suffer from opportunistic infections of the oral cavity.[1] Necrotizing ulcerative periodontal diseases and opportunistic virus infections, such as acute HSV1 or HSV2 infection, hairy leukoplakia (an Epstein–Barr virus infection) or papilloma virus infection, do occur more frequently in HIV seropositive patients than in the general population. Further suspicious findings may be treatment-resistant linear erythema of the gingiva (due to candidosis) and neoplasms such as Kaposi's sarcoma. In any of these cases, an HIV test should be arranged.

*Note*: Because even careful history-taking does not always reveal a patient's infectious status, standard precautions for avoiding cross-infection must be adopted with all patients.

### Increased Risk of Infective Endocarditis

Infective endocarditis is a life-threatening disease. It is an infection of hemodynamically exposed endocardial structures, especially native or prosthetic cardiac valves. It may occur after transient bacteremia. In a patient at highest risk of endocarditis (**Table 8.1**), appropriate antibiotic prophylaxis[2] is required.

*Note*: Since periodontal probing inevitably leads to bacteremia, in cases at highest risk for infective endocarditis antibiotic prophylaxis should be initiated before thorough periodontal examination.

Depending on bacterial virulence and the patient's resistance, various forms of endocarditis may be differentiated according to the course of the disease:
- ➤ *Acute infective* endocarditis:
  - Septic disease, high fever
  - Rapid destruction of the endocardium, fatal within less than six weeks
  - Causative are *Staphylococcus aureus, Streptococcus pneumoniae, Streptococcus pyogenes*
- ➤ Intermediate *acute–subacute* forms are more frequently caused by enterococci.

**Table 8.1** Cardiac conditions associated with the highest risk of adverse outcome from infective endocarditis for which antibiotic prophylaxis with dental procedures is reasonable[2]

| Cardiac conditions |
| --- |
| • Prosthetic cardiac valve or prosthetic material used for cardiac repair |
| • Previous infective endocarditis |
| • Congenital heart disease (CHD)<br>– Unrepaired cyanotic CHD, including palliative shunts and conduits<br>– Completely repaired congenital heart defect with prosthetic material or device, whether placed by surgery or by catheter intervention, during the first 6 months after the procedure<br>– Repaired CHD with residual defects at the site or adjacent to the site of a prosthetic patch or prosthetic device (which inhibits endothelialization) |
| • Cardiac transplantation recipients who develop cardiac valvulopathy |

➤ *Subacute* forms:
  – Slight fever, night sweat, loss of weight
  – If left untreated, fatal within six weeks to three months
➤ *Chronic infective* endocarditis:
  – Symptoms similar to the subacute form
  – If left untreated, fatal after more than three months
➤ *Note*: Subacute and chronic cases of endocarditis are usually caused by oral viridans streptococci.

In persons with *congenital* and *acquired heart anomalies* the risk of infective endocarditis is considerably increased. It is highest in patients with *prosthetic cardiac valves* and those who have a *previous history of endocarditis*.
➤ Predisposing conditions are abnormal blood flow with eddy formation and congenital or rheumatic valve disease.
➤ Blood starts to clot on surface alterations of the valves and forms fibrous and thrombotic vegetations (nonbacterial thrombotic endocarditis).
➤ These appositional thrombi are subsequently colonized by bacteria during transient bacteremia.

Lesions in areas of high turbulence are particularly prone to bacterial colonization:
➤ Atrial surface of the mitral valve
➤ Ventricular surface of the aortic valve

Bacteria have different affinities to the thrombus, which is primarily free from any bacteria:
➤ Viridans streptococci, enterococci, *Staphylococcus aureus*, *S. epidermidis*, and *Pseudomonas aeruginosa* adhere better than *Escherichia coli*, *Klebsiella pneumoniae*, and *Aggregatibacter actinomycetemcomitans*.
➤ Adhesion of oral streptococci *Streptococcus mutans*, *S. bovis*, *S. mitis*, and *S. sanguinis* depends on production of the extracellular polysaccharide dextran.

In addition to *A. actinomycetemcomitans*, further gram-negative bacteria of the oral cavity and upper respiratory tract may cause infective endocarditis: *Haemophilus* spp., *Cardiobacterium* spp., *Eikenella corrodens*, *Kingella* spp. (so-called HACEK group), *Capnocytophaga* spp., and *Neisseria* spp.
  *Note:* All dental procedures that involve manipulation of gingival tissue or the periapical region of teeth or perforation of the oral mucosa require antibiotic prophylaxis in patients at highest risk for infective endocarditis. Bacteremia must be expected during all dental measures that result in bleeding of the tissues, for example:
➤ Tooth extraction, surgical tooth removal, placing implants
➤ Apicoectomy
➤ Suture removal
➤ Calculus removal
➤ Periodontal probing, in particular of highly inflamed gingival tissues

According to the current recommendations of the American Heart Association,[2] antibiotic prophylaxis is not needed for the following procedures and events:
➤ Routine anesthetic injections through non-infected tissue
➤ Taking dental radiographs
➤ Placement of removable dental prostheses or orthodontic appliances
➤ Adjustment of orthodontic appliances
➤ Placement of orthodontic brackets
➤ Shedding of deciduous teeth
➤ Bleeding from trauma to the lips or oral mucosa

Current recommendations of the AHA for antibiotic prophylaxis of infective endocarditis for dental procedures[2] suggest a simplified regime (**Table 8.2**). In addition to antibiotic prophylaxis, preoperative rinsing with 0.2% chlorhexidine digluconate mouthwash or application of 1% chlorhexidine gel (see Chapter 10) on dried mucosa may largely reduce bacterial load. Furthermore, during periodontal treatment the patient is advised to use 1% chlorhexidine gel for toothbrushing rather than toothpaste.
  *Note*: Treatment appointments should be carefully planned so that as few antibiotic prescriptions as possible are necessary. A period of 10 to 14 days should be kept between subsequent appointments to allow recovery of the resident flora.
  Spontaneous bacteremia in patients with severe gingival inflammation and poor oral hygiene is an additional risk for infective endocarditis. Healthy periodontal conditions are therefore regarded an important aspect of endocarditis prophylaxis.

**Table 8.2** Antibiotic prophylaxis of infective endocarditis: regimens for dental procedures[2]

| Situation | Agent | Regimen: single dose 30–60 min before the procedure | |
| --- | --- | --- | --- |
| | | **Adults** | **Children** |
| Oral | Amoxicillin | 2 g | 50 mg/kg |
| Patient is unable to take oral medication | Ampicillin *or* | 2 g intramuscular (IM) or intravenous (IV) | 50 mg/kg IM or IV |
| | Cefazolin *or* Ceftriaxone | 1 g IM or IV | 50 mg/kg IM or IV |
| Patient is allergic to penicillins or ampicillin—oral | Cephalexin*† *or* | 2 g | 50 mg/kg |
| | Clindamycin *or* | 600 mg | 20 mg/kg |
| | Azithromycin *or* Clarithromycin | 500 mg | 15 mg/kg |
| Patient is allergic to penicillins or ampicillin and unable to take oral medication | Cefazolin *or* Ceftriaxone † *or* | 1 g IM or IV | 50 mg/kg IM or IV |
| | Clindamycin | 600 mg IM or IV | 20 mg/kg IM or IV |

\* Or other first- or second-generation oral cephalosporin in equivalent adult or pediatric dosage.
† Cephalosporins should not be used in individuals with a history of anaphylaxis, angioedema, or urticaria with penicillins or ampicillin.

### Further Indications for Antibiotic Prophylaxis

Antibiotic prophylaxis may be indicated in any patient with impaired host defense, any surgery with a high rate of associated infectious complication, and any surgery for which the associated infectious complications are rare (low rate) but serious.[3]

➤ Patients with *organ transplants.* Immunosuppressive medication with, for example, cyclosporin, tacrolimus, sirolimus, and/or glucocorticosteroids for suppression of T cell functions:
  – The patient's physician should be consulted. For example, for any procedures in which bacteremia are expected (see above), long-term prophylaxis with 1,500 mg/day amoxicillin for 3 days (1 day before and 2 days after the procedure) should be arranged. Patients with penicillin allergy should take 200 mg doxycycline the day before the intervention, thereafter 100 mg/day. Alternatively, erythromycin (1,000 mg/day) may be prescribed.
  – *Note:* During, in particular, immune-suppressive therapy with cyclosporin or tacrolimus, respectively 60% and 30% of patients may develop gingival enlargement,

which in some cases needs to be treated by gingivectomy (see Chapter 11).
➤ *Radiation of the head and neck.* Vascular damage with hypovascularity, degeneration of bone marrow, and more or less complete destruction of osteoblasts and osteoclasts lead to increased risk for osteoradionecrosis.
  – Following any oral surgery, including tooth extraction, primary wound closure is required. Antibiotic prophylaxis should be arranged with 1,500 mg/day amoxicillin or 600 mg/day clindamycin on the day of the procedure and up to two days thereafter.
  – Larger operations should be done in hospital.
  – As far as possible, any periodontal treatment should be carried out before radiation. *Caution:* Osteoradionecrosis has been observed also after spontaneous exacerbation of chronic periodontitis.
➤ *Antibiotic prophylaxis according to physician's instructions:*
  – Patients on dialysis; patients with blood dyscrasias, neutropenia, or impaired function of polymorphonuclear granulocytes. Patients with rheumatic disorders usually have to take corticosteroids. In any of

these cases, the patient's physician should be consulted about antibiotic prophylaxis.

– The American Academy of Orthopedic Surgeons (AAOS) and the American Dental Association (ADA) recently pointed to the fact that evidence for antibiotic prophylaxis to prevent orthopedic implant infection in patients undergoing dental procedures is largely lacking.[4] Given the potential adverse outcomes and cost of treating an infected joint replacement, dentists may consider antibiotic prophylaxis for all patients with joint implants prior to any procedure that may cause bacteremia —for example, prescription of 2 g cephalexin 1 hour before the procedure and 1 g after 4 hours (erythromycin or clindamycin in patients who are allergic to β-lactam antibiotics).

## Bleeding Disorders, Anticoagulant Therapy

Periodontal treatment of patients with vascular and platelet disorders, *congenital hemophilia* or, more frequently, those under *anticoagulant medication* (e. g., coumarin derivatives or heparin after myocardial infarction, stroke, or for thrombosis prophylaxis) can only be carried out after consultation with the patient's physician:

➤ Life-threatening bleeding may occur after any oral surgical procedure, for example, tooth extraction, flap surgery, gingivectomy, and even calculus removal.

➤ In a patient with an International Normalized Ratio (INR, which is based on the patient's prothrombin time) of 3.0 to 3.4, only minor oral surgical procedures can be carried out without any problems.

➤ If the INR is ≥ 3.5, only minor emergency surgery is possible.

➤ Comprehensive treatment should ideally be carried out during few appointments scheduled closely together.

*Pharmacological interactions with anticoagulant drugs* have to be considered as well. For example, an anticoagulant effect is enhanced by salicylates and nonsteroidal anti-inflammatory drugs, corticosteroids, or certain antibiotics. It is reduced by barbiturates, resulting in an increased risk of thrombosis.

*Note*: Hemophilic patients have a considerably increased risk of hepatitis and HIV infections.

## Atherosclerosis, Cardiovascular Diseases

Oral surgery represents an increased risk of adverse effects in patients with a history of *myocardial infarction, angina pectoris, heart insufficiency, stroke*, or *peripheral vascular disease*.

➤ In any case, the patient's physician should be consulted and all prescribed medications carefully checked.

➤ In particular after myocardial infarction, any dental treatment, except emergency treatment, should be postponed for 6 months.

➤ Diazepam premedication may be given if required. Nitroglyceride should be at hand.

➤ Only short sessions should be planned.

➤ There is no general contraindication regarding local anesthetics with an adrenaline content of up to 10 µg/mL (1:100,000).

➤ *Note:* In patients with a pacemaker implant, use of ultrasonic and electrosurgical devices and electric pulp vitality testing are contraindicated.

➤ Antihypertensive medication should be maintained during dental therapy. Calcium antagonists (nifedipine, diltiazem, verapamil, etc.), which are frequently prescribed in cases of coronary artery disease, lead in about 20 % of cases to gingival enlargement. In some cases surgical correction is required (see Chapter 11).

➤ *Note*: Patients who have had a myocardial infarction or stroke are frequently under anticoagulant therapy (see above).

## Associations between Periodontitis and Cardiovascular Diseases

At the outset of new interest in an interrelationship between periodontitis and systemic disease, early reports on associations between cardiovascular diseases and certain chronic infections with, for example, *Chlamydia pneumonia, Helicobacter pylori* or Cytomegalovirus has been extended to dental infections,[5] especially chronic periodontitis.

➤ In prospective cohort studies weak associations between the incidence of cardiovascular events (myocardial infarction, death due to myocardial infarction, coronary revascularization) were observed (**Box 8.1**).

➤ While DNA of periodontal pathogens *A. actinomycetemcomitans, Porphyromonas gingivalis, Prevotella intermedia*, and *Tannerella forsythia* have consistently been detected in atheromatous plaques, it is unclear whether frequent bacteremia is actually causal in atherogenesis.

Chronic infections at large seem to increase the risk for atheroma development and thromboembolic events:

➤ Increased serum concentrations > 3 mg/L of C-reactive protein (CRP), which is a potent marker of systemic inflammation, has been shown to be a risk factor for cardiovascular disease.[13]

➤ In that regard it may be noteworthy that in periodontitis patients, CRP levels are commonly increased.[14]

It has been speculated that atherosclerosis and periodontitis are both linked to a *hyperresponsive monocyte/macrophage phenotype* (**Fig. 8.1**; see Chapter 3) with excessive release of proinflammatory cytokines and mediators (IL-1β, TNF-α, PGE2) after contact of macrophages with LPS of gram-negative bacteria.[15] This hyperreactive trait may largely be genetically de-

termined but might be modified by environmental and behavioral factors such as:

➤ High-fat diet: Low density lipoproteins (LDL) and triglycerides may lead to an increased secretion of proinflammatory and catabolic cytokines.

➤ Stress, distress, insufficient stress coping strategies.

In several genome-wide studies and a meta-analysis, increased linkage disequilibrium in the chromosomal region 9p21.3 has been weakly associated with coronary artery atherosclerotic disease and a number of other chronic diseases.[16] Linkage disequilibrium in this particular region was also associated with generalized and localized aggressive periodontitis (see Chapter 3).[17]

In intervention studies it has been shown that systematic periodontal treatment with the aim of resolution of gingival inflammation also had systemic effects (**Box 8.1**):

➤ Transient increase of serum concentrations of CRP and IL-6.

➤ Short-term endothelial dysfunction (lower flow-mediated vasodilatation of the brachial artery as measured by the ankle-brachial pressure index).

➤ In the long term, however, endothelial function improved.[18]

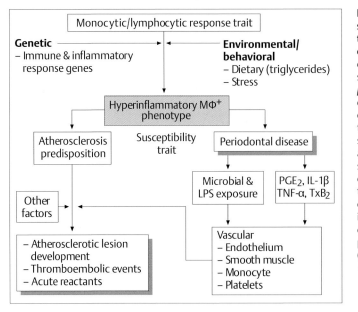

Fig. 8.1 **A proposed model describing the possible link between vascular diseases and chronic periodontitis** was based on the hypothesized existence of a so-called *hyperreactive macrophage phenotype*, which might be genetically controlled and modified by environmental and behavioral factors. In persons with increased susceptibility for development of atherosclerotic vascular lesions, such lesions could develop after excessive release of proinflammatory mediators in the wake of chronic systemic exposure of the individual to bacteria and/or LPS during a chronic infection such as periodontitis. MΦ: macrophage. (Adapted from Beck et al.[15])

**Box 8.1 Does established periodontitis increase the risk for atherosclerotic events and what is the effect of periodontal therapy on clinical atherosclerotic disease parameters and markers related to atherosclerosis and cardiovascular disease risk?**

Based on recent systematic reviews and meta-analyses of prospective cohort studies[6–10] at least weak associations with periodontitis are undeniable. When further established risk factors were considered and proper confounder adjustment was done in longitudinal cohort studies, significant relative risks for coronary heart disease of about 1.14 to 1.34 have been calculated in meta-analyses. Although observational studies do support weak associations between cardio-/cerebrovascular disease and periodontitis, which seem to be independent of known confounders, they do not support a causal relationship.

In order to address the effect of periodontal treatment on clinical cardiovascular disease parameters and/or markers related to atherosclerosis and cardiovascular disease risks, Teeuw et al[11] conducted a systematic review of 25 intervention trials, 7 where otherwise healthy periodontitis patients had been enrolled, and 18 which dealt with patients with co-morbidity: cardiovascular disease, metabolic disorders such as diabetes, or a combination thereof. The effects of periodontal treatment on primary or secondary markers of inflammation and thrombosis, lipid and glucose metabolism were analyzed in a series of meta-analyses. While periodontal treatment may improve endothelial function, alternative measures of vascular function did not change after periodontal therapy. When all studies were considered, significantly more favorable weighted mean differences of the groups receiving periodontal treatment were calculated for high sensitive CRP (−0.50 mg/L, 95% confidence interval [CI] −0.78; −0.22), IL-6 (−0.48 ng/L, 95% CI −0.90; −0.06), TNF-α (−0.75 pg, 95% CI −1.34; −0.17) and fibrinogen (−0.47 g/L, 95% CI −0.76; −0.17); as well as total cholesterol (−0.11 mmol/L, 95% CI −0.21; −0.01) and HDL-cholesterol (0.04 mmol/L, 95% CI 0.03; 0.06). Notably, patients with co-morbidity seemed to benefit more from periodontal treatment. None of the included trials used a primary cardiovascular event (i.e., angina pectoris, myocardial infarction, stroke, or death) as outcome. Moreover, considerable heterogeneity of studies was observed. Quality of evidence: low.

Although periodontal interventions have resulted in short-term reduction of systemic inflammation and endothelial dysfunction, there is no evidence that they can prevent atherosclerotic vascular disease or modify its outcomes. In a recommendation statement on nontraditional risk factors for coronary heart diseases (CRP serum levels, ankle-brachial index, leukocyte count, fasting blood glucose level, periodontal disease, carotid intima-media thickness, coronary artery calcification, etc.) the US Preventive Services Task Force[12] concluded that the current evidence was insufficient to assess the balance of benefits and harms of using respective nontraditional risk factors to screen asymptomatic men and women with no history of coronary heart disease to prevent coronary heart disease events.

## Pulmonary Diseases

Chronic periodontitis may also be related to the development of pulmonary disease.[19]
➤ Colonization of the oral cavity with respiratory pathogens, particularly in patients with poor oral hygiene and periodontitis, may lead to nosocomial pneumonia. Dental intervention aimed at reducing intraoral bacterial load may attenuate the risk for lung infections in susceptible patients. Quality of evidence: low.

➤ An observed weak association between chronic periodontitis and chronic obstructive pulmonary disease (COPD) cannot currently be causally explained.

*Note:* Any disease, which is mostly initiated by or worsens when smoking tobacco, may be associated with chronic periodontitis even in carefully adjusted statistical models:
➤ In an exemplary analysis of NHANES I longitudinal data (see Chapter 5), an observed association between periodontitis and lung cancer[20] was certainly spurious and may be

explained by insufficient adjustment for smoking as confounder which is strongly implicated in both diseases.

➤ The cumulative effect of decade-long smoking on the development and progression of complex chronic diseases has not been properly addressed in older longitudinal studies.

## Diabetes Mellitus

Diabetes mellitus (DM) is a heterogeneous group of diseases. Common characteristics are impaired glucose tolerance and altered lipid and carbohydrate metabolism. Two main forms of DM are differentiated:

➤ *Type 1:* Cell-mediated autoimmune destruction of insulin-producing β-cells of the pancreas. There is a genetic predisposition. The onset may be triggered by virus infection. Typical features are:
  – High susceptibility to ketoacidosis
  – Early onset in children and adolescents
  – Mandatory insulin substitution
  – Patients are underweight or have a normal stature

➤ *Type 2:* Alteration of insulin receptors with increase in insulin resistance of target tissues. Characteristics are:
  – Genetic predisposition
  – Onset usually in adults; increasing incidence in adolescents
  – Usually adequate insulin production
  – Resistance to ketoacidosis
  – Hypertriglyceridemia
  – Patients are frequently obese. They often have a flushed appearance of the face and neck (diabetic rubeosis).
  – Therapeutic control is achieved by (1) diet and weight reduction, (2) diet and orally administered antidiabetic drugs; or (3) a combination of diet, oral antidiabetic drugs, and insulin.

In addition, numerous *further diagnoses* related to diabetes may be made:

➤ Gestational diabetes:
  – May be the primary manifestation of type 1 diabetes mellitus
  – Resembles in most cases type 2 diabetes mellitus, in particular as regards inadequate insulin secretion and resistance
  – Affects about 2 to 5% of pregnant women
  – About 20 to 50% of patients later develop type 2 diabetes mellitus

➤ Genetic defects of β-cell function (e.g., maturity onset diabetes of the young, or MODY)
➤ Genetic defects in proinsulin conversion or insulin action
➤ Exocrine pancreatic defects (e.g., chronic pancreatitis, cystic fibrosis, hemochromatosis)
➤ Endocrinopathia (e.g., acromegaly, Cushing's syndrome, hyperthyroidism)
➤ Pancreas infections (e.g., infections with cytomegalovirus, Coxsackievirus B)
➤ Drug-induced pancreatic disorder

The *Prevalence* of diabetes mellitus in industrialized countries is about 8% but increases to 18 to 20% above the age of 60 years. About one-third of cases are undiagnosed. Type 2 is far more common (85–90%) than type 1.

Classic symptoms typically result from *hyperglycemia*:
➤ Triad of polyuria, polydipsia, and polyphagia
➤ In addition itching, weakness, and fatigue
➤ Increased susceptibility to infections

Hyperglycemia leads to:
➤ Osmotic diuresis
➤ Worsening of tissue oxygen supply and perfusion
➤ Impaired chemotaxis, phagocytosis, and adhesion of neutrophilic granulocytes
➤ Effect on *collagen metabolism*:
  – Synthesis, maturation, and homeostasis of collagen are strongly influenced by glucose concentration in the tissue.
  – Collagenolytic activity in gingival exudate is increased in diabetics.[21]

Further important *pathogenic mechanisms*:
➤ Hyperglycemia leads to reversible glycation of lipids and proteins. Prototype is glycated hemoglobin, $HbA_{1c}$, an important marker of diabetic control.
➤ If hyperglycemia is sustained, irreversible nonenzymatic formation of advanced glycation end products (AGEs) occurs.
  – AGEs alter form and function of numerous extracellular matrix components, including collagen.
  – AGEs react with specific receptors (RAGE) on diabetic target cells: endothelial and

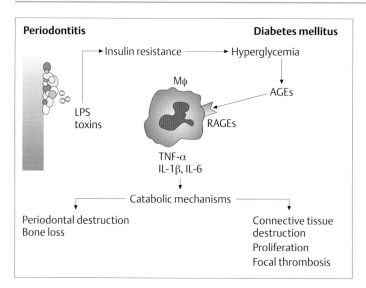

Periodontitis       Diabetes mellitus

Insulin resistance → Hyperglycemia

Mφ

AGEs

LPS
toxins

RAGEs

TNF-α
IL-1β, IL-6
↓
Catabolic mechanisms

Periodontal destruction
Bone loss

Connective tissue
destruction
Proliferation
Focal thrombosis

**Fig. 8.2 Bidirectional relationship between periodontitis and diabetes mellitus.** Chronic infection with gram-negative bacteria in dental plaque leads, in diabetic patients, to increasing insulin resistance of the tissues and increasing hyperglycemia. This may result in an accumulation of irreversibly altered proteins (advanced glycated end products, AGEs), which bind to respective receptors (RAGEs) on macrophages (MΦ) and may induce excessive release of proinflammatory cytokines, giving rise to a more catabolic situation.

mesangial cells, neuronal cells, as well as monocytes and macrophages.

– This may lead to vascular dysfunction (vasoconstriction, focal thrombosis), impaired wound healing, and excessive reactivity of monocytes which release large amounts of proinflammatory mediators and insulin-like growth factor (IGF).

– *Note*: AGE-mediated processes play a central role in the pathogenesis of diabetic complications (**Fig. 8.2**):

• Retinopathy
• Nephropathy and, consequently, renal hypertension
• Neuropathy
• Macroangiopathy (atherosclerosis and, subsequently, cardiovascular, cerebrovascular, and peripheral vascular disease)
• Impaired wound healing
• Periodontal alterations—the "sixth complication" of diabetes mellitus[22]

Glycemic control is therefore prevention of complications.

Diabetes mellitus and *periodontitis*[21]:

➤ Periodontal alterations (**Fig. 8.3**) usually occur in patients with poorly controlled or undiagnosed diabetes mellitus. Some characteristics are:

– Tendency to enlargement/proliferation of the gingiva
– Increased bleeding tendency

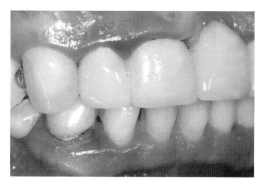

**Fig. 8.3 Periodontal disease in a patient with type 2 diabetes mellitus.** Hemorrhagic, thickened, and proliferative gingiva with a tendency for abscess formation.

– Tendency to periodontal abscess formation
– Increased progression rate of periodontal destruction

➤ Overall, diabetics have three-times higher risk of periodontitis than nondiabetics (see **Table 7.1**). In particular, poorly controlled diabetic individuals have a much higher risk of progressive periodontitis, where the relative risk may be > 10.

➤ There is some evidence that the relationship between diabetes mellitus and periodontitis may be bidirectional.[23] Since all chronic infections impair metabolic control, insulin resistance of the tissues does increase also in patients with periodontitis. Moreover, periodontal treatment may have favorable, albeit limited, effects on metabolic control (**Box 8.2**). Adjunctive systemically administered doxycycline may be considered, which may reduce proteinuria in patients with diabetic nephropathy[29] and inhibits tissue collagenase (see Chapter 13).

If diabetes is suspected, appropriate tests should be arranged (**Table 8.3**). Rapid and cost-effective self-monitoring glucometers may be used in the dental office—to confirm an initial suspicion or to check blood glucose levels in known diabetics, for example. Quality control is mandatory.

---

**Box 8.2   Does periodontal therapy improve glycemic control in patients with diabetes mellitus?**

After a systematic search for randomized clinical trials (RCTs) in which patients with diabetic mellitus and periodontitis either received periodontal therapy or were left untreated for at least 3 months, Engebretson and Kocher[24] did a meta-analysis which basically confirmed the results of previous systematic reviews.[25,26] They identified nine studies in which a significantly more favorable mean treatment effect of −0.36 % HbA1 c (95 % confidence interval −0.54; −0.19) was calculated as compared to groups where periodontal therapy was postponed. The studies in this meta-analysis were basically single-center and small-scale. In a more recent large multicenter RCT by

Engebretson et al,[27] in which more than 500 diabetic patients were enrolled and randomized for receiving or not receiving nonsurgical periodontal therapy, glycemic control was not improved 6 months after periodontal therapy. This study has been criticized for limited clinical improvement of periodontal parameters after nonsurgical periodontal therapy. When the results of this study and another small-scale study[28] were included in a new meta-analysis employing a random effects model, a mean reduction of HbA1 c of −0.26 (95 % CI −0.43, −0.09) was calculated. Significant and substantial heterogeneity among studies was noted (unpublished). Quality of evidence: low.

---

### Obesity, Metabolic Syndrome

In cross-sectional and case–control studies, periodontitis had been associated with obesity.[30]

Metabolic syndrome, which includes obesity, insulin resistance, hypertension, and atherogenic dyslipidemia, is a strong risk factor for diabetes mellitus and cardiovascular events. It is defined by the International Diabetes Federation as:

➤ Visceral (central) obesity (e. g., in Caucasians waist circumference > 94 cm in men and > 80 cm in women; or body mass index > 30 kg/m$^2$) and any two of the following:
  – Raised fasting blood glucose of > 100 mg/dL (5.6 mmol/L), or confirmed type 2 diabetes mellitus
  – Raised triglyceride levels of > 150 mg/dL (1.7 mmol/L)
  – Reduced HDL cholesterol of < 40 mg/L (1.03 mmol/L) in men and < 50 mg/L (1.29 mmol/L) in women
  – Raised blood pressure (> 130 systolic, > 85 diastolic, mmHg) or treatment of previously increased blood pressure

In a systematic review of studies which had addressed the possible relationship between periodontitis and metabolic syndrome, rather strong associations (odds ratio 1.71, 95 % CI 1.42; 2.03) were calculated in meta-analyses of 20 basically cross-sectional and case–control studies.[31] Moreover, based on observations made in a longitudinal study,[32] periodontitis may in fact increase the risk for conversion of one or more components of so-called metabolic syndrome during a 4-year period.

### Pregnancy

During pregnancy, various alterations of the periodontal condition may be observed, which frequently lead patients to consult a dentist:

➤ Usually in the second trimester pregnancy gingivitis develops.

**Table 8.3** Diabetes diagnosis

| Patient with suspected undiagnosed diabetes mellitus | Known diabetic patient |
|---|---|
| • Symptoms of diabetes mellitus: polyuria, polydipsia, polyphagia, unexplained weight loss **and**<br>• Plasma glucose ≥ 200 mg/dL or ≥ 11.1 mmol/L, respectively (not fasting) | Glycated hemoglobin: reflects average blood glucose level of the last four to six weeks:<br>• Normal HbA1: 5.5–8.4 %<br>• Normal HbA1c: 4.4–6.7 %<br>• Well controlled: < 8 % (aim is < 7 %)<br>• Moderately controlled: 8–10 %<br>• Poorly controlled: > 10 %<br>*Note:* % HbA1c may be recalculated in IFCC units (mmol/mol) according to the following formula: HbA1c (mmol/mol) = (HbA1c [%] – 2.15) × 10.929. Normal range is 29–42 mmol/mol |
| Assessment of fasting blood glucose:<br>• Diabetic: ≥ 126 mg/dL (≥ 7 mmol/L)<br>• Increased: ≥ 110 to < 126 mg/dL (≥ 6.1 to < 7 mmol/L)<br>• Normal: 70–110 mg/dL (3.9–6.1 mmol/L) | |
| Assessment of glucose intolerance: Plasma glucose 2 h after intake of an equivalent of 75 g anhydrous glucose dissolved in water<br>• Intolerance: ≥ 200 mg/dL (≥ 11.1 mmol/L)<br>• Impaired tolerance: ≥ 140 to < 200 mg/dL (≥ 7.8 to < 11.1 mmol/L)<br>• Normal glucose tolerance: < 140 mg/dL (< 7.8 mmol/L)<br>*Note:* As a rule, the findings should be confirmed on another day using any of these three methods. | |

➤ Existing periodontitis may worsen. In certain cases, a pyogenic granuloma (**Fig. 8.4**) may develop.
➤ Towards the end of pregnancy tooth mobility is largely increased.

In pregnant women, both dental caries and periodontal infections should be carefully controlled. To avoid emergency situations, open carious lesions should be treated, proper oral hygiene established, and periodontal disease treated. Routine dietary habits should be modified and supportive periodontal care provided.

One important aim may be the reduction of oral pathogens such as *S. mutans*, *A. actinomycetemcomitans*, and *P. gingivalis* in the expectant mother. This so-called primary primary prevention (see Chapter 7) may in fact attenuate the likelihood of early transmission of oral pathogens to the child. Development of dental caries and inflammatory periodontal diseases may be delayed or prevented.

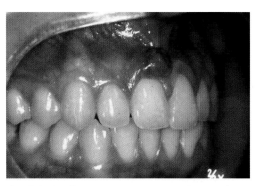

**Fig. 8.4  During pregnancy a pyogenic granuloma may develop as a response to local irritation.**

*Note*: There are no objections to an intraoral adjunctive use of chlorhexidine-containing mouthwash and gels during pregnancy.

Severe periodontal disease of the expectant mother seems to increase the risk for preterm labor and *low birth weight* (below 2,500 g):

➤ Consistent observations have been made in various populations and after adjustment for established risk factors[33] of low birth weight such as previous preterm delivery, young and older age, intrauterine infection and ethnicity.[34]

➤ *Note:* In several large intervention studies the risk for low birth weight was not reduced after periodontal treatment (**Box 8.3**).

---

**Box 8.3    Can periodontal therapy reduce the risk for preterm birth and low birth weight?**

Several recent systematic reviews have addressed the question of the effect of periodontal therapy on pregnancy outcome.[35–38] Chambrone et al[37] included 11 randomized controlled studies in a meta-analyses in which a total of 7,107 pregnant women had been screened or enrolled. All except those in one study presented with periodontitis. Only five trials were considered to be at low risk of bias and meta-analyses yielded no effect of periodontal treatment on either preterm birth at less than 37 weeks of gestation (risk ratio 1.05, 95% CI 0.84; 1.30) or low birth weight less than 2,500 g (risk ratio 1.07, 95% CI 0.86; 1.33). Moderate and low heterogeneity

was observed, respectively. Quality of evidence: high.

Pregnancy commonly leads to enhanced gingival inflammation and may aggravate pre-existing periodontitis, which might be difficult to abolish completely. Despite evidence from large randomized controlled trials that periodontal treatment has no overall effects on pregnancy outcomes, it cannot be ruled out that risk attenuation for preterm birth may depend on the quality of periodontal treatment.[39] Moreover, treatment may have to be provided early during pregnancy or prior to conception.

---

## Osteopenia, Osteoporosis

Osteopenia and osteoporosis most often affect women after the menopause. A relationship between osteoporosis and periodontitis has been suggested, but according to a recent systematic review[40] conclusive data are presently missing.

➤ If osteopenia or osteoporosis is suspected, the patient should be referred to her gynecologist for bone density measurement.
➤ Management of osteoporosis may include:
  – Lifestyle prevention: smoking cessation and moderation of alcohol consumption, weight-bearing endurance exercise, etc.
  – Dietary supplements: combinations of vitamin D and calcium, vitamin K (see Chapter 13)
  – Medication: bisphosphonates (*caution:* osteoradionecrosis of the jaw), parathyroid hormone teriparatide
➤ In view of new evidence regarding considerable other risks, the benefits of hormone substitution therapy with estrogen have been seriously questioned.[41]

## Smoking

Smoking is the most important avoidable risk factor for many serious and life-threatening diseases, for example:
➤ Chronic obstructive lung disease
➤ Lung, bladder, oral, and throat cancer
➤ Cardiovascular diseases

In particular in Western countries, smoking prevalence has declined in recent decades (see Chapter 7):
➤ In Germany, in 2005, 27.2% of 15-year-olds and older people currently smoked cigarettes (32.2% men and 22.4% women).
➤ In Norway, smoking prevalence is still very high. In 2004, 37% of 14 to 74-year-olds currently smoked cigarettes, 39% men and 35% women.
➤ According to recent estimates in 2012, 18.1% of the adult population (≥ 18 years) in the United States smoked cigarettes (from 20.9% in 2005), 20.5% of adult men and 15.8% of adult women.[42]

Smokers may easily be identified during dental examination (**Fig. 8.5**):
➤ Typical breath odor.
➤ *Smoker's melanosis* of the gingiva which affects about 20 to 30% of such patients, especially heavy smokers.
➤ Externally stained teeth and marked *calculus* formation.
➤ Only minor signs of gingival inflammation in the presence of plaque. Smokers have less redness and edematous swelling of the gingiva and a reduced tendency to bleed on probing. Smoking appears to be an independent risk factor for gingival bleeding on probing.[43]

*Note*: In order to detect early signs of cancer or precancerous conditions (leukoplakia, smoker's leukokeratosis) in heavy smokers, a careful inspection of the oral cavity is mandatory (see **Fig. 6.2**).

Pathogenic mechanisms of smoking on periodontal tissues include the following[44]:
➤ Tobacco smoke affects the first line of defense against infection. For example, chemotaxis and phagocytosis of neutrophil granulocytes may be reduced. Moreover, antibody production may be impaired.
➤ On the other hand, monocytic release of proinflammatory mediators is stimulated.
➤ At high doses, nicotine damages gingival and desmodontal fibroblasts.
➤ While prevalence of periodontal pathogens in smokers and nonsmokers was not found

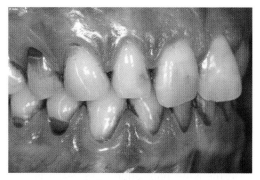

**Fig. 8.5 Typical clinical appearance of the dentition of a heavy smoker.** Note melanosis of the attached gingiva, in particular in the mandible, hyperkeratosis of the gingiva, recession, heavy extrinsic stain, and calculus formation, but no overt cardinal signs of gingival inflammation.

to be different in comparative studies, proportions of obligately anaerobic periodontal pathogens such as *T. forsythia* and *P. gingivalis* in subgingival plaque may in fact be increased. Furthermore, beneficial commensals (see Chapter 2), which are mainly associated with periodontal health, may be reduced.[45]

Epidemiological data confirm the role of smoking as the main risk factor for the development and progression of periodontal disease:
➤ For periodontitis, a relative risk of cigarette smoking of 2.5 to 6 has been reported (see Chapter 7). In adolescents the relative risk may be considerably higher.[46]
➤ Cigarette smoking is responsible for more than 50% of observed periodontitis in age groups up to 45 years. If smoking could totally be eliminated, the prevalence of periodontitis might be reduced by 30 to 60%.[47,48]

Results after periodontal therapy may be suboptimal in smokers.[49] Whereas proper periodontal treatment leads to a reduction in probing depth, attachment gains may be 25 to 60% less than those achievable in nonsmokers. This holds true for all forms of treatment, be it adjunctive antibiotic, nonsurgical, or surgical, including regenerative methods and plastic periodontal surgery. Moreover, the predictability of treatment outcome, especially after guided tissue regeneration (see Chapter 11), is considerably reduced in heavy smokers.

A **meta-analysis** of 12 controlled clinical trials on clinical effects of nonsurgical periodontal therapy in smokers and nonsmokers with chronic periodontitis[50] revealed:
➤ Studies, in which all gingival units were considered, yielded a significantly less mean reduction (0.13 mm) of periodontal probing depth (six studies) in smokers but no significant difference of clinical attachment gain (four studies).
➤ Likewise, in studies in which only periodontal sites with a baseline probing depth of ≥5 mm were considered, significant less mean reduction (0.43 mm) of periodontal probing depth was calculated for smokers (eight studies) but no difference in attachment gain (six studies). Significant hetero-

geneity among studies was observed. Quality of evidence: moderate.

After smoking is quit, positive, albeit limited, effects may occur rapidly.[51] The progression rate of periodontitis slows down. Wound healing after periodontal surgery improves.

*Note*: Contemporary dentistry with its special focus on prevention of oral diseases must include advice to the patient and, especially, medical support of the patient's attempts to definitively quit smoking:

➤ Regular assessment and documentation of the patient's smoking status. A special smoking questionnaire (**Table 8.4**) may be useful.
➤ Medical counseling about smoking.
➤ Consistent nicotine replacement: Nicotine patches, nicotine chewing gums.
➤ *Note*: Less than 7% of individuals who attempt to quit smoking are abstinent after a year. However, 25% of smokers who are abstinent after one week of using nicotine replacement are still abstinent after a year.[53]
➤ Whether E-cigarettes are safe and can have overall beneficial effects is currently not clear.[54]

➤ A close cooperation with the general practitioner, psychologist, etc. should be sought. If required, antisympathetic, antidepressants, or anxiolytic drugs may be prescribed.

A first goal should be to give up smoking at least during, and for several weeks after, periodontal surgery. In heavy smokers, who are unwilling or unable to quit, early extraction of questionable teeth may be indicated:

➤ The patient should be informed about considerably lower success rates after, in particular, regenerative measures or implant placement.
➤ In any case, rigorous attempts have to be made to control periodontal infections.

**Alcohol Consumption**

In cross-sectional studies a moderate, dose-dependent association between alcohol consumption and periodontal attachment loss has been reported.[55]

If systemic metronidazole is to be prescribed as an adjunct to periodontal therapy (see Chapter 13) possible alcohol intolerance should be mentioned.

**Table 8.4** Smoking questionnaire.[52]

| Are you now or have you ever been a smoker? | Yes<br>No |
|---|---|
| At which age did you first smoke regularly (at least once a day)? | ☐ years of age |
| For how many years altogether have you smoked/did you smoke regularly? | ☐ years smoked regularly |
| Do you currently smoke at least once a day? | Yes<br>No |
| On average, how many cigarettes do you smoke a day? | ☐ cigarettes per day |
| On average, how many cigars do you smoke a day? | ☐ cigars per day |
| On average, how much tobacco (pipe or roll-ups) do you smoke a day? | ☐ ounces of tobacco per week |
| In the last 12 months, have you seriously tried to give up smoking? | Yes<br>No |
| In the last 12 months, has a doctor or nurse advised you to give up smoking? | Yes<br>No |
| Do you think the amount you smoke is harmful to your health? | Yes<br>No |
| Would you like to give up smoking? | Yes<br>No<br>Don't need to |

In abstinent living patients suffering from alcoholism, ethanol-containing mouthwash is contraindicated. Note that alcohol-free rinsing solutions of chlorhexidine (0.12 % chlorhexidine digluconate, 0.05 % cetylpyridinium chloride, Perio-aid, Dentaid, Cerdanyola, Spain) or Listerine (Johnson & Johnson, New Brunswick, New Jersey, USA) are meanwhile available (see Chapter 10).

## Impact of Periodontal Therapy on General Health

Periodontal diseases cause considerable morbidity in the population. How and to what extent periodontitis can be prevented (see Chapter 7) and, in most cases, successfully treated (see upcoming Chapters) has been well established for decades. Without question, periodontal treatment has its own outstanding benefits, but as a matter of fact, due to widespread distribution and rather high costs, only a minor portion of any population received proper therapy so far.

Since periodontitis is associated with a plethora of other systemic diseases and conditions (see above and ref. [56]) it is only logical to ask questions about the impact of periodontal therapy on general health (see **Boxes 8.1–8.3**).

In a large-scale retrospective intervention cohort study[57], the hypothesis was tested that periodontal treatment reduces medical costs and inpatient hospital admissions. Five systemic diseases and conditions were considered, namely type 2 diabetes mellitus, coronary artery disease, cerebral vascular disease, rheumatoid arthritis, and pregnancy; apart from that all patients had periodontitis. Records from more than 300,000 individuals with both medical and dental insurance coverage and one of the above diseases/conditions were considered. Patients were categorized according to whether they had completed periodontal treatment in the baseline year. Outcomes were (1) total allowed medical costs and (2) number of hospitalizations per subscriber and per year in the following 5 years. Periodontal treatment significantly reduced costs for diabetes by 40.2 %, cerebrovascular disease by 40.9 % and coronary artery disease by 10.7 % and pregnancy by 73.7 %. The authors concluded that, based on their observation, simple and noninvasive periodontal therapy may improve health outcomes in pregnancy and other systemic conditions. Quality of evidence: moderate.

# 9  Emergency Treatment

## ■ Periodontal Emergencies

Only a few periodontal diseases and conditions are associated with acute pain and require urgent treatment; in particular, necrotizing periodontal diseases and the periodontal abscess. Due to infrequent occurrence of either type of disease, treatment strategies are still not really based on hard evidence, but usually straightforward since both are caused by bacteria resident in dental biofilm.[1]

In addition, not infrequent gingival trauma, certain infectious diseases unrelated to dental plaque, and mucocutaneous disorders (see Chapters 4 and 13) may cause considerable discomfort and have to be considered in certain cases as differential diagnoses.

### Traumatic Injury

Main causes are improper use of oral hygiene aids (brushing trauma, **Fig. 9.1**; clefts after misuse of dental floss), or thermal (e. g., hot cheese on pizza) or chemical injuries of the gingiva.
➤ Differential diagnoses:
  – Necrotizing ulcerative gingivitis/periodontitis
  – Herpesvirus infection
➤ Treatment of traumatic injuries:
  – Mechanical oral hygiene measures should be suspended.

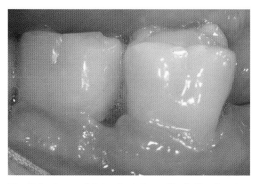

**Fig. 9.1  Loss of interdental papilla following improper use of interdental brush.**

  – The injured area may be covered by periodontal pack (CoePak, see Chapter 11) for a week.
  – Chemical plaque control with 0.1 to 0.2 % chlorhexidine digluconate mouthwash (see Chapter 10) twice daily.

A follow-up appointment should be arranged after one week.

### Necrotizing Ulcerative Periodontal Diseases

Various forms may be distinguished depending on the extent of the disease and the topography of the lesions:
➤ Acute necrotizing ulcerative gingivitis (**Fig. 9.2a, b**)
➤ Necrotizing ulcerative periodontitis (**Fig. 9.2c, d**)
➤ Necrotizing stomatitis

Differential diagnoses:
➤ Herpesvirus infection, especially herpetic gingivostomatitis
➤ Traumatic injury

Diagnosis and treatment of necrotizing periodontal diseases:
➤ Differential blood count should be arranged to rule out hematological disorders, in particular agranulocytosis and leukemia. It is also recommended to test the patient for HIV.
➤ Local treatment:
  – Careful supragingival debridement
  – Removal of pseudomembranes, which cover necrotic areas, with 3 % $H_2O_2$
  – Chemical plaque control with chlorhexidine preparations: 0.1 to 0.2 % mouthwash, 1 % gel for cautious toothbrushing
➤ Daily follow-up until complaints subside.
➤ The usual recommendations for adjunct antibiotic therapy should be followed (see Chapter 13):
  – Acute necrotizing ulcerative gingivitis (ANUG) can in most cases easily be con-

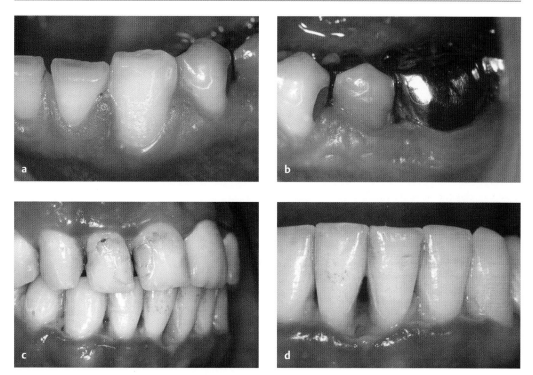

**Fig. 9.2 Necrotizing ulcerative periodontal diseases**
**a, b** Acute necrotizing ulcerative gingivitis (ANUG). Loss of papilla tip between teeth 33 and 32 and another painful interdental ulcer mesial of tooth 36 in a HIV-seropositive 36-year-old patient.
**c, d** Generalized necrotizing ulcerative periodontitis (NUP) in HIV-seropositive 26-year-old patient.

trolled by mechanical removal of dental plaque and adjunct antiseptics.
- Rather chronic, necrotizing ulcerative periodontitis (NUP) mostly requires adjunct systemic antibiotic therapy, in particular if complaints persist. After contraindications have been ruled out, metronidazole (3 × 250 mg per day) may be prescribed for 7 days.
- *Note*: There is a high potential for regeneration of lost interdental papillae after ANUG, in particular in young persons performing good oral hygiene. Use of dental floss should be preferred to interdental brushes or tooth picks. If interdental craters persist, gingivoplastic correction (see Chapter 11) may be indicated.

## Herpetic Gingivostomatitis

Herpetic gingivostomatitis is the primary infection with herpes simplex virus (HSV-1 or HSV-2).
➤ It is typically a childhood disease with a peak incidence at age 2 to 4 years.
➤ However, it may occur in young adults as well (**Fig. 9.3a**).

Differential diagnoses may include:
➤ Necrotizing ulcerative gingivitis
➤ Erythema multiforme

Treatment of herpetic gingivostomatitis:
➤ Any superinfection with pathogenic bacteria should be prevented. Since lesions are very painful, local debridement of teeth should be supplemented with 0.1 to 0.2% chlorhexidine digluconate mouthwash (see Chapter 10).

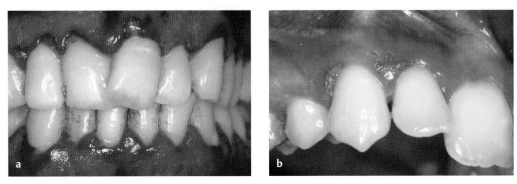

**Fig. 9.3   HSV-1 infection of gingiva.**
**a** Herpetic gingivostomatitis. Primary infection with HSV-1 in a 22-year-old HIV-seronegative patient. Note ulcerative lesions in the attached gingiva.
Similarly burst vesicles were found on tongue and lips.
**b** Herpetic lesions of the gingiva. Secondary infection with HSV-1. Vesicles have burst, leaving painful ulcerations. In this patient typical lesions were also seen on the upper lip (orolabial herpes, cold sore).

➤ Depending on the extent of the disease, the patient may be referred to a pediatrician or physician for virustatic medication (acyclovir).
➤ If appropriate, an HIV test should be arranged.

Recurrent herpes lesions (orolabial herpes, so-called cold sores; **Fig. 9.3b**) are secondary infections by virus particles which have persisted in sensory dorsal root ganglia. Such lesions usually do not require any special therapy.

**Periodontal Abscess**

Differential diagnoses include:
➤ Acute apical periodontitis
➤ Dentoalveolar abscess
➤ Langerhans' cell histiocytosis

Diagnosis and treatment of a periodontal abscess (**Fig. 9.4**):
➤ Careful periodontal probing to identify the bottom of the lesion
➤ Vitality testing
➤ Periapical radiograph, preferably with an inserted endodontic gutta-percha point (ISO 35)
➤ Local anesthesia
➤ Drainage can frequently be accomplished by careful subgingival scaling. If necessary, a marginal incision through the entrance of the pocket (**Fig. 9.4b**) is made.

➤ Instillation of 3% hydrogen peroxide (**Fig. 9.4c**)
➤ Adjunct antibiotics in case of systemic symptoms like fever and/or lymphadenitis: Metronidazole or azithromycin, or amoxicillin in combination with a β-lactamase inhibitor (e. g., clavulanic acid or sulbactam) (see Chapter 13)

Multiple periodontal abscesses have been described after prescription of non-β-lactamase-resistant antibiotics[2]:
➤ A differential blood count should be arranged and antibiotic treatment terminated.
➤ Microbiological diagnosis, preferably using cultivation and antibiotic susceptibility testing (see Chapter 2) should be instigated.
➤ Daily follow-up continues until complaints subside.
➤ Proper systematic periodontal treatment should be initiated.

**Combined Periodontal–Endodontic Lesions**

Differential diagnosis and treatment[3]:
➤ *Endodontic cause:*
  – Acute spread of an apical infection along the periodontal ligament.
  – The tooth does not respond to vitality testing and is presumably not vital.
  – Proper root canal treatment should be initiated. If the prognosis is guarded, root canal preparation should be carried out in

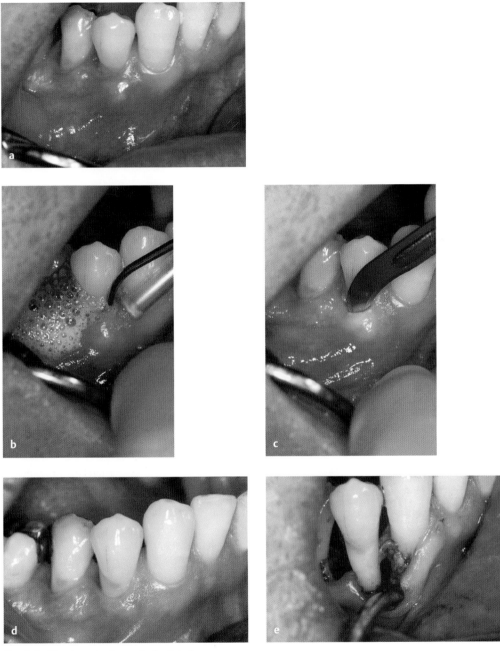

**Fig. 9.4 Treatment of a periodontal abscess.**
**a** Hemispherical swelling at vital tooth 44.
**b** Marginal incision through the pocket entrance. Note that pus emanates.
**c** Rinsing with 3% $H_2O_2$.
**d** Follow-up after 1 week. The patient should be scheduled for access flap/regenerative surgery.
**e** Situation during flap surgery. Note the connective tissue bridge mesial at tooth 44.

due order, but temporary dressing with calcium hydroxide may suffice.

– It is important to avoid using root surface instrumentation, since bone loss may rapidly revert after elimination of apical infection.

– Radiographic follow-up is scheduled after 3 and 6 months.

➤ *Periodontal cause:*

– Possibly retrograde pulpitis; in that case, sensitivity testing would still yield a vital tooth.

– A decision has to be made as regards tooth preservation. *Note*: Bone loss up to the apex usually indicates a hopeless case.

– If considered reasonable, proper root canal treatment should be initiated. A temporary dressing may be applied (calcium hydroxide).

– Thorough root surface instrumentation.

– Radiographic follow-up is scheduled after 3 and 6 months.

➤ In cases of longstanding combined periodontal-endodontic lesions the cause is often unclear and tooth preservation highly questionable.

# 10 Phase I—Cause-Related Treatment

## ■ Mechanical Plaque Control

The aim of cause-related therapy (see **Fig. 6.32**) is to significantly reduce the load of oral pathogens in the mouth. For that reason, cause-related therapy is sometimes called the hygienic phase of periodontal treatment, but its effects go far beyond that.[1]

First, the ecological conditions in the oral cavity have to be altered (see Chapter 2):
➤ Hopeless teeth should be extracted in an early phase of the treatment. Sometimes temporary dentures have to be incorporated in order to restore/maintain function and esthetics.
➤ Open carious lesions should be treated and defective restorations (marginal gaps, overhanging fillings, crowns) corrected or exchanged. Endodontic treatment, if needed, should be initiated.
➤ As soon as the patient's ability to practice oral hygiene has been restored (see below), motivation and instructions are given.
➤ Supra- and subgingival scaling, which should always be considered definitive, is carried out in one or several sessions.

Due to open interdental embrasures and large exposed root surfaces, effective oral hygiene may be particularly complicated in patients with severe periodontitis. That usually requires a revision of the patient's ideas of the time it takes to properly clean the teeth.

Thorough tooth cleaning should be performed once per day; for example, before going to bed:
➤ Methodical toothbrushing with fluoride-containing (1,450 ppm) toothpaste. Cleaning of interdental tooth areas (see below).
➤ Highly motivated patients will want to check remaining plaque with a disclosing agent (e. g., Disclotabs, Colgate-Palmolive, New York, USA) followed by its removal after careful inspection with a plastic mouth mirror.
➤ Note: All patients should in addition perform simple toothbrushing and mouth rinsing after each meal, optionally chewing xylitol-containing chewing gum.

Improvement of oral hygiene and decrease of bleeding tendency after probing should be recorded on appropriate forms (see **Fig. 6.13**).

### Toothbrushing Techniques

Dental plaque is the main cause of both dental caries and inflammatory alterations of the periodontium. Therefore, at the start of every periodontal treatment, oral hygiene has to be checked and usually improved.
➤ Dental plaque is a biofilm, similar to that found on all surfaces of standing or streaming water and water supplies, sewage, and sanitary installations (see Chapter 2).
➤ As a rule, biofilms can only be removed mechanically.

One should not forget, however, that oral hygiene is commonly practiced for other reasons as well; for instance, getting a pleasant mouth feel, gaining self-confidence, showing a winning smile and, not least, fighting bad breath.

As far as changing the patient's behavior is concerned, a major aspect of communication is an appropriate explanation of the problem—what is called *motivating the patient*. Hardly visible plaque should be revealed with a disclosing agent:
➤ Colored agents should be used, for example, aqueous solutions of 1.5% D&C Red #28 (phloxine B).
➤ *Note*: Before using a plaque-disclosing agent informed consent has to be obtained.
➤ The mouth should be rinsed with water first to remove any viscous saliva from the tooth surfaces. The disclosing agent is then applied with soaked cotton pellets.

After acclaiming already-clean tooth surfaces (e. g., anterior teeth in the maxilla), problematic areas should be inspected together with the patient who holds a hand mirror: lingual surfaces in the mandible, interdental embrasures, and cervical areas.

In order to convince the patient to change his or her behavior, the close relationship between dental plaque and bleeding gums after cautious probing and, if applicable, pockets may be visualized. That gingiva does not bleed at clean areas should be demonstrated as well.

Numerous *toothbrushing techniques* have been developed for various purposes and situations:

➤ Most patients prefer the *scrub technique* (horizontal brushing). While this technique may lead to injury, plaque removal is not very effective.
➤ The rather complicated *modified Bass technique* is still recommended by many dentists:
  – It is best practiced with a dry, multi-tufted brush with a short head.
  – A small amount of toothpaste (pea size) is applied.
  – The head of the brush is placed on the tooth surface at an angle of 45° to the tooth axis, while the bristles are directed towards the gingival margin.
  – Small vibrations of the brush are supposed to loosen cervical and sulcus plaque (**Fig. 10.1**).
  – The brush is then coronally rotated to wipe the plaque off the tooth surface.
➤ *Charters technique:*
  – This technique is particularly recommended for patients with wide interdental embrasures.

– The brush is directed towards the crown at an angle of 45° (the opposite way to the Bass technique).
➤ *Modified Stillman technique:*
  – The brush is directed at an angle of 45° towards the gingiva and rolled towards the crown (roll technique).
  – The technique is particularly suitable for patients with gingival recessions since there is virtually no risk of injury.
➤ Rather than laying stress on learning a completely new and unaccustomed technique, the emphasis should at first be on becoming *methodical*:
  – It makes sense to commence brushing in difficult-to-reach, habitually unclean areas, for instance lingual tooth surfaces in the mandible. Cleaning should then proceed from one tooth group to the next, for example:
    • Start lingually at the left side of the lower jaw and move to subsequent tooth groups: left wisdom tooth → molars → premolars → canine → incisors → right canine → premolars → molars → wisdom tooth.
    • Continue at the palatal surfaces in the upper jaw. Start on the right side in the wisdom tooth/molar region and proceed to the left side.
    • Change to the buccal surfaces in the upper jaw. Start on the left side and proceed to the right side.

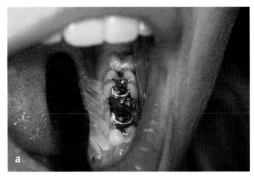 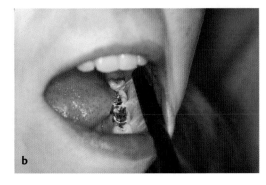

**Fig. 10.1  The modified Bass technique.**
**a** Patients are advised to start at lingual surfaces in the mandible. The head of the toothbrush is placed at an angle of 45° to the tooth axis towards the gingiva in order to remove, in particular, plaque in the gingival sulcus.
**b** Placing the toothbrush at buccal surfaces. Note that bristles reach the interdental areas.

- Continue at the buccal surfaces of the lower jaw. Start on the right side and proceed to the left.
- Finally, brush occlusal surfaces.
➤ Innovative brushes with longer oblique bristles are supposed to improve interdental cleaning.
➤ *Note:* In order to achieve the desired effect—that is, far-reaching cleaning of dental plaque from supragingival parts of the tooth—the design of toothbrushes or the brushing technique are of secondary importance. Pivotal rather is individual skills, which should be professionally trained in each treatment session. Audiovisual media may be useful.

In general, *electric toothbrushes* make oral hygiene more effective, easier, and faster.
➤ In particular, oscillating and rotating brush heads (e. g., Oral-B ProfessionalCare Smart-Series 4000, Procter & Gamble, Ohio, USA) have proved particularly successful. Features are:
  - Round, slightly tilted brush head
  - Longer outer bristles for reaching interdental areas
  - 450° oscillation angle. Rotation frequency 147/s, vertical pulsating frequency 667/s

- Possible undesired side effects (abrasion, recession) seem no longer to be an issue (**Box 10.1**)
➤ Some electric toothbrushes make use of acoustic energy (e. g., Sonicare, Philips, Koninklijke, Netherlands; Oral-B Sonic complete):
  - Disruption of the biofilm and possibly killing of fastidious periodontal pathogens.
  - Effectiveness corresponds to that of oscillating toothbrushes.

*Note:* Innovative electric toothbrushes and economically priced models have led to a paradigm shift when it comes to recommending oral health aids. Rather than confronting patients with unfamiliar and complicated brushing techniques, electric toothbrushes should be consequently considered. Oscillating and rotating or sonic toothbrushes are highly interesting, quasi-professional alternatives for patients (**Fig. 10.2**) and facilitate more effective, easier, and faster cleaning than conventional, hand-held toothbrushes.

*Irrigating devices* (e. g., Water Pik, Water Pik Inc, Ford Collins, Colorado, USA) cannot remove structured plaque from tooth surfaces. If recommended, they should be used only in combination with antimicrobial agents.

---

**Box 10.1   Are modern powered toothbrushes more effective than hand brushes?**

A systematic review by Yaacob et al[2] considered 51 clinical trials with more than 4,600 volunteers for meta-analyses. The following results were reported for short (up to 3 months) and long-term periods (greater than 3 months). There is evidence that powered toothbrushes provide a statistically significant benefit compared with manual toothbrushes as regards plaque reduction in the short and long term, about 11 % and 21 % for the Turesky modification of the QHI,* respectively. The same applies for gingivitis reduction in the short and long term (6 % and 11 % when using the Löe and Silness GI,* respectively). Quality of evidence: moderate.

The greatest body of evidence pertained to rotation oscillation brushes which demonstrated a statistically significant reduction in plaque and gingivitis at both time points. In both meta-analyses, significant and substantial heterogeneity of studies was observed which could not be explained by different toothbrush types. Moreover, cost, reliability, and side effects were inconsistently reported.

According to a systematic review by van der Weijden et al,[3] electric toothbrushes are safe and do not pose a clinically relevant concern for soft and hard tissues. Quality of evidence: moderate.

*See Chapter 5 for explanation of the respective indices.

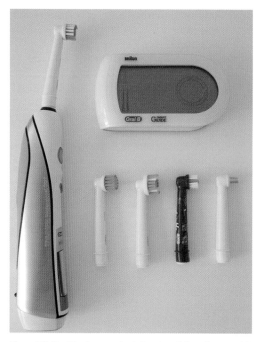

**Fig. 10.2 Modern electric toothbrushes** with highly developed designs make daily oral hygiene considerably more effective, easier, and faster.

## Interdental Hygiene

Interdental areas are usually not adequately reached by normal or electric toothbrushes. Therefore, additional *special aids* are required for interdental cleaning:
➤ Dental floss
➤ Interdental brushes
➤ Tooth picks

*Note*: Interdental cleaning can only be performed if the interdental embrasures are free and open. It must be very frustrating for patients, and even discouraging, if dental floss tears in a certain area because of a restoration overhang, for example. Thus, before introducing dental floss, any supragingival calculus should be removed. Likewise, marginal imperfections should be corrected, if possible, with fine (40 µm) and extra-fine (15 µm) diamond-coated spatulas (Lamineer Set) in the Profin handpiece (Dentatus, Spånga, Sweden).

The interdental aid with the broadest range of applications is certainly *dental floss* (**Fig. 10.3**). Basically, dental floss may be unwaxed or

waxed. The following methodical technique may be recommended:
➤ Start on the right side of the maxilla between the most posterior and second most posterior tooth.
➤ About 40 cm of dental floss is wound around the middle fingers of both hands.
➤ With thumbs and index fingers the floss is cautiously guided across and beyond the contact area of the teeth.
➤ The floss is moved up and down in contact with the proximal tooth surface to be cleaned,
➤ *Note*: After five to six movement cycles, unwaxed floss may make a squeaking sound—a sign that the tooth surface is clean. Waxed floss and Teflon floss (Glide, Oral-B) will not squeak.

Special dental floss (Superfloss, Oral-B) is recommended for patients with fixed dental prostheses and orthodontic retainers. It consists of three parts: a stiff end to thread; a spongy intermediate part to clean (e. g., the gingival side of a pontic); and a longer part of normal dental floss.

The risk of papilla injury is negligible. Flossing is regarded by some patients as a rather demanding technique; such patients may prefer *dental floss holders*.

In patients with wide open interdental embrasures and, in particular, exposed concave root areas *interdental brushes* (e. g., GUM Proxabrush, Sunstar, Chicago, Illinois, USA, **Fig. 10.4a**; TePe, Malmö, Sweden, **Fig. 10.4b**) should be recommended:
➤ Since interdental embrasures usually vary in size in a given patient, more than one interdental brush may be needed.
➤ After careful analysis of existing conditions (passage, friction), specific advice should be given.
➤ *Note*: More than two interdental brushes should not be recommended. Having too many aids must always be regarded as counterproductive.

*Interdental sticks* may be used instead of dental floss.
➤ Sticks are made of birch wood, which does not splinter, and have an increasing, triangular profile.

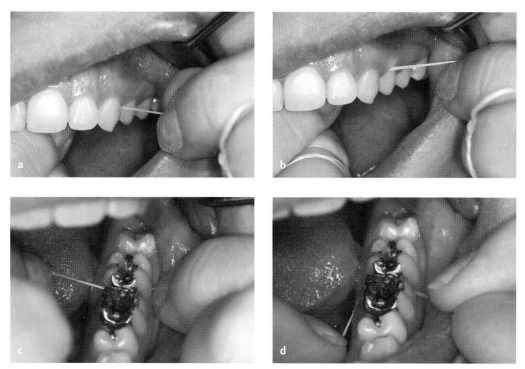

**Fig. 10.3   Dental flossing technique.**

**a** Dental floss is wound around the middle fingers and cautiously guided between thumbs and index fingers beyond the contact area with sawing movements.

**b** Here, the mesial surface of the first premolar is cleaned first by moving the floss up and down, keeping tight contact. Then, the distal surface of the canine is cleaned accordingly.

**c, d** Interdental cleaning of teeth in the mandible. A methodical approach is recommended.

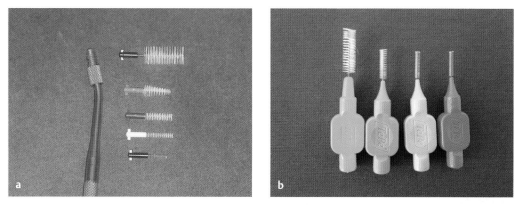

**Fig. 10.4   Interdental brushes** are nowadays easily available and offered by various companies in different sizes and designs. The presence of interdental embrasures of different sizes may cause some problems since more than two different interdental brushes are generally not accepted by the patient. Using an improper brush may increase the risk for injuries (see **Fig. 9.1**).

➤ They are supposed to be inserted interdentally until friction is felt.
➤ Note that correct application in posterior areas is hardly possible, and there is a high risk for papilla height reduction if used on a daily basis.

## ■ Chemical Plaque Control

Antimicrobial agents may be incorporated into oral health remedies to support the effects of daily mechanical plaque control; these are basically toothpastes and gels, and mouthwash solutions. Toothpastes are particularly suitable, since most people commonly brush their teeth at least once a day. Moreover, the importance of fluoride application as an active compound in toothpastes for dental caries prevention has been well known in the population for decades. *Note*: The wide distribution of fluoride-containing toothpastes is probably the most important reason for the observed decline in caries in most Western industrialized nations.

The rather complicated *composition of toothpastes* may interfere with antibacterial additives. In general, toothpastes contain the following constituents:
➤ *Abrasive components:* calcium carbonate and phosphate, metaphosphate, silica, aluminium oxide
➤ Suspension media: water, glycerin, propylene glycol, sorbitol syrup
➤ *Thickening, stabilization, and binding agents:* gels, starch, alginate, oily substances
➤ *Detergents* such as sodium lauryl phosphate
➤ *Aromatic compounds:* essential oils such as menthol or peppermint oil to improve taste which also exert antibacterial effects (see below)
➤ A large array of *medical and chemical ingredients* may be added:
  – Fluorides
  – Antimicrobial agents such as metal salts
  – Anti-inflammatory compounds such as triclosan
  – Enzymes (e.g., amyl glucosidase, glucose oxidase)
  – Tartar (calculus)-inhibiting substances such as diphosphonate, pyrophosphate, triclosan

– Desensitizing substances such as potassium and strontium salts, hydroxyapatite, calcium carbonate, and arginine
– Vitamin A
– Dyes

There is usually a limit as to what can be achieved by merely mechanical plaque control. Breakthroughs in individual oral hygiene may be expected by employing different kinds of chemical plaque control, so-called "soft chemoprophylaxis" (**Table 10.1**). The following factors should be considered:
➤ *Substantivity*: The active substance should adhere to surfaces of the oral cavity as strongly as possible, so that it is released slowly at concentrations that interfere with de novo plaque formation.
➤ *No adverse interaction* with other components of the toothpaste. *Note*: Despite excellent retention and subsequent sustained release, the plaque-inhibiting effect of cationic chlorhexidine (see below) in customary toothpaste formulations may be neutralized by anionic detergents and calcium ions.

### Chlorhexidine

1,1'-Hexamethylene-bis[5-(*p*-chlorphenyl)-biguanide]. As digluconate, acetate, or (less water-soluble) hydrochloride, it is the most efficacious oral antiseptic. Chlorhexidine has been firmly established in dentistry for several decades. In clinical studies for the development of new mouthwash formulations, it is commonly used as a positive control.

Chlorhexidine exerts antimicrobial action against a broad spectrum of microorganisms including:
➤ Gram-positive and gram-negative bacteria
➤ Fungi and yeasts, including *Candida* spp.
➤ Some viruses (hepatitis B virus, HIV)

Mouth rinse solutions usually contain 0.05 to 0.2% chlorhexidine digluconate. A gel containing 1% chlorhexidine but no detergents and abrasives and a spray with 0.1% chlorhexidine for disinfection of the tonsillar region (Corsodyl, GlaxoSmithKline, Brentford, UK) are also available. Note that chlorhexidine mouthwash may contain up to 12% ethanol. If contraindicated (e.g., for abstinent rehabilitated alcohol addicts) an ethanol-free solution of 0.12% chlorhexidine

**Table 10.1** Some antimicrobial compounds and related products to reduce plaque and gingivitis

| Compounds | Examples | Mechanism of action | Products |
|---|---|---|---|
| Bisbiguanides | Chlorhexidine | Antimicrobial | Toothpastes, gels, mouthwash, spray, chewing gum, varnish |
| Quarternary ammonium compounds | Cytylpyridinium chloride, benzalconium chloride | Antimicrobial | Mouthwash |
| Phenolic compounds, essential oils | Thymol, menthol, methylsalicylate, eucalyptol | Antimicrobial | Mouthwash, toothpastes |
| | Triclosan | Antimicrobial, anti-inflammatory | |
| Metal salts | Tin, zinc Strontium, potassium | Antimicrobial Desensitizing | Mouthwash, toothpastes |
| Fluorides | Sodium fluoride, sodium monofluorophosphate, stannous fluoride, amine fluoride | Dental caries inhibiting, antimicrobial, desensitizing | Toothpastes, gels, mouthwash, varnish |
| Amino alcohols | Delmopinol | Interferes with biofilm formation | No product available |
| Oxygen-releasing compounds | Hydrogen peroxide, sodium perborate, sodium percarbonate, sodium hypochlorite | Antimicrobial | Mouthwash |
| Enzymes | Glucose oxidase, amyloglucosidase | Antimicrobial | Toothpaste |

digluconate with 0.05% cetylpyridinium chloride (see below)[4] is available (Perio-aid, Dentaid, Cerdanyola, Spain).

Indications for chemical plaque control with 0.1 to 0.2% chlorhexidine as mouthwash include:
➤ Painful infections of the oral cavity if effective mechanical oral hygiene is not possible, for example, necrotizing ulcerative periodontal diseases, periodontal abscess, and herpetic gingivostomatitis (see Chapter 9).
➤ Postoperative infection control after periodontal or oral surgery (see Chapter 11).
➤ Intellectually disabled retarded and/or physically handicapped, and hospitalized, patients.

Chlorhexidine mouthwash at 0.1 to 0.2% should be used only for a few weeks since comparatively mild adverse effects may occur:
➤ Discoloration of teeth and restorations
➤ Hairy tongue
➤ Taste alterations
➤ Occasionally, desquamation of the epithelium
➤ Rarely, swelling of the parotid gland

Note that chlorhexidine mouthwash at 0.05% (Corsodaily) may be used for prolonged periods to supplement toothbrushing.

**Essential Oils**

Under the brand name Listerine, antiseptic mouthwash preparations containing essential oils have been marketed since 1915 in the United States, in particular for fighting halitosis and to control dental calculus.
➤ Currently, variously flavored alcoholic (22–26%) solutions of menthol (0.042%), thymol (0.064%), methyl salicylate (0.06%), and eucalyptol (0.092%) are available. Note that ethanol is toxic to bacteria only at concentrations of greater than 40%.

➤ Regular rinses with Listerine mouthwash for 30 seconds after toothbrushing significantly reduced plaque and gingivitis levels, notably in interdental areas (**Box 10.2**).

➤ Due to enduring concerns about an increasing risk for oral cancer when continually using alcoholic mouthwash, a solution with essential oils but no alcohol is currently marketed as well (Listerine Total Care Zero, Johnson & Johnson, New Brunswick, New Jersey, USA).

➤ Moreover, due to concerns about increasing the risk for dental caries when using mouthwash after toothbrushing with fluoride-containing toothpaste,[10] an essential oil-containing mouthwash with relatively high fluoride content has been introduced mainly for Nordic countries (226 ppm, equivalent to 0.05% w/v; Listerine Total Care Tooth Guard, Johnson & Johnson Consumer Nordic, Stockholm, Sweden). *Note:* In particular, patients with active dental caries are recommended to use mouthwash solutions containing a higher content of fluoride after toothbrushing

➤ Due to its strong taste (and possibly, high content of ethanol), Listerine is not suitable for children under the age of 14 years. *Note:* Listerine Smart Rinse for children of 6 years and older does not contain essential oils, but cetylpyridinium chloride (see below).

---

**Box 10.2  Should oral hygiene measures be supplemented with antiseptic mouthwash to further reduce plaque and gingivitis?**

Three systematic reviews of clinical studies of at least 6 months duration were compiled by Gunsolley.[5] Mouth rinsing with 0.12% chlorhexidine (6 studies), Listerine (25 studies) and cetylpyridinium chloride (7 studies) resulted in a lower mean gingival index of about 29, 18, and 13%, respectively, when compared with placebo mouthwash. Respective mouthwash solutions yielded a lower mean plaque index of 40, 27, and 15%.

According to meta-analyses of 11 controlled clinical trials,[6] when used as an adjunct to unsupervised oral hygiene, Listerine mouthwash provides considerable additional benefit as regards plaque and gingivitis reduction as compared to placebo or control. The effect was particularly pronounced in interproximal areas. Plaque and gingivitis reductions were comparable with those when dental floss is regularly used. Authors noted considerable issues with study design and large heterogeneity of the studies. Quality of evidence: low.

A meta-analysis of 19 randomized clinical long-term studies (≥ 4 weeks), in which plaque and gingivitis reduction after use of essential oil (Listerine) or 0.1 to 0.2% chlorhexidine mouthwash were compared[7] revealed slightly better plaque reductions after rinsing with chlorhexidine mouthwash. As regards reduction of gingival inflammation, differences were not significant. Quality of evidence: moderate.

In a meta-analysis by the same authors[8] four studies were identified in which the effects of essential oil mouthwash on plaque and gingivitis were compared with alcohol vehicle solution. Data suggested that the effect of essential oils on plaque and gingivitis extends beyond that of alcohol vehicle solution, which did not differ from water-based control. Quality of evidence: moderate.

Recommendations should take into account various undesired side effects of 0.1 to 0.2% chlorhexidine mouthwash, in particular when permanently used (discoloration of teeth and restorations, hairy tongue, taste alterations, desquamation of epithelium, parotid gland swelling). Both the American Dental Association and the US National Cancer Institute currently regard alcohol-containing mouthwash as safe. The available evidence does not support a connection between oral cancer and alcohol-containing mouthrinse. Nevertheless, based on a re-evaluation of the evidence[9] it is recommended to restrict mouthwash with high alcohol content to short-term therapeutic situations if needed.

## Cetylpyridinium Chloride

A cationic quaternary ammonium compound, 1-hexadecylpyridiniumchloride. This is a readily water-soluble antiseptic with a broad range of applications in the oral cavity: mouthwash, toothpaste, lozenges, spray. Substantivity is low; therefore, limited effects on plaque and gingivitis reduction have to be expected.[11]

## Triclosan

5-Chloro-2-(2,4-dichlorphenoxy)-phenol. Triclosan is a nonionic, lipid-soluble, antimicrobial substance with a broad range of action, which does not interfere with detergents and other toothpaste components. It is added to cosmetics and soaps as a preservative.

Since substantivity is low, various strategies have been employed to increase oral retention:
➤ Lipid-soluble triclosan is incorporated into a copolymer of polyvinylmethylether and maleic acid (PVM/MA, Gantrez), which has considerable retention capacity on oral surfaces.
➤ Triclosan is dissolved in polydimethylsiloxane (silicon oil).
➤ Triclosan is combined with zinc citrate (additive plaque-inhibiting effect).

An observed anti-inflammatory effect appears to be independent of its antimicrobial effect[12]:
➤ Triclosan interferes with arachidonic acid metabolism.
➤ After topical application, production of proinflammatory mediators $PGE_2$ and leukotriene $B_4$ (see Chapter 3) is reduced.

Even short-term use of toothpaste containing 0.3% triclosan may lead to an attenuation of the otherwise relatively strong association between the amount of supragingival plaque and the tendency of gingival bleeding.[13] In the long run, use of triclosan-containing toothpaste may influence the composition of subgingival plaque which in turn might slow-down the progression of periodontitis.[14]

A meta-analysis of 30 controlled clinical trials of at least 6 months duration[15] in which the effects on plaque and gingivitis of triclosan-containing toothpaste (0.3% triclosan, 2% Gantrez) were compared with those of fluoride-containing toothpaste revealed significantly lower plaque levels and gingival inflammation when triclosan-containing toothpaste was used. Quality of evidence: moderate.

Concerns have been raised as regards possible risks for individual health and the environment[16]:
➤ Triclosan may be degraded by microorganisms or react with sunlight to form chlorphenols and dioxin.
➤ Triclosan may cause bacterial resistance and cross-resistance (e. g., as regards doxycycline or ciprofloxacin).

## Metal Salts

Stannous fluoride, zinc citrate, and other metal salts have low toxicity but do have plaque-inhibiting effects.[17] They may be used as components of toothpastes and mouthwashes:
➤ Metal ions interfere with bacterial metabolism. For example, $SnF_2$ inhibits bacterial glycolysis.
➤ Zinc, tin, and copper ions eliminate volatile sulfur compounds of gram-negative bacteria ($H_2S$, $CH_3SH$), which are responsible for halitosis.

Moreover, strontium chloride and potassium nitrate or potassium citrate have been incorporated into toothpastes against dentin hypersensitivity.

## Other Additives

The aminoalcohol *delmopinol* (morpholinoethanol derivative) is a third generation plaque-inhibiting agent. It is neither bactericidal nor bacteriostatic. Instead, adherence of pioneer colonizers of the tooth surface (see Chapter 2) is inhibited. Based on a meta-analysis of eight randomized clinical studies,[18] rinsing for 60 seconds after toothbrushing with 0.2% delmopinol-containing mouthwash leads to significant more plaque and gingivitis reduction than placebo preparations. Quality of evidence: low and very low, respectively.

*Calculus formation* may be influenced by pyrophosphate, triclosan in combination with Gantrez or zinc citrate (see above), or diphosphonates.

*Dentin hypersensitivity* is a consistent problem in particular for periodontally diseased and treated patients. Numerous agents have been incorporated in toothpastes.[19] There are different hypotheses about the mode of action of desensitizing compounds:

➤ Occlusion of dentinal tubules
➤ Coagulation or precipitation of tubular fluids
➤ Stimulate secondary dentin formation
➤ Blocking pulpal neural responses

Metal salts (strontium chloride, potassium salts, sodium citrate) or formaldehyde have also been incorporated into special toothpastes for the treatment of hypersensitive teeth, with varying results. Limited effects may be expected for potassium salts (nitrate or citrate), which may be superior to fluoride application.

*Note*: High concentrations of fluoride lead to precipitation of calcium fluoride and occlusion of dentinal tubules. This still appears to be the safest treatment for dentin hypersensitivity. A similar mechanism of action is provided by a combination of 8% arginine and calcium carbonate.

Further developments in the oral hygiene sector of health care require frequent revisions of current concepts. As usual, differing problems in different patients require individual solutions. *Note*: The patient's oral hygiene in particular offers multiple opportunities for intensive communication.

## ■ Local Anesthesia

The most important part of the first stage of periodontal therapy is supra- and subgingival scaling and root planing, which should be definitive. *Note*: The latter usually requires local anesthesia. Local anesthesia involves the regionally limited, reversible block of pain receptors or their afferent nerves.[20] The mode of action is based on blocking sodium ion influx during afferent nerve conduction.

Local anesthetics are quite toxic for the organism, so resorption should be kept to the minimum:

➤ Vasoconstrictors prolong resorption time and reduce toxicity.
➤ Surgical procedures may be carried out more easily under conditions of local ischemia.
➤ Topical application may reduce pain from injection needle penetration.

Local anesthetic agents are either amino-esters of *p*-aminobenzoic acid or aminobenzoic amides. The respective residues of the molecule determine pharmacological properties and metabolism in the tissue:

➤ Esters of benzoic acid: procaine, tetracaine
➤ Amino amides: lidocaine, prilocaine, butanilicaine, mepivacaine, articaine, bupivacaine
➤ Procaine, tetracaine, and to some extent also articaine, may be hydrolyzed in the tissue. After some time, further injections exceeding the threshold dose may be possible.
➤ All other anesthetics mentioned are either secreted unchanged or metabolized in the liver. *Note*: The threshold dose must not be exceeded in these cases.

### Adverse Effects of Local Anesthetics

*Maximum admissible dose.* An adult patient with a body weight of 70 kg may tolerate subcutaneous injections of up to 400 mg lidocaine (20 mL of 2% solution, or 10–12 carpules). Note that at usual epinephrine concentration of 10 µg/mL, 20 ml anesthetic solution would be the maximum admissible dose for epinephrine as well (which is 0.2 mg). Since resorption is much higher in oral mucosa due to greater vascularization, this maximum dose **must not be exploited** in dentistry. It has been recommended to place a venous line whenever 25% of the maximum admissible dose is to be surpassed.

*Intoxications* affect the central nervous system and the cardiovascular system:

➤ Initial excitation phase: restlessness, tremor, anxiety, nausea, vomiting, visual deficits, tachycardia, rise in blood pressure
➤ Later: loss of orientation, tonic spasms, and dyspnea
➤ If not treated immediately: loss of consciousness, drop in blood pressure, bradycardia, finally circulation arrest and asphyxia

Under unfavorable circumstances (high endogenous release and exogenous supply of catecholamines, or accidental intravascular injection), *adrenaline intoxication* is possible despite careful consideration of any contraindications which may lead to:

➤ Increase in blood pressure
➤ Tachycardia

➤ Extra systoles, to the point of ventricular fibrillation

## Regional Infiltration and Block Anesthesia

An adequate depth of anesthesia is essential for subgingival scaling and periodontal surgery. Root instrumentation usually leads to very unpleasant dentinal pain. Ischemia after local anesthesia facilitates sufficient visualization of the surgical site. Therefore, small amounts of quite highly concentrated anesthetics (2–4%) containing adrenergic vasoconstrictors (10–12.5 µg/mL) are injected.

Procedure:

➤ Most suitable are carpule systems equipped with a fine (∅ 0.4 mm for block anesthesia, 27 G) or extra fine needle (∅ 0.3 mm for infiltration, 30 G). Respective needles are either 40 mm or 25 mm long.

➤ **In the maxilla**: Infiltration anesthesia of the *dental plexus* is done in the buccal vestibular fold. Two or three injections of about 0.5 mL each (e. g., 2% lidocaine with 10–12.5 µg/mL epinephrine) are required for groups of not more than two teeth. The tip of the needle should be adjacent to bone covering the apices of the teeth.

– If the operation is extended to one quadrant, block anesthesia of the *greater palatine nerve* and the *nasopalatine nerve* is necessary. The greater palatine nerve is blocked by carefully injecting, after aspiration, 0.5 mL anesthetic solution about 0.5 to 1 cm from the gingival margin at the second molar at a right angle to the mucosa. *Note:* Masticatory mucosa of the hard palate in this region contains a submucosa with loose connective tissue, elastic fibers and minor salivary glands (see Chapter 1). Careful injection of the anesthetic solution should therefore be rather painless. More anterior injections should generally be avoided.

– Block of the *nasopalatine nerve* at the incisive foramen may be somewhat painful because of dense fibrous tissue of the incisive papilla. The patient should be informed accordingly. On bone contact, the needle is withdrawn about 0.5 to 1 mm and, after aspiration, 0.2 mL is carefully injected.

➤ **In the mandible**: Except for subgingival scaling and root planing, or surgical treatment of lower anterior teeth where infiltration anesthesia may be sufficient, due to the thick cortical bone of the mandible, block anesthesia of the inferior alveolar nerve including the buccal, lingual and mental nerves is usually necessary.

– Several techniques for block anesthesia of the *inferior alveolar nerve* have been described. For example, the coronoid notch is palpated with the thumb of the nondominating hand while the index finger is placed behind the ramus below the ear. The mandibular foramen is then probably situated in a line between thumb and index finger. The syringe is directed parallel to the posterior teeth and the needle is inserted at the level of the thumb. In adults, the injection point lies about 1 cm above the occlusal surface of the most posterior molar. The needle is advanced dorsally by 1.5 to 2 cm under contact with the ramus and then rotated towards premolars of the opposite side. The needle is slightly further advanced until it meets resistance from the middle section of the ramus. The needle is then withdrawn by 1 to 2 mm and, after careful aspiration, 1.5 mL anesthetic solution is injected.

– The *lingual nerve* is blocked by further withdrawing the needle by about 1 cm and injecting 0.5 mL solution. Since the location of the injection is rather ill-defined it may be necessary to do further injections in the lining mucosa of the floor of the mouth in the molar and premolar regions.

– The *buccal nerve* is blocked by infiltration above the buccal fold right to the first molar.

– In addition, block of the *mental nerve* may be necessary when premolars are treated and the operation extends to the anterior teeth. A mental block is accomplished by injecting a small volume of 0.5 mL close to the mental foramen.

*Note*: The following techniques *should be avoided* because of the danger of traumatizing the gingiva and, especially, the periodontal ligament, as well as the likelihood of deep implantation of plaque bacteria:

➤ Intrapapillary injections of small amounts to the base of the bony pocket.
➤ So-called intraligamentary anesthesia. In fact, the anesthetic solution is rather spread out via spongy bone.
➤ A technique by which the needle is advanced through the buccal part of the interdental papilla to reach the incisive foramen, which is rather unreliable and may be overly traumatic.

An anesthetic gel (e.g., 25 mg/g lidocaine and 25 mg/g prilocain in an elastic gel at body temperature; Oraqix, Dentsply, York, Pennsylvania, USA) may be used for painless scaling in certain patients who are afraid of injection pain. Plasma concentrations are far below threshold doses and mild local adverse effects are very rare.

## ■ Supragingival and Subgingival Scaling and Root Planing, Subgingival Curettage

The most decisive procedure for the control of periodontal infections is definitive supra- and subgingival scaling and root planing.[21] Supragingival and subgingival scaling should be carried out in the same session. Working more or less only by tactile sensation requires considerable experience in assessing tooth and, especially, pocket morphology and in using the instruments.

### Definitions

*Scaling*: Mechanical removal of plaque, calculus, and stain from coronal parts of the tooth and root surface.
  *Root planing*: Removal of bacterially or toxically contaminated root cementum or dentin and leveling irregularities of the surface.
  *Curettage*: Removal of pocket epithelium and gingival granulation tissue, usually using curettes.

### Aims

Major aims are far-reaching reduction of bacterial load in the oral cavity and control of pocket infection by:

➤ Removal of bacterial deposits and endotoxin from the root surface
➤ Removal of necrotic and bacterially infiltrated root cementum
➤ If considered necessary, removal of pocket epithelium

Furthermore, an optimum healing result after creation of a biocompatible root surface should be achieved.

### Indication

Subgingival scaling is indicated in any periodontal pocket with a depth of more than 3 mm.

### Contraindication

Subgingival scaling in shallow pockets up to 3 mm may result in attachment loss (see below) and should be avoided.

### Instruments

The following hand- and machine-driven instruments are used for mechanical debridement (**Table 10.2**):

➤ *Scalers:*
  – Straight, sickle-shaped scaler H6/7 for the anterior and premolar region
  – Angled scaler Cl2/3 for the molar region
  – Taylor scaler 2/3: as Cl2/3 but smaller
➤ *Universal curettes* (**Fig. 10.5a**): The face of the blade is honed at a 90° angle to the terminal shank. Both cutting edges can be used for all surfaces of each tooth, for example:
  – Columbia 4 R/4 L
  – LM-Syntette
➤ *Intermediates*: Langer curettes combine the shank design of Gracey curettes (see below) with a universal blade honed at 90°. Both sides of the blade are cutting.
  – Langer 1/2 is less angled and adapts to mesial and distal surfaces of posterior teeth in the mandible.
  – Langer 3/4 is distinctly angled for scaling posterior teeth in the maxilla.

**Table 10.2** Standard instruments in tray for mechanical debridement of teeth

| Instruments | Description | Article no., manufacturer |
|---|---|---|
| Mouth mirror | Plane, front surface rhodium-coated, Ø 22 mm | M4C, Hu-Friedy |
| Dressing pliers | | DP18 or DP17, Hu-Friedy |
| Explorer | For subgingival calculus detection | EXD 56, Hu-Friedy |
| Periodontal probes<br><br>Furcation probe | • Calibration in 1-mm steps<br>• Color coded 3-3-2-3 mm<br>• Nabers' probe | • PCPUNC156<br>• PCP116, Hu-Friedy<br>• PQ2N6, Hu Friedy |
| Scalers | Sickle scalers<br>• Anterior teeth and premolars: H6/7<br>• Molars: CI2/3 or T 2/3 | • SH6/76, Hu-Friedy<br>• SCI2/36 or ST2/36, Hu-Friedy |
| Curettes | *Universal curettes*<br>• LM-Syntette<br>• Columbia 4 R/4 L<br>• Posterior teeth in the lower jaw: Langer 1/2<br>• Posterior teeth in the upper jaw: Langer 3/4<br>• Anterior teeth: Langer 5/6<br><br>*Area-specific curettes*<br>• Anterior teeth: Gracey 1/2 or 5/6<br><br>• Buccal/lingual surfaces of posterior teeth: Gracey 7/8<br>• Mesial surfaces of posterior teeth: Gracey 11/12 or 15/16<br>• Distal surfaces of posterior teeth: Gracey 13/14 or 17/18 | • 215–216, LM<br>• SC4R/4L6, Hu-Friedy<br>• SL1/26 or SL1/2AF, Hu-Friedy<br><br>• SL3/46 or SL3/4AF, Hu-Friedy<br><br>• SL5/66 or SL5/6AF, Hu-Friedy<br><br>• SG1/26 or SAS1/26, or SG5/66 or SAS5/66, Hu-Friedy<br>• SG7/86 or SAS7/86, Hu-Friedy<br><br>• SG11/126 or SRPG11/126, or SRG15/166, Hu-Friedy<br>• SG13/146 or SRPG13/146, or SG17/186, Hu-Friedy |
| Sharpening stone | Arkansas stone | SS4, SS299, Hu-Friedy |

- Langer 5/6 is straight and designed for anterior teeth.
➤ *Area-specific curettes* (**Fig. 10.5b**): The face of the blade is honed at about 70° to the terminal shank. Area-specific curettes have one cutting edge only. Gracey curettes comprise a variety of numerous area-specific curettes for all purposes. Usually a limited set is used, for example:
  - Gracey 1/2 or 5/6 for anterior teeth; 7/8 for buccal and lingual surfaces of posterior teeth; 11/12 (or 15/16) for mesial surfaces of posterior teeth; 13/14 (or 17/18) for distal surfaces of posterior teeth.
  - Further Gracey curettes are available with flexible terminal shanks for finishing; or more rigid shank for removal of larger amounts of calculus. Tactile sensation is usually better with flexible curettes.
  - Both Gracey and Langer curettes are available with terminal shanks extended by

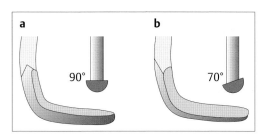

**Fig. 10.5  Design differences of universal and area-specific curettes.**
**a** The face of the blade of universal curettes is honed at a 90° angle to the terminal shank, and there are two cutting edges.
**b** In area-specific curettes, the angle is 70°, and there is only one cutting edge.

3 mm ("after-five") for deep pockets, and considerably shortened blades ("mini-five") for more slender incisor roots and tight pockets (**Fig. 10.6**).

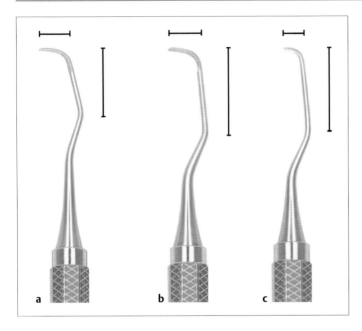

**Fig. 10.6  Area-specific curettes.**
**a** Common Gracey curette.
**b** After-five curette with a terminal shank extended by 3 mm.
**c** Mini-five curette with extended shank and blade shortened by about 50%.

➤ *Rotating instruments* (Perio-Set, Intensiv, Montagnola, Switzerland):
  – Diamond-coated (75 or 40 μm) burs for smoothing the root surface after odontoplasty (see Chapter 11).
  – Extra-fine diamonds (15 μm) for root planing. *Caution:* Undesired removal of larger amounts of root cementum and dentin must be avoided.

➤ *Periodontal files* are only of historical importance. They may be of use in rare cases—narrow furcation entrances, for example. Orban files are relatively wide while Hirschfeld files are more slender.

➤ *Airflow* has previously been used for removal of stain on tooth surfaces (tea, red wine, tobacco stain) and employs a relatively abrasive sodium bicarbonate-water spray. A novel device (Airflow Master, EMS, Nyon, Switzerland) uses slightly abrasive glycine powder (PerioFlow Powder, EMS; ClinPro Prophypowder, 3 M ESPE, St. Paul, Minnesota, USA), which may facilitate removal of subgingival biofilm in pockets up to 5 mm in size.

➤ *Ultrasonic instruments* (magnetostrictive, piezoelectric, **Table 10.3**) make the removal of subgingival deposits considerably easier. In clinical studies ultrasonic scaling was as effective as scaling with hand instruments,

in particular at single-rooted teeth (see below). Innovative slim, micro-ultrasonic tips allow instrumentation of deep, subgingival areas including furcations with sufficient water cooling.

– The cavitation effect of the water spray has a plaque-removing action. Acoustic energy may even destroy sensitive bacteria.

– Antimicrobial agents may be used for rinsing.

– *Caution:* Damage of the root surface depends on tip angle and, especially, lateral force. Important issues to be considered are:
  • A very shallow tip angle should be employed; the tip should work parallel to the root surface.
  • Virtually no active force should be applied (≈0.5 N).
  • Especially for piezoelectric devices, the power setting may adversely influence hard tissue removal.

– Because of the aerosol created while operating, special precautions for *cross-infection control* are necessary:
  • Patients should rinse with povidone–iodine (Betadine, Mundipharma, Cambridge, UK) or 0.1 to 0.2% chlorhexidine

**Table 10.3** Advantages and disadvantages of hand and ultrasonic instruments for root debridement

|  | Advantages | Disadvantages |
|---|---|---|
| Hand instruments | • Superior tactile sensation<br>• Good access to tight pockets, particularly with miniaturized blades<br>• Good adaptation to different root morphologies<br>• No aerosol<br>• No heat development | • Correct angulation of the blade of about 80° to root surface is necessary<br>• Frequent sharpening required<br>• Considerable working force for calculus removal<br>• Tiring of the operator<br>• Negative time factor |
| Ultrasonic instruments | • Current tips are very slender<br>• Instrumentation virtually without pressure<br>• Most surfaces can be reached, especially furcation areas<br>• Destruction of the biofilm by cavitation<br>• Possible bactericidal effect of acoustic energy<br>• Little soft tissue damage<br>• Pocket irrigation with antimicrobial agents<br>• Requires less time<br>• No sharpening of tips<br>• Higher patient acceptance<br>• Less tiring for the operator | • Poorer tactile sensation<br>• Produces microscopic rippling of the root surface<br>• Aerosol is highly contaminated<br>• Possible risk for patients with pacemakers<br>• Contraindication in infectious patients |

solution for germ reduction before any treatment.

- Face mask and face-shield should be worn.
- Adequate suction has to be ensured.
- *Note*: Ultrasonic instrumentation should not be used in known infectious patients (HIV, hepatitis) and patients with pacemaker implants.
  - For *sonic scalers*, which are driven by compressed air and fit to the turbine handpiece, similar recommendations may apply as for ultrasonic devices.
- ➤ A novel, *"smart" ultrasonic device* (Perioscan, Sirona, Bensheim, Germany) claims to be able to detect remnants of calculus on root surfaces which are visually indicated on the handpiece. Promising results have been reported after laboratory experiments.[23] Currently, no randomized clinical study has shown superior efficacy of the device.
- ➤ *Note:* Scaling and root planing mainly aims at disrupting the bacterial biofilm. Sole calculus removal does not usually assure clinical success.

Based on 13 randomized clinical studies on the efficacy of ultrasound/sonic scaling as compared to scaling and root planing with hand instruments, a **systematic review** revealed the following[24]:

- ➤ For single-rooted teeth, clinical results did not differ; however, the evidence for comparable efficacy of machine-driven scaling was not very strong.
- ➤ Ultrasonic/sonic scaling requires less time. Quality of evidence: high.
- ➤ There was no difference in undesired side effects when comparing machine-driven scaling with hand instrumentation.

After scaling, any surface roughness should be leveled by careful *polishing*:

- ➤ Nylon brushes or silicon cups with appropriate polishing paste may be used.
- ➤ Polishing pastes with different RDA (relative dentin abrasion) values may be applied dependent on intensity of external stain.
  - After having used pastes with rather high RDA, for example, 83 or 36 (Proxyt, Ivoclar Vivadent, Schaan, Liechtenstein), teeth

need to be re-polished with low-abrasive paste (RDA 7) or toothpaste.
  – A special prophylaxis paste containing perlite crystals (Cleanic, KavoKerr, Charlotte, North Carolina, USA) is especially abrasive in the beginning. Due to rounding off during polishing, abrasiveness of the crystals rapidly ceases and polishing effects prevail.

Interdental spaces should be polished with special plastic spatulas (EVA Tips, Dentatus, Stockholm, Sweden) for the Profin handpiece (Dentatus). Finally, a 1% fluoride gel (Elmex Gelée, GABA, Basel, Switzerland) is applied to all tooth surfaces.

### Procedure

*Subgingival scaling* and root planing consists of the following treatment steps:
➤ Disinfection: mouth rinsing with 0.1 to 0.2% chlorhexidine solution for germ reduction.
➤ Local anesthesia.
➤ Scaling: removal of any soft and hard deposits from the root surface.
➤ Root planing: smoothing of the root surface and leveling of resorption lacunae in cementum which might be colonized by bacteria.
➤ If necessary, soft tissue curettage for removal of granulation tissue and pocket epithelium.
  *Note:* Intentional removal of pocket epithelium is not regularly performed. It has not been shown in clinical studies that routinely performed subgingival curettage (i.e., scaling, root planing, and soft tissue curettage), was superior to scaling and root planing alone. While routine curettage is obsolete, it may be justified in certain cases, for example:
  – Pronounced inflammatory swelling of gingival tissue
  – Targeted tissue removal in case of a subgingival restoration margin

Four areas of concern have to be considered when root surfaces are to be debrided:
➤ Adequate access to the bottom of the pocket
➤ Good fit between the curette and root morphology
➤ Correct blade angle
➤ Thoroughness, that is, complete root coverage

*Note:* An intraoral fulcrum close to the working area, as traditionally recommended, may actually hamper correct blade angulation of 70 to 80 degrees[21]:
➤ Traditional techniques may prevent adequate access to the bottom of the pocket.
➤ More flexibility of the operator, alternative fulcrums, and alternative operator positioning are required:
  – In posterior areas of the maxilla, use of the mandible as an extraoral fulcrum is recommended (**Fig. 10.7a**).
  – Posterior areas of the right mandible are operated on from a 1 o'clock position using the posterior teeth of the maxilla as fulcrum. The mandible is stabilized with the dominant hand (**Fig. 10.7b**).
  – Posterior areas of the right maxilla are instrumented from a 2 or 3 o'clock position. The patient's head is tilted backwards (**Fig. 10.7c**).
  – Fingers of the nondominant hand may serve as a fulcrum (**Fig. 10.7 d**).
  – In certain cases, an extraoral, reinforced fulcrum may be necessary. The curette is activated with the index finger of the nondominant hand (**Fig. 10.7e**).

After intensive training, advanced scaling techniques may soon be exerted more or less unconsciously:
➤ The instrument is held in a modified pen grasp.
➤ The blade of the curette is inserted, toe down, into the pocket for an exploratory stroke (e. g., to identify subgingival calculus).

---

**Fig. 10.7   Advanced techniques for subgingival scaling.**                              ▶
**a** Mandible as extraoral fulcrum during instrumentation of posterior areas of the maxilla.
**b** Maxillary teeth as fulcrum during instrumentation of posterior teeth in the mandible. The nondominant hand stabilizes the mandible.
**c** Instrumentation of posterior areas of the right maxilla from a 2 or 3 o'clock position.
**d** Fingers of the nondominant hand used as fulcrum.
**e** Reinforcement of the curette with the index finger of the nondominant hand.
**f** Horizontal stroke.

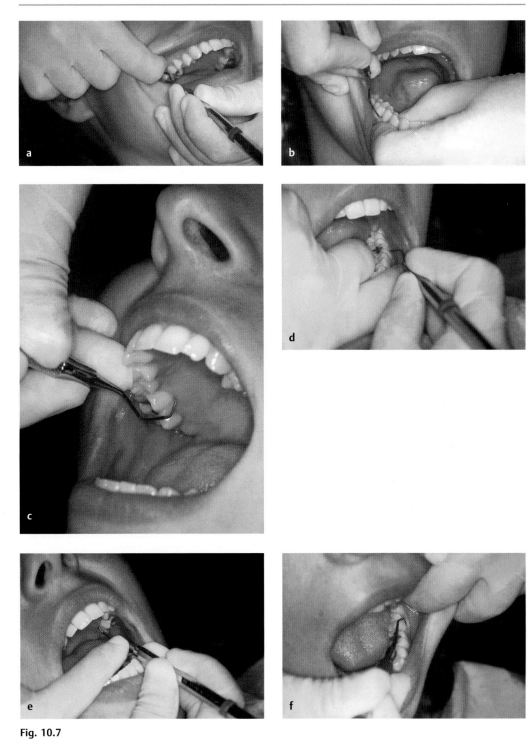

**Fig. 10.7**

➤ The correct working angle of 70 to 80° between the cutting edge of the curette and the root surface is established.
➤ Handle and shank position of the instrument determine whether an intra- or extra-oral fulcrum is necessary.
➤ An appropriate fulcrum and firm grasp are established.
➤ The body is positioned according to the fulcrum.
➤ Then, the working stroke is activated.
➤ In deep and narrow bony pockets and at line angles, for example, between distal and buccal surfaces, horizontal strokes at the bone level are performed across the root surface (**Fig. 10.7f**).
➤ After removal of mineralized and nonmineralized deposits (*scaling*), *root planing* is carried out with universal and area-specific curettes:
  – Bacteria generally colonize resorption lacunae in pathologically altered root cementum. These can only be leveled by thorough instrumentation.
  – Note that complete removal of root cementum is generally not desired. Opening of dentinal tubules may increase the risk of bacterial penetration and dentin hypersensitivity. Moreover, any reattachment is prevented.
  – Instrumentation is carried out in an overlapping pattern for complete removal of biofilm.
  – In practice, no distinction is made between scaling and root planing.
➤ *Soft tissue curettage* (e. g., in cases of slightly hypertrophic gingiva):
  – After thorough scaling and root planing, a universal curette is inversely inserted into the pocket and the inner surface of the pocket is carefully peeled.
  – *Note*: There is no evidence that routinely performed gingival curettage has any therapeutic benefit over scaling and root planing alone.
➤ While subgingival scaling may be carried out with both ultrasonic and hand instruments, finishing is always done with Gracey curettes.

Smoothness of the root surfaces is checked with an explorer. Not-instrumented areas with remaining biofilm can, of course, not be identified with dental explorers. Whether the procedure was effective can only be assessed during re-evaluation after healing has occurred (see below).

After subgingival scaling, teeth are rinsed and widened gingival margins compressed with gauze. In some cases periodontal pack (CoePak, PeriPak, see Chapter 11) may be applied for a couple of days.

### Critical Assessment

With a continuing trend of more elaborate and expensive new treatments being developed (many of which have quickly vanished), any therapist has to ask pertinent questions about efficacy, effectiveness, and efficiency of treatment methods:
➤ *Efficacy* measures the extent to which an intervention does more good than harm under ideal conditions: Is there scientific evidence (systematic reviews or randomized clinical trials) for superiority (or at least equivalence) of the new method when compared to conventional means?
➤ *Effectiveness* measures the same (as just listed) under general practice circumstances: Is the new method feasible?
➤ *Efficiency* measures the effect of intervention in relation to the resources it consumes: Is it worth it?

Invariably all clinical studies have proved efficacy of nonsurgical periodontal therapy (supra- and subgingival scaling and root planing) as regards resolution of gingival inflammation, decrease of periodontal probing depth, and gain of clinical attachment. A **systematic review** of 26 clinical studies on the efficacy of subgingival debridement[25] revealed that, in patients with chronic periodontitis, supra- and subgingival scaling in combination with oral hygiene improvement is an effective treatment in reducing probing depths and improving clinical attachment levels. It is in fact more effective than supragingival plaque control alone. Quality of evidence: high.

Moreover, nonsurgical periodontal therapy, for instance one or more sessions of subgingival scaling per year in the dental office, may reduce the risk for tooth loss (a true end point) by about 50%.[26]

While efficacy of subgingival scaling has been proved in clinical studies to be excellent, effectiveness in the dental office may be anything else than impressive. The therapist has to develop a certain "feeling" about his or her effectiveness. Prerequisites are technical skills as well as sharp instruments. Note that very hard subgingival calculus usually cannot be removed but rather is burnished with dull instruments. Subsequent removal is then even harder. Moreover, the risk for fracture of the instrument increases as well. Routine maintenance of periodontal scalers and curettes is therefore indispensable (see below).

Meticulous supra- and subgingival debridement often needs to be done in several weekly sessions (see **Table 6.3**). At re-evaluation after about 6 weeks (see below), considerable improvement of the clinical periodontal situation may be expected:

➤ A reduced number of gingival units that bleed on probing.
➤ Reduced periodontal probing depths (**Fig. 10.8**):
  – Pockets with a probing depth of ≥6 mm may respond with a combination of gain in clinical attachment and gingival recession. As a rule of thumb, the deeper the pocket the more gain in clinical attachment may be expected.
  – *Note*: Subgingival scaling in shallow pockets (≤3 mm) may result in undesired gingival recession and attachment loss.

➤ The number of pockets for which periodontal surgery (e.g., flap surgery; see Chapter 11) would be indicated should be largely reduced.

After 6 to 12 months, partial bone-fill of infrabony lesions may be seen on highly standardized intraoral radiographs (see Chapter 6), even after nonsurgical periodontal therapy (**Fig. 10.9**).

As to the subgingival microflora, some striking alterations have been observed after supra- and subgingival scaling and root planing as well (**Fig. 10.10**)[28]:

➤ Increase of periodontally inert *Actinomyces* spp., which have been shown to be antagonists of some periodontal pathogens (see Chapter 2).
➤ Reduction of established periodontal pathogens *Tannerella forsythia*, *Porphyromonas gingivalis*, and *Treponema denticola*.
➤ Most interestingly, prevalence of other bacteria remains more or less unchanged.

### One-Stage, Full-Mouth Disinfection

Conventionally, subgingival scaling is done in several weekly sessions. In particular in generalized severe cases of periodontitis, quadrant- or even sextant-wise scaling seems to be most appropriate. Before each session, the patient should be remotivated and further instructed in oral hygiene measures.

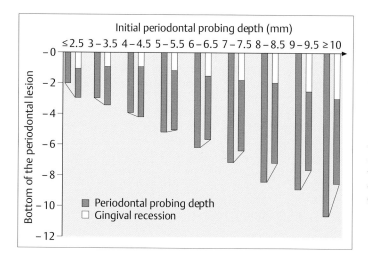

Fig. 10.8 **Average changes of probing parameters** (periodontal probing depth, clinical attachment level, gingival recession) two years after subgingival scaling in relation to initial periodontal probing depth. (Adapted after Badersten et al.[27]) Sixteen adults with severe periodontitis were treated. Scaling in shallow pockets up to 4 mm led to considerable attachment loss. In deep pockets (6 mm or more), attachment gain was observed—the deeper the pocket, the greater the gain, for example, about 2 mm in 10-mm deep pockets, on average.

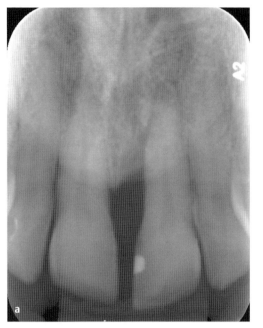
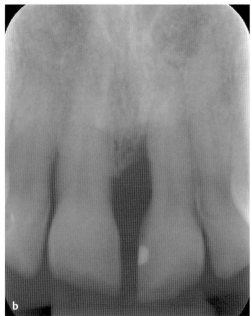

**Fig. 10.9   Bone-fill in deep infrabony lesion.**
**a** Deep, well accessible bony lesion mesial at tooth 21.
**b** Partial bone-fill 20 months after thorough subgingival scaling. Note considerable loss of tooth substance. Probing pocket depth was reduced from 11 mm to 4 mm, while 5 mm clinical attachment was gained. No bleeding on probing.

In order to intercept recolonization of already debrided root surfaces with periodontal pathogens from deep pockets and other areas of the oral cavity (tongue, tonsils), so-called one-stage *full-mouth disinfection* has been suggested:

➤ Definitive supra- and subgingival scaling is completed preferably within 24 hours.
➤ Instillation of 1% chlorhexidine gel (Corsodyl, GlaxoSmithKline, Brentfort, UK) into scaled pockets.
➤ In addition, disinfection of extracrevicular oral ecosystems (see Chapter 2) is done at home: Continuous and consistent application of chlorhexidine preparations for about 6 weeks:
  – 0.1 to 0.2% mouthwash, toothbrushing with 1% chlorhexidine gel.
  – Chlorhexidine spray (Corsodyl) for tonsil areas.
  – Tongue coatings should be removed with a special tongue cleaner.
  – *Note*: After cessation of chemical plaque control, all stain is to be removed and mechanical plaque control reinforced.

As compared to the traditional approach of quadrant-wise debridement over several weeks, one-stage full-mouth disinfection over a short period yielded slightly better clinical results in particular at single-rooted teeth (**Box 10.3**).

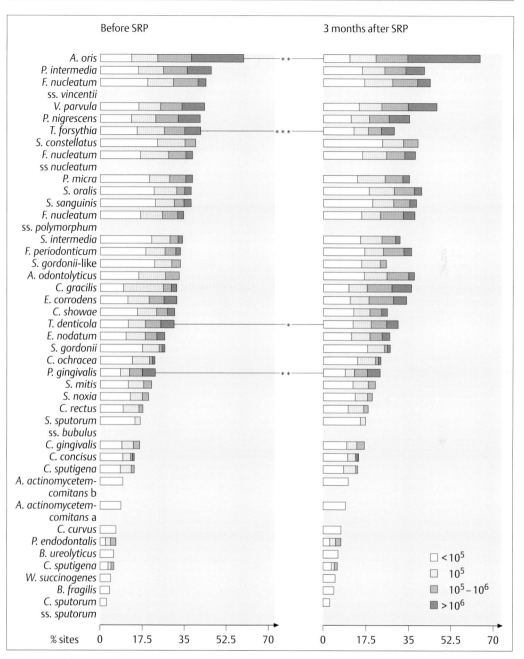

**Fig. 10.10** Alterations in subgingival microflora after subgingival scaling and root planing (SRP). (Adapted after Haffajee et al.[28]) Prevalence of the 40 most frequent bacterial species of the oral cavity was studied at each tooth of 57 adult patients with chronic periodontitis. Checkerboard DNA-DNA hybridization (see Chapter 2) was employed. Significant alterations (*: $p < 0.05$, **: $p < 0.01$, ***: $p < 0001$) occurred for *Actinomyces oris* (↑), *Tannerella forsythia*, *Treponema denticola*, and *Porphyromonas gingivalis* (↓). The prevalence of other bacteria was not significantly changed. Concomitantly, reductions of bleeding after probing and probing depth as well as gain in clinical attachment in pockets of 6 mm or more were registered.

**Box 10.3    Is full-mouth disinfection of the oral cavity superior as compared to conventional quadrant-wise scaling?**

Eberhard et al[29] identified seven randomized clinical studies, in which subgingival scaling within 24 hours with and without adjunct chlorhexidine was compared with conventional quadrant-wise scaling in patients with chronic periodontitis. The authors conducted several meta-analyses.

At least 3 months after treatment, all treatment modalities revealed significant improvements of the clinical situation. Disinfection of the oral cavity including application of chlorhexidine preparations to 5 to 6 mm deep pockets of single rooted teeth resulted in significantly more pocket reduction (mean difference 0.53 mm,

95% confidence interval [CI] 0.28; 0.77) than quadrant-wise scaling. In 5 to 6 mm deep pockets of single- and multi-rooted teeth, the difference in clinical attachment gain was 0.33 mm (95% CI 0.04; 0.63). Quality of evidence: moderate.

According to the authors, these rather small differences, which had only been observed in moderately deep pockets in a limited number of studies, limit general conclusions about the clinical benefits of full-mouth disinfection. In practice, patient's preferences and convenience of the treatment schedule should be taken into account.

## Photodynamic Therapy, Laser

The fundamental principle of photodynamic periodontal therapy is activation and excitement of a photosensitizer (e.g., thiazine dye) by light of a specific wavelength, which is applied, for example, by a fiber optic diode laser (e.g., Periowave, Odine Biomedical, Toronto, Canada).

➤ The photosensitizer undergoes transition to a higher triplet state and may react with oxygen by producing highly reactive singlet oxygen, $^1O_2$, which irreversibly damages viruses, bacteria, and fungi.
➤ Since singlet oxygen has a short lifetime and a very short radius of action (0.02 μm), the reaction is largely limited in space and time and thus considered safe.

In a **systematic review**, Azarpazhooh et al[30] identified five randomized clinical studies, in which photodynamic therapy was compared with conventional nonsurgical periodontal therapy.

➤ Based on a meta-analysis, the combined therapy of subgingival scaling and photodynamic therapy, in particular, resulted in slightly more reduction of periodontal probing depth (mean difference 0.25 mm) and somewhat more gain of clinical attachment (mean difference 0.34 mm). Quality of evidence: moderate.

➤ Owing to the currently low number of small-scale studies, routine application of sole photodynamic therapy or its combination with scaling and root planing cannot be recommended.

Laser therapy with, for example, the Nd:YAG (neodymium-doped yttrium-aluminium garnet) laser has been propagated as an alternative to, or in combination with, nonsurgical periodontal therapy. Laser light may penetrate (pigmented) soft tissue up to a depth of 0.5 to 4 mm. Laser energy is supposed to kill bacteria in dental biofilm.

In a **systematic review** by Slot et al,[31] eight studies were identified in which application of a pulsed Nd:YAG laser during initial periodontal therapy was compared with conventional nonsurgical periodontal therapy using ultrasonic and/or hand instruments. In the majority of studies, laser therapy was not superior over conventional periodontal therapy. Quality of evidence: very low.

Recently, the laser-assisted new attachment procedure (LANAP) used a different protocol in which a pulsed Nd:YAG laser is claimed to selectively remove pocket epithelium from underlying connective tissue. Some periodontal regeneration has in fact been shown in a few studies of human biopsy material (see Chapter 11).

## Re-evaluation

Depending on extent and severity of periodontitis, about 4 to 6 weeks after cause-related therapy has been completed, including oral hygiene improvement, subgingival scaling, and root planing, periodontal conditions are carefully re-evaluated (see **Table 6.3**):
➤ Periodontal probing depths and clinical attachment levels are assessed.
➤ Decisions are made regarding further therapeutic measures (see Chapter 11).
➤ An oral hygiene check is carried out.

## ■ Sharpening of Instruments

Apart from the operator's skill, one important prerequisite for success is sharp instruments:
➤ Dull instruments burnish subgingival calculus rather than remove it. Subsequent removal is then almost impossible.
➤ Furthermore, there is an increased risk of fracture of a dull instrument because higher pressure is exerted on it.
➤ For these reasons, periodontal instruments need to be regularly sharpened with, for example, Arkansas or ceramic sharpening stones. Oil or water is used as a lubricant.

Moreover, in particular after successful periodontal therapy, tighter pockets may require curettes with narrow blades. Dental hygienists usually prefer sets with various sharpened-down Gracey curettes.

Instrument sharpness should be assessed *after* thermo-disinfection and sterilization:
➤ The easiest way to do this is to turn the instrument and assess whether the cutting edge reflects light, a reliable sign that the instrument is dull. A sharp cutting edge does not reflect light.
➤ Plastic sticks are commonly used to test sharpness.

Preferably, specially trained dental assistants should sharpen all instruments. Sharpening machines are generally preferred (e. g., LM-RondoPlus, LM, Parainen, Finland). Before using a sharpening machine, however, knowledge about different designs of periodontal instruments and basic principles about sharpening are necessary.

*Note*: Sharpening of dull instruments shortly before the treatment session or even in front of the patient should be avoided.

Whenever periodontal instruments are sharpened, maintaining the original design of the instrument is most important.

The terminal shank of the instrument, which is the area between the blade and the first angle, is a key element for each scaler or curette (**Fig. 10.11**).
➤ By holding the instrument in a way that the terminal shank is in an upright position, the cutting edge of an area-specific curette can easily be identified as the lower edge.
➤ Furthermore, proper alignment of the terminal shank will automatically place the instrument in the correct position for sharpening.

### Sickle Scalers

The instrument with its tip *towards the body* is held with the nondominant hand and a secure palm grasp. The top shank is braced with the index finger to counterbalance the pressure. The elbow is placed on the table.
➤ The terminal shank is held in an upright position.
➤ The lower half of the lubricated sharpening stone (oil for Arkansas stone, water for ce-

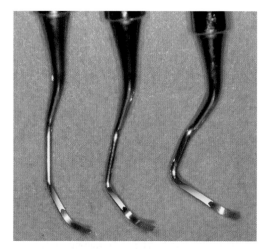

**Fig. 10.11 The terminal shank** (red) is a key element of any scaler and curette. Proper alignment of the terminal shank may facilitate identification of the cutting edge of an area-specific curette and automatically place the instrument in the correct position for sharpening.

ramic stone) is grasped by the dominant hand. It is pressed against the right blade of the scaler at an angle of slightly less than 30°.

➤ The stone is moved up and down with moderate pressure:
  – first, against the lateral surface of the heel of the blade;
  – then gradually moving forwards to grind the middle part;
  – finally, the stone is advanced to the third part of the blade towards the tip.

The tip of the scaler is then rotated *away from the body* with the terminal shank upright. The sharpening stone is pressed at an angle of slightly less than 30° to the blade. The heel, middle and tip thirds are gradually sharpened by moving the stone up and down with moderate pressure. Any wire edges may be removed from the face of the scaler with a conical sharpening stone.

Sharpness is tested with a plastic stick:
➤ The stick is held upright with the thumb and the index finger of the nondominant hand.
➤ The scaler is held with the dominant hand in a modified pen grasp.
➤ The blade of the scaler is slightly tilted by 20°. The blade must bite into the plastic stick. A metallic sound may be heard.

### Universal Curettes

The same principles as for scalers apply for universal curettes (e. g., LM-Syntette, Columbia 4 R/4 L, see **Fig. 10.5a**). Note that the rounded toe of the curettes also has to be sharpened.
➤ The terminal shank is held upright.
➤ The lubricated sharpening stone is pressed against the right blade of the curette at an angle of slightly less than 30°.
➤ The stone is moved up and down with moderate pressure, starting at the heel third of the blade. The stone is continuously moved along the entire length of the blade.

The curette is then rotated so that the toe points away from the body. The terminal shank is held upright. The sharpening stone is tilted at an angle of slightly less than 30° to the blade.
➤ Grinding motion is activated at the heel third of the blade.
➤ Up and down movements proceed to the middle, then the toe third of the curette.

To maintain the rounded shape of the toe, the face is held horizontally. The position of the stone is about 30° to the toe. The stone is moved in a slight and consistent up and down motion, rotating around the toe. Any wire edges are removed from the face of the curette with a conical stone.

Sharpness is tested with a plastic stick. The stick is held upright, whereas the blade of the curette is slightly tilted by about 20°. The blade has to bite into the plastic stick. A metallic sound may be heard.

### Area-Specific Curettes

Area-specific curettes have only one cutting edge. The face of the blade is honed at the terminal shank at 70° (**Fig. 10.5b**). Sharpening is done as follows:
➤ The instrument is held with a firm palm grasp, the right lateral surface being the cutting edge. For all odd-numbered Gracey curettes the toe points to the body, for even-numbered curettes it points away from the body.
➤ The terminal shank is tilted to the left by 20° until the face of the curette is parallel to the table.
➤ The lubricated stone is positioned to the right lateral surface (blade) and tilted to the right by 30°.

The stone is moved up and down with moderate pressure, starting at the heel third of the blade. The stone is continuously moved along the entire length of the blade.

To maintain the rounded shape of the toe it is held horizontally. The position of the stone is about 30° to the toe. The stone is moved in a slight, regular up and down motion, rotating around the toe. Any wire edges need to be removed from the face of the curette with a conical stone.

To sharpen the blade of the corresponding working end, the curette is turned. The toe now points in the opposite direction.

To test sharpness the plastic stick is held upright. The terminal shank of the blade is held parallel to the stick. The cutting edge is pressed against the test stick. It must bite into the stick. A metallic sound may be heard.

After sharpening, instruments need to be sterilized again.

# 11 Phase II—Corrective Procedures

## ■ Periodontal Surgery

About 4 to 6 weeks after cause-related therapy (see Chapter 10) has been completed, periodontal conditions are carefully re-evaluated for the first time. Decisions have to be made as regards further therapeutic measures. *Note:* In the majority of cases, particularly as regards mild or localized moderate periodontitis, no further active therapy is necessary and patients may be scheduled for supportive periodontal therapy (see Chapter 12).

Periodontal surgery may be indicated in cases of gingival enlargement, infrabony osseous lesions and/or furcation involvement, or recession (see Chapter 6). Within the framework of comprehensive dental care, surgical measures are part of various corrective measures (see **Table 6.3**), including the restoration of esthetics and function with dental prostheses. The latter can only be completed after results of the surgical phase have been carefully re-evaluated. *Note:* The comprehensive, so far preliminary, treatment plan has to be revised and possibly adjusted depending on the outcome of periodontal surgical measures.

Surgical periodontal procedures have the following objectives:
➤ Treatment of persisting periodontal lesions under visual control
➤ In some cases, alteration of tooth morphology and/or morphology of the gingiva and the alveolar bone in order to achieve a more physiological form
➤ Attempts to regenerate lost periodontal structures

Resective measures are differentiated from more or less regenerative procedures:
➤ Gingivectomy/gingivoplasty (resective)
➤ Flap operations (resective, sometimes regenerative)
➤ Guided tissue regeneration (regenerative)

During the corrective phase, further surgical procedures may be performed as well:

➤ Plastic periodontal surgery to correct developmental and acquired deformities and conditions around teeth and on edentulous alveolar ridges
➤ Oral surgical measures
➤ Placement of implants

Definitive restorative treatment should be carried out not earlier than 4 to 6 months after surgical measures have been completed (see **Table 6.3**). In some cases, orthodontic treatment is also necessary and needs to precede restorative measures.

## ■ Gingivectomy

Nowadays, gingivectomy is a rather outdated concept for the treatment of periodontitis lesions. Nevertheless, there are still certain indications (see below).

During gingivectomy, all of the pathological tissue is surgically removed while maintaining the physiological form of the gingiva. The main advantage of this quick and simple but rather radical procedure is pocket elimination. Disadvantages include a high risk of undesired root exposure which may lead to esthetic problems, especially in the anterior region. There is also an increased risk of dentin hypersensitivity.

### Aims

➤ Excision of thick, fibrotic gingiva
➤ Pocket elimination

### Indications

The few, largely restricted, indications may include:
➤ Supra-alveolar pockets of more than 4 mm in the presence of fibrotic, thick gingiva; for example:
 – Drug-induced gingival enlargement
 – Hereditary gingival fibromatosis
 – Thick periodontal phenotype

➤ Pre-prosthetically, to expose a subgingival preparation line before taking an impression
➤ To surgically expose impacted teeth in cases of eruption anomaly

## Contraindications

Contraindications mainly exist whenever there are indications for alternative treatment procedures:
➤ Particularly in esthetically sensitive areas— for example, anterior teeth in the maxilla with a thin periodontal phenotype characterized by rather delicate and narrow gingiva (see Chapter 6)
➤ Infrabony pockets
➤ Bulged thickening of the bone margin with a risk of surgical exposure

## Instruments

A suitable surgical tray may be equipped with the following instruments (**Table 11.1**), which are commonly used for gingivectomy procedures:
➤ Tweezers:
  – Special tweezers for pocket marking
  – Anatomical and surgical tissue pliers

➤ Scalpel blades (**Fig. 11.1a**):
  – No. 11: lancet-shaped
  – No. 12: sickle-shaped, blade on one side only; no. 12D: cutting blades on both sides
  – No. 15, no. 15C: curved
➤ Scalpel handle:
  – Straight blade handle
  – Universal 360° blade handle (**Fig. 11.1b**)
➤ Gingivectomy knives (for local gingivectomy), for example:
  – Hatched-shaped Kirkland knife (**Fig. 11.1c**)
  – Lancet-shaped Orban knife (**Fig. 11.1 d**)
➤ Scissors:
  – Goldman–Fox gingival scissors
  – LaGrange gingival scissors

## Procedure

External gingivectomy consists of the following *treatment steps*:
➤ Disinfection—for example, mouth rinsing with 0.1 to 0.2% chlorhexidine solution for 2 minutes
➤ Local anesthesia
➤ Creating bleeding points with pocket marker
➤ Incision

**Table 11.1** Standard instruments for gingivectomy

| Instruments | Description | Article no., manufacturer |
|---|---|---|
| Mouth mirror | Plane, front surface rhodium-coated, ∅ 22 mm | M4C, Hu-Friedy |
| Periodontal probe | Calibration in 1-mm steps or color coded 3–3–2–3 mm | PCPUNC156 or PCP116, Hu-Friedy |
| Pliers | • Dressing pliers<br>• Periodontal pocket marker left, right<br>• Anatomical tissue pliers<br>• Surgical tissue pliers | • DP18 or DP17, Hu-Friedy<br>• PMGF1 + 2, Hu-Friedy<br>• TP31 or TPG1, Hu-Friedy<br>• TP33 or TPG3, Hu-Friedy |
| Surgical retractors | • Langenbeck retractor<br>• Middeldorpf retractor | • SR2, Hu-Friedy<br>• RSMID 2, Hu-Friedy |
| Scalpel holder | • Straight scalpel holder<br>• Universal 360° blade handle | • 10-130-05E, Hu-Friedy<br>• K360, Hu-Friedy |
| Scalers | Sickle scaler CI2/3 | SCI2/36, Hu-Friedy |
| Curettes | • Posterior teeth in the lower jaw: Langer 1/2<br>• Posterior teeth in the upper jaw: Langer 3/4<br>• Anterior teeth: Langer 5/6 | • SL1/29, Hu-Friedy<br>• SL3/49, Hu-Friedy<br>• SL5/69, Hu-Friedy |
| Scissors | • Goldman–Fox gingival scissors<br>• LaGrange gingival scissors | • S16, Hu-Friedy<br>• S14, Hu-Friedy |

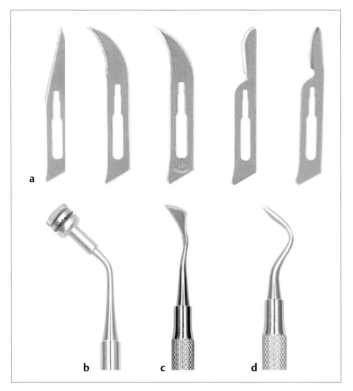

**Fig. 11.1 Scalpel blades and blade handles.**
**a** Disposable scalpel blades (from *left* to *right*): nos. 11, 12, 12D, 15, 15C.
**b** Universal 360° blade handle.
**c** Hatched-shaped Kirkland knife (15/16).
**d** Lancet-shaped Orban knife (1/2).

➤ Tissue excision
➤ Scaling and root planing
➤ Re-contouring of the gingival margin
➤ Cleaning of the wound area
➤ Periodontal dressing

*Bleeding points* are created with special pocket markers (Goldman–Fox or Crane–Kaplan):
➤ One arm of the tweezers is inserted into the pocket, while the one with the sharp inward point remains on the outside (**Fig. 11.2a**).
➤ By pinching the tweezers, a bleeding point is made on the gingiva, marking the level of the bottom of the pocket.

For the *incision*, mainly disposable scalpel blades are used:
➤ No. 11 or no. 12D scalpel blades are mounted in a universal 360° handle perpendicular to the handle. *Note*: In lingual and distopalatal areas, incisions cannot be made with straight scalpel handles.

➤ Gingivectomy knives (**Fig. 11.1c, d**) are only used for small, regionally limited interventions. A main disadvantage is that blades must be sharpened after every use.
➤ Continuous incision across the entire surgical site (**Fig. 11.3**):
  – The incision angle to the tooth axis is about 120° (**Fig. 11.2b**, incision line 3).
  – Note that the incision should end apical to the bleeding points but coronal to the mucogingival border.
  – A horizontal incision is not recommended (**Fig. 11.2b**, incision lines 1 and 2) because of resulting balcony-like contours.
  – Bone exposure has to be avoided because of delay in wound healing, possible attachment loss and pain.

Interdental separation and excision of the tissue may be carried out with the CI2/3 scaler.
Re-contouring of the incision edge may be done with gingival scissors (**Fig. 11.2b**, incision line 4).

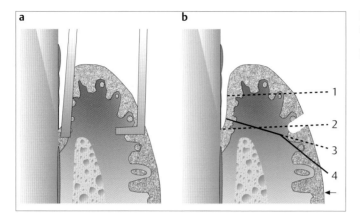

**Fig. 11.2   External gingivectomy.**
**a** Bleeding points are created with pocket-marking tweezers.
**b** Incision lines 3 and 4 are recommended for gingivectomy. Incision line 1 does not remove the pocket, while line 2 leads to balcony-like contours. Note that the mucogingival border (←) should not be affected and alveolar bone exposed.

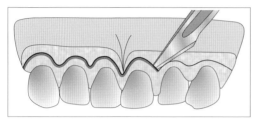

**Fig. 11.3   Gingivectomy.** Continuous, scalloped incision at an angle of 120° to the tooth axis.

The exposed tooth surfaces are carefully scaled and any tissue remains are removed with gauze soaked in saline. A soft periodontal dressing (CoePak, GC Europe, Leuven, Belgium, see below) has to be applied, which should be renewed after 1 week. In case of full-mouth gingivectomy (which should preferably be performed under general anesthesia), a vacuum-formed acrylic splint may serve as a tray for the periodontal pack.

Gingivectomy may also be conducted with pulsed infrared laser (Nd:YAG or $CO_2$ laser, see Chapter 10). While it is questionable whether this provides any advantage over gingivectomy performed with a scalpel, it may be an important option for hemophilic patients and patients receiving anticoagulant therapy. Laser light reflection at metallic restorations or metal instruments must be avoided.

### Postoperative Care

To prevent postoperative infection, chemical plaque control is performed twice daily with a 0.1 to 0.2% chlorhexidine mouthwash solution until normal oral hygiene measures become possible. A follow-up session is scheduled after one week when the periodontal dressing is removed:

> The wound surface is cleaned with gauze soaked in saline, and fibrin and desquamated epithelial cells are removed.
> Usually, a new periodontal dressing is applied for another week.

### Critical Assessment

Postoperative complications are more likely after gingivectomy procedures than after other periodontal surgical interventions:

> Secondary wound healing generally requires a periodontal dressing (CoePak).
> Epithelialization starts from incision edges. Thus, interdental areas are epithelialized last, that is, after at least 10 to 14 days.

Extra care should be taken in esthetically demanding areas, especially the anterior teeth in the maxilla, where gingivectomy may be contraindicated. Successful gingivectomy depends on strict observance of the above-mentioned indications and contraindications. *Note:* In cases of hereditary gingival fibromatosis (see Chapter 4) recurrent enlargement should be expected as long as body growth has not come to an end (**Fig. 11.4**). Likewise, if medication cannot be changed (see below), gingival enlargement will inevitably recur.

Contrary to the situation about 30 or 40 years ago, gingivectomy is nowadays hardly relevant in surgical treatment of periodontitis. In any

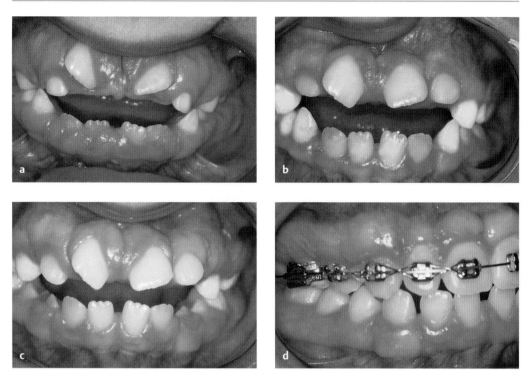

**Fig. 11.4 Gingival fibromatosis.**
**a** Eight-year-old child with hereditary gingival fibromatosis and severe eruption anomaly of permanent teeth.
**b** Following gingivectomy and extraction of the deciduous lateral incisors in the maxilla, orthodontic treatment commenced.
**c** Situation after 2 years.
**d** Three years after commencement of orthodontic therapy, shortly before completion. Although gingivectomy procedures were repeated, gingiva remained thick and bulgy.

case, the periodontal phenotype has to be considered (see **Fig. 6.9**). Extremes are:
➤ Highly-scalloped, thin and narrow gingiva which tends to recede after traumatic injury or chronic inflammation. In such cases a gingivectomy is absolutely contraindicated.
➤ Wide and thick gingiva usually associated with rather square anterior teeth in the maxilla. This phenotype tends to pocket formation and represents a possible indication for gingivectomy.
➤ *Note*: Since the periodontal phenotype is largely genetically determined, it can hardly be altered by surgical procedures.

Today, gingivectomy is quite frequently indicated in patients with drug-induced gingival enlargement, in particular in patients taking calcium antagonists, cyclosporin (frequently in combination) or tacrolimus (see Chapter 4).[1]

Nowadays, medical prescriptions of anticonvulsive drugs phenytoin and phenobarbital, which have been associated with gingival enlargement as well, are rather uncommon. *Note:* Due to considerable risk for recurrence after sole surgical excision in cases where medication has to continue, the responsible physician should be consulted and possible drug substitution discussed:
➤ Sirolimus instead of cyclosporin or tacrolimus
➤ Alternative antihypertensive drugs
➤ New generation of antiepileptic drugs (e. g., lamotrigin, gabapentin, topiramate)

## ■ Gingivoplasty

### Definition

Minor plastic surgical correction of the gingiva.

### Aim

To reshape the gingiva in order to obtain a more physiological contour.

### Indications

Gingivoplasty, which is by and large a limited intervention, may be indicated in cases of:
➤ Regionally limited thickening of the gingiva without presence of pathologically deepened pockets.
➤ Persistent interdental soft tissue craters after healing of necrotizing ulcerative gingivitis/periodontitis (see Chapter 9). *Note:* In young individuals the potential for papilla regeneration is high and a wait-and-see strategy is preferred before a gingivoplasty procedure is asserted.
➤ As an additional surgical step during gingivectomy (**Fig. 11.2b**, incision line 4). Smoothing of the incision edge to avoid balcony-like contours.
➤ Pre-prosthetic measures; for example, to expose preparation lines before impression taking and to reshape the gingiva in the area of the later pontic.

### Contraindications

Consequently, contraindications are:
➤ Generalized bulgy and thick, fibrous gingiva
➤ Periodontal pockets

### Instruments

Gingiva may be modeled with various instruments:
➤ Scalpel blades no. 11 or no. 12 D
➤ LaGrange or Goldman–Fox gingival scissors
➤ Diamond-coated burs
➤ Electrosurgical device

### Electrosurgery

Dental electrosurgical devices usually have a power of 50 W:
➤ Monoterminal use; no neutral electrode is required.
➤ Current setting "rectified and filtered" (unmodulated high-frequency current, about 2 MHz).
➤ *Note:* Strongly modulated high-frequency current for electrocoagulation, electrofulguration, or electrodesiccation is not used in dentistry. *Caution:* Injuries of the pulp (by touching metal restorations), cementum, periodontal ligament or, in particular, bone have to be avoided in any case.
➤ Preferably, needle-shaped, rhomboid, elliptic, or round sling electrodes are used (**Fig. 11.5**).

### Procedure

Fast, determined working is recommended. Only the superficial surface of the tissue is to be removed.
➤ *Note:* Heat development depends mostly on the length of time the electrode is moved through the tissue.
➤ Electrical spark formation represents extreme energy density and leads to tissue carbonization.
➤ Contact with the tooth or, especially, bone *must* be avoided at any rate.
➤ Smoke formation has very negative psychological effects, so excellent suction has to be ensured.

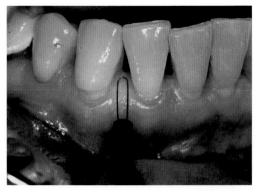

**Fig. 11.5  Sling electrode for electrosurgical contouring of the gingiva.**

## Critical Assessment

Certain advantages of electrosurgery have been claimed:
➤ Use of tiny electrodes which do not need sharpening
➤ Largely ischemic conditions because of immediate coagulation of small vessels and capillaries
➤ Excellent visual control

Disadvantages, which ultimately outweigh possible advantages, are:
➤ High risk of deep tissue injury
➤ Risk of postoperative infection, delayed wound healing, sequestrum formation
➤ Unpleasant smell

*Note*: Electrosurgical procedures do not play an important role in periodontal surgery. On the other hand, as a pre-prosthetic measure, gingiva may easily be modeled electrosurgically in the area of the later pontic and for exposure of preparation lines.
   *Note*: Before taking an impression of subgingival preparation lines, the (inflammation-free) gingival margin should be rather carefully retracted with a retraction cord. Unlike electrosurgery, this procedure does not lead to attachment loss.[2]


## ■ Flap Operations

### Aims

Periodontal flap surgery is performed for the following reasons:
➤ To gain access to the infected root surface when the morphology of bony lesions is complicated and/or furcation involvement is present.
➤ To facilitate careful debridement of root surfaces under visual inspection.
➤ To surgically alter unfavorable morphology of the alveolar bone (osteoplasty) or tooth (odontoplasty).
➤ To regenerate lost periodontal tissues.

### Indications

Flap operations may be indicated in the following cases:
➤ Persisting pockets deeper than 5 mm at re-evaluation after cause-related therapy (see Chapter 10)
➤ In particular, bony pockets and interdental craters, furcation involvement
➤ Need for surgical crown lengthening

*Note*: Whether to raise a flap for better access to a periodontal lesion with complicated morphology is mainly a technical question, for example:
➤ Difficulty to insert the curette to the bottom of the bony lesion in a deep and narrow pocket or furcation
➤ Problematic to achieve a correct angle between the blade of a curette and the root surface
➤ Loss of control while working on the root surface in deep pockets

### Contraindications

Flap operations are not indicated in the following cases:
➤ Rather shallow (up to 5 mm), supra-alveolar pockets at single-rooted teeth, and especially in esthetically demanding areas, where subgingival scaling and root planing can easily be repeated.
➤ Thick, fibrous gingiva, where gingivectomy might result in more favorable tissue morphology.

### Instruments

In addition to the surgical instruments already mentioned, the following instruments may be used (**Table 11.2**):
➤ An appropriately small elevator for mobilizing a mucoperiosteal flap
➤ Universal curettes for removing granulation tissue, particularly from bony pockets and furcations
➤ Needle holders and suture material

Some supplementary instruments, which are not regularly used, should be kept at hand:
➤ Sugarman and/or Schluger bone files for osteoplasty (see **Fig. 11.36**)
➤ Special furcation curettes (see **Fig. 11.32**)

**Table 11.2** Standard instruments for periodontal flap surgery

| Instruments | Description | Article no., manufacturer |
| --- | --- | --- |
| Mouth mirror | Plane, front surface rhodium-coated, Ø 22 mm | M4C, Hu-Friedy |
| Periodontal probe | Calibration in 1 mm steps or color coded 3–3–2–3 mm | PCPUNC156 or PCP116, Hu-Friedy |
| Pliers | • Dressing pliers<br>• Anatomical tissue pliers<br>• Surgical tissue pliers | • DP18 or DP17, Hu-Friedy<br>• TP31 or TPG1, Hu-Friedy<br>• TP33 or TPG3, Hu-Friedy |
| Surgical retractors | • Langenbeck retractor<br>• Middeldorpf retractor | • SR2, Hu-Friedy<br>• RSMID 2, Hu-Friedy |
| Scalpel holder | Straight scalpel holder | 10-130-05E, Hu-Friedy |
| Periosteal elevator | | P24GSP or P8 D, Hu-Friedy |
| Scalers | Sickle scalers CI2/3 and T 2/3 | SCI2/36 and ST2/36, Hu-Friedy |
| Curettes | *Universal curettes*<br>Goldman–Fox 4 or Columbia 4 R/4 L<br>*Area-specific curettes*<br>• Anterior teeth: Gracey 1/2<br>• Buccal/lingual surfaces of posterior teeth: Gracey 7/8<br>• Mesial surfaces of posterior teeth: Gracey 11/12 or 15/16<br>• Distal surfaces of posterior teeth: Gracey 13/14 or 17/18 | SGF46 or SC4R/4L6, Hu-Friedy<br><br><br>• SG1/26 or SAS1/26, Hu-Friedy<br>• SG7/86 or SAS7/86, Hu-Friedy<br><br>• SG11/126 or SRPG11/126, or SRPG15/166, Hu-Friedy<br>• SG13/146 or SRPG13/146, or SRPG17/186, Hu-Friedy |
| Bone files | • Schluger<br>• Sugarman | • FS 9/10S, Hu-Friedy<br>• FS 1/2S, Hu-Friedy |
| Scissors | • Goldman–Fox gingival scissors<br>• LaGrange gingival scissors | • S16, Hu-Friedy<br>• S14, Hu-Friedy |
| Needle holder | Olson–Hegar | NH5068, Hu-Friedy |
| Suture material | • C 6 reverse cut, 3/8 circle, 5-0 polyester or polypropylene<br>• C 6 reverse cut, 3/8 circle, 4-0 polyester or polypropylene | • PSNR698L or PSN8698P, Hu-Friedy<br>• PSNR683L or PSN8683P, Hu-Friedy |

### Various Techniques

Historically, surgical techniques employing flap operation had been described between 1912 and about 1920 by R. Neumann, A. Cieszynski, and L. Widman. These pioneers described rather radical operations regularly involving bone resection. As a rule, the bottom of the bony pocket became the new alveolar crest.

In 1931 Kirkland described a *modified flap operation*[3] which was supposed to largely preserve the periodontal tissues. Only interdental papillae were raised, and carefully replaced and sutured after root debridement.

During the 1950s and 1960s, rather radical methods were propagated again, for example, the *apically repositioned flap*[4–6]:

➤ After bone resection to remove intrabony pockets, the flap was apically repositioned and fixed by periosteal sutures.

➤ Of advantage was that pockets were totally eliminated while, in contrast to the gingivectomy procedure, keratinized tissue was more or less preserved.

➤ As a disadvantage, considerable bone was sacrificed after leveling bony pockets.

Nowadays, this technique is performed only when osteoplasty is required: for surgical crown lengthening; tunnel preparation of mandibular molars with furcation involvement (see below); or surgical exposure of impacted teeth.

➤ Procedure:
- Elevation of buccal and lingual mucoperiosteal flaps and mobilization beyond the mucogingival border.
- Cautious osteoplasty with, for example, universal curettes (Columbia 4 R/4 L) and/ or bone files (Schluger, Sugarman, see **Fig. 11.36**), or rose head burs with constant cooling with saline.
- Meticulous root planing to prevent undesired reattachment.
- Securing the flaps with periosteal, or vertical mattress, sutures in their new position (see **Fig. 11.11**).
- In some cases only a buccal flap is apically repositioned and secured with a periosteal sling suture (**Fig. 11.6**). At lingual/palatal aspects either gingivectomy may be performed or the flap is shortened.

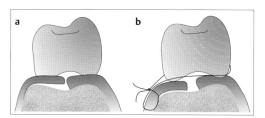

**Fig. 11.6a, b  Periosteal sling suture for fixation of a buccal flap in an apical position.** Note in (**b**) that some bone has been surgically removed buccally (surgical crown lengthening).

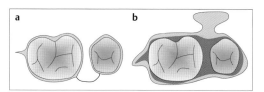

**Fig. 11.7  Incision lines for the papilla preservation flap described by Takei et al.[7]** Semilunar circumcision of the papilla palatally (**a**). Mobilization of the papilla in buccal direction (**b**). Inflammation-free gingiva and adequate width of the papilla (> 2 mm) are prerequisites.

A *papilla preservation flap* has been described by Takei et al[7] to cover interdentally placed graft material; for example, implantation of bone substitutes or membranes for guided tissue regeneration. As a prerequisite, wide (> 2 mm) and inflammation-free interdental gingiva was mentioned.

➤ Procedure:
- The papilla is *palatally/lingually* circumcised and mobilized in buccal direction (**Fig. 11.7**).
- After thorough root debridement, the buccal periosteum has to be dissected to advance the flap coronally and cover the graft material.
- Since blood supply is compromised, there is a certain risk that the palatal part of the papillae may become necrotic.

➤ Cortellini et al[8] modified the papilla preservation flap (see **Fig. 11.26**):
- *Buccal* semilunar circumcision of the papilla facilitates blood supply via the greater palatine artery.
- The vestibular flap is coronally mobilized after dissection of the periosteum at its base, allowing coverage of, for example, a space-keeping membrane.

Recently, further papillae preserving flap operations[9] and *minimally invasive surgical techniques*[10] have been described (see below), which

may facilitate the application of regeneration promoting proteins (e.g., Emdogain, see below) and/or bone substitutes:

➤ Only the buccal papilla is mobilized to gain access to the interdental osseous lesion.
➤ Primary stabilization is by internal mattress suture.
➤ Note that indications, which largely depend on defect morphology, are very much limited: isolated deep interdental bony lesions, especially in esthetically demanding areas.

In particular in the 1980s the *modified Widman flap*[11] was widely applied for gaining access to bony lesions. One explicit aim was preservation of soft and hard tissues as much as possible. In light of current minimally invasive techniques, the accomplishment of this aim might be questioned. In any case, the flap allows excellent inspection of the surgical site. Instrumentation under direct visual control is possible, and correct suturing may allow primary wound healing.

### Procedure for the Modified Widman Technique

The following steps are applied:
➤ Disinfection
➤ Local anesthesia
➤ Several methodical incisions are made (**Fig. 11.8**), preferably with a no. 12 D scalpel blade:
   – First, a *paramarginal incision* is done up to the bone crest (so-called reverse bevel incision, sometimes also called *internal gingivectomy*; **Fig. 11.8a**). Particularly palatally, in case of thick, fibrous gingiva, the incision is made about 1 to 2 mm lateral to the gingival margin. *Note*: Paramarginal incisions should be avoided in esthetically sensitive areas and in patients with thin gingiva.
   – Next, an *intracrevicular incision* is made again up to the bone crest (**Fig. 11.8b**).
   – The flap is then carefully mobilized and a *horizontal incision* is done perpendicular to the tooth axis (**Fig. 11.8c**). As a result, the inflamed tissue is circumcised.
   – In cases of isolated bony pockets, one or two *vertical releasing incisions* may be necessary, which confine the surgical site laterally. The paramedian incisions (i.e., 1–2 mm lateral to the root prominence) should diverge into the vestibule to avoid postoperative recession or papilla necrosis. *Note:* Vertical releasing incisions should be avoided in esthetically demanding areas.
➤ A mucoperiosteal flap is carefully mobilized with a periosteal elevator. The circumcised tissue is removed with the CI2/3 sickle scaler and any granulation tissue with a Goldman-Fox 4 universal curette (**Fig. 11.8 d**).
➤ Root surfaces are carefully scaled and planed with area-specific curettes and, if appropriate, periodontal files (Orban, Hirschfeld).
➤ Remaining granulation tissue at the inner surface of the flap is removed with LaGrange gingival scissors.

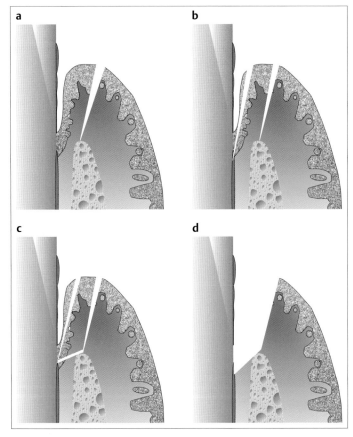

**Fig. 11.8 Incisions of the modified Widman flap technique.**
**a** Paramarginal incision (reverse bevel incision) at a distance of about 0.5 mm from the gingival margin. In esthetically demanding areas and in case of thin gingiva, this incision has to be skipped.
**b** Intracrevicular incision to the bottom of the defect.
**c** Incision that is as near horizontal as possible. The granulation tissue has now been circumcised.
**d** After removal of the circumcised tissue, scaling and root planing can be performed under direct sight.

➤ After rinsing with saline and meticulous final inspection of the root surfaces, the flap is secured and sutured in its original position:
  – Note that this may only be possible if the flap was not mobilized beyond the mucogingival border. Otherwise it will collapse at the alveolar crest.
  – In order to sufficiently close the wound, sometimes coronal displacement of the buccal flap may be necessary, which can be accomplished after dissection of the periosteum at its base.
➤ Suturing:
  – In general, synthetic suture material is preferred. If sutures are placed for 10 to 14 days, monofilament polypropylene or polytetrafluoroethylene is recommended.
  – Interrupted sutures (**Fig. 11.9**) are done, for example, with needle C6, reverse cut, 3/8 circle, atraumatic, 5-0. About six sutures may be placed with one thread of 45 cm.
  – A clockwise double knot (friction knot) is placed first, followed by a counterclockwise single knot and another clockwise single knot on top.
  – If a periodontal dressing is required (see below), all knots should be placed lingually, which makes removal of dressing and sutures easier. Otherwise, all knots should be placed buccally. *Note:* Exposed lingual knots might be disturbing.
  – Horizontal (**Fig. 11.10**) and vertical *mattress sutures* (**Fig. 11.11**) are used to tightly approximate interdental wound margins.
  – Some surgeons prefer *continuous sutures* (**Fig. 11.12**). A C6 needle is used. The suture starts from the anterior region and secures first the buccal flap with tooth-embracing sling sutures. Then, sling sutures secure also the lingual flap. Only one anterior knot is placed.
  – Finally, vertical releasing incisions, if any, are sutured (C3, 5-0).
➤ If needed, a periodontal dressing (CoePak) is placed to protect the surgical site.

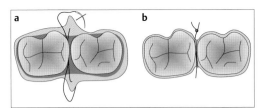

**Fig. 11.9  Simple interrupted suture.**
**a** The flap is secured and sutured in its original position.
**b** If no periodontal dressing is planned, knots are generally placed buccally (lingual placement is very disturbing for the patient's tongue). If a periodontal dressing is to be placed, knots are placed lingually/palatally. For suture removal, the buccal part of the dressing is removed first. Sutures are cut with scissors. The palatal part of the dressing embedding the knots can then easily be removed together with the sutures.

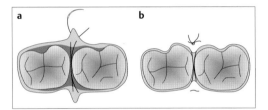

**Fig. 11.10  Horizontal mattress sutures for tight interdental wound approximation.**

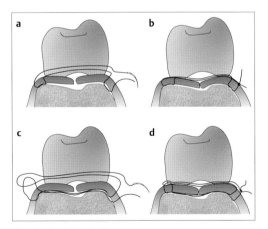

**Fig. 11.11  Vertical mattress sutures.**
**a, b** Simple vertical mattress suture.
**c, d** Vertical mattress suture additionally secured.

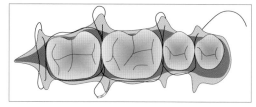

**Fig. 11.12 Continuous suture.** The suture starts in the anterior region of the surgical site in the first buccal papilla. Tooth-embracing sling sutures secure the buccal flap. Continuing distal to the most posterior tooth, the palatal/lingual flap is now also secured with sling sutures. There is only one anterior knot, which is placed buccally.

**Wedge operation.** In cases of thick and fibrotic gingiva of the maxillary tuberosity a distal wedge operation may be indicated, in particular if a distal furcation involvement of the most posterior molar is present (**Fig. 11.13**). Another indication may be surgical crown lengthening of a wisdom tooth or second molar as a pre-prosthetic measure:

➤ Circumcision and removal of a tissue wedge distal to the last tooth.
➤ Sharp preparation and removal of additional palatal and, if needed, buccal wedges (so-called internal gingivectomy).
➤ Careful instrumentation of the root surface, particularly in the distal furcation area.
➤ Tight adaptation of the flaps to the alveolar crest with interrupted sutures (**Fig. 11.9**) or, if the surgical site is more extended, continuous suture (**Fig 11.12**).

## Postoperative Care

A *periodontal dressing* should protect the wound area from chemical, thermal, and mechanical irritation during healing. If interdental wound closure could be achieved, a periodontal dressing is usually not necessary. Further indications may include stabilization of highly mobile teeth and psychological reasons.

A periodontal dressing should have the following properties:
➤ It is easily applied in a soft condition and should set rapidly.
➤ It should be sufficiently firm after setting.
➤ Its surface should be smooth.
➤ It should not interfere with wound healing.
➤ Antimicrobials may be added if necessary.

The following dressings may be used:
➤ CoePak (GC Europe, Leuven, Belgium) is a eugenol-free synthetic dressing, which remains quite soft after setting and has a very smooth and pleasant surface.
➤ Nobetec (Nordiska Dental, Ängelholm, Sweden) is based on zinc oxide and eugenol. After setting, it becomes very firm.
➤ PeriPac (Dentsply, York, Pennsylvania, USA) is based on calcium sulfate and sets after saliva exposure.

Postoperative infection control:
➤ While the usual mechanical oral hygiene measures should be practiced in nonoperated areas, *chemical plaque control* is necessary as long as effective oral hygiene with toothbrushes is compromised in the wound area, that is, for about 4 to 6 weeks.

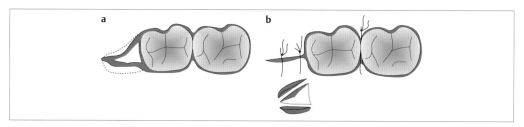

**Fig. 11.13 Distal wedge operation with excision of thick, fibrotic gingiva** (e.g., in the maxillary tuberosity).
**a** A central wedge is first circumcised and removed. The palatal and, if required, also the buccal flap are thinned with the scalpel, which results in further one or two wedges.
**b** After removal of these wedges and thorough root planing, the flaps are tightly approximated to the alveolar crest with circular sutures.

- Mouth rinsing with 0.1 to 0.2% chlorhexidine solution for 1 to 2 minutes, twice daily.
- The patient needs to be informed about possible, usually mild, adverse effects:
  - Black staining of the dorsum of tongue (hairy tongue)
  - Discoloration of teeth and restorations
  - Taste alterations
  - Epithelial desquamation
  - Infrequently, swelling of the parotid glands
➤ *Suture removal* should be scheduled after 7 to 10 days:
  - If a periodontal dressing was placed, a second dressing is usually not necessary.
  - Note that suture removal may be difficult after continuous (**Fig. 11.12**) and secured vertical mattress suture (**Fig. 11.11c, d**).
  - After implantation of foreign material (autogenous bone or bone substitute, membrane for guided tissue regeneration) or root coverage (see below), sutures should remain in place for an extended period. In these cases use of monofilament polypropylene or polytetrafluoroethylene is recommended.
➤ Further *follow-up inspections* should be conducted every second week until re-evaluation after two to three months.

## Critical Assessment

Following healing after flap surgery, the inflammatory infiltrate in the gingiva will be largely reduced in size. The bleeding tendency upon probing attenuates while gingiva shrinks. Some gingival recession may lead to esthetic deficits (**Fig. 11.14**) and dentinal hypersensitivity.

The resistance of the soft tissues to probing pressure increases. The periodontal probe may not be inserted between tooth and gingiva as deeply as before therapy:

➤ Periodontal probing depth is reduced.
➤ Seemingly, (clinical) attachment gain has occurred (**Fig. 11.15**):
  - *Note*: The amount of clinical attachment gain may be related to the number of bony walls of the periodontal lesion (see Chapter 6), that is, the more bony walls, the better the result which may be expected.

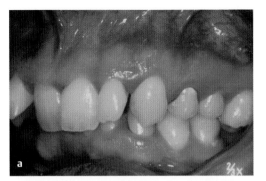
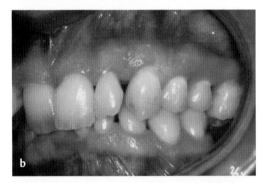
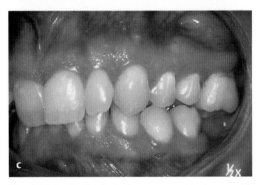

**Fig. 11.14  Particularly in young patients, considerable regeneration after flap surgery may be expected.**
**a** A 28-year-old woman with advanced periodontitis.
**b** Situation 6 weeks after surgical therapy. Considerable recession of the gingiva had occurred. Note in particular loss of the papilla between the lateral incisor and the canine in the maxilla.
**c** Situation after 3 years. Gingiva shows no sign of inflammation. Note complete regeneration of papillae.

  - Considerably more clinical attachment gain may be expected in plaque-free dentitions.

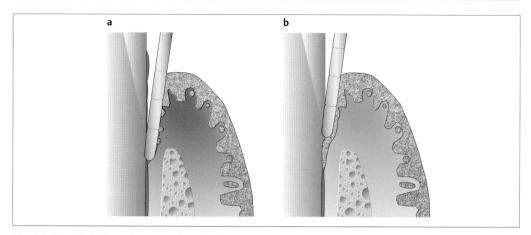

**Fig. 11.15   Clinical attachment gain after flap surgery.**
**a** Situation before surgery. The periodontal probe passes the remnants of junctional epithelium at the bottom of the pocket and is stopped only by the supra-alveolar connective tissue.
**b** After treatment, the inflammatory infiltrate has disappeared. A long junctional epithelium has formed, which attaches to the root surfaces at about the same level as the bottom of the former periodontal lesion. At an appropriate probing force of about 0.25 N, the probe cannot pass the entire long junctional epithelium, suggesting some gain of attachment.

Due to mechanical trauma during surgery, teeth may become more mobile. Usually, tooth mobility decreases gradually during the healing period. By the time of re-evaluation after therapy, teeth should have become at least as firm as before surgery.

Postoperative results after flap surgery may be differentiated as follows:

➤ In shallow pockets up to 3 mm, slight attachment loss may be noted.
➤ In moderately deep pockets of 4 to 6 mm, clinical attachment gain of about 1 mm may be recorded.
➤ Considerable greater clinical attachment gain of more than 2.5 mm, on average, may occur in deep pockets of 7 mm or more (**Fig. 11.16**).[12]

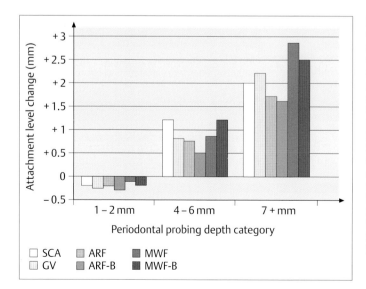

**Fig. 11.16   Average alterations of attachment levels 6 months after treatment.** Results after various treatment modalities. SCA: scaling and root planing; GV: gingivectomy; ARF(-B): apically repositioned flap (with bone recontouring); MWF(-B): modified Widman flap (with bone recontouring). In shallow pockets (up to 3 mm) slight attachment losses were observed. In moderately deep pockets (4–6 mm), attachment gain averaged 0.5 to 1 mm. In deep pockets (7 mm or more), the modified Widman flap performed best with an average attachment gain of more than 2.5 mm. (After Westfelt et al.[12])

➤ After conventional flap surgery, no new *connective tissue attachment* can be expected. Rather, a long epithelial attachment will form in most of the cases, which is not regarded a *locus minoris resistentiae*.[13]

➤ Six to twelve months after surgery, some bone-fill in intrabony lesions may be observed on standardized periapical radiographs (**Fig. 11.17**):

– The more bony walls there are, the more bone-fill may be expected.

– Whether bone-fill actually occurs, strongly depends on a plaque-free dentition (**Fig. 11.18**).[14]

– *Note:* The vast majority of periodontal lesions are associated with largely irreversible horizontal bone loss.

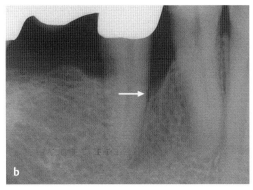

**Fig. 11.17 Bone-fill in deep intrabony pockets.**
**a** Three-wall bony pocket at second premolar, which extends up to the apex.
**b** About 70 % bone-fill 12 months after flap surgery. Tooth remained vital. *Arrows* indicate the bottom of the bony lesion.

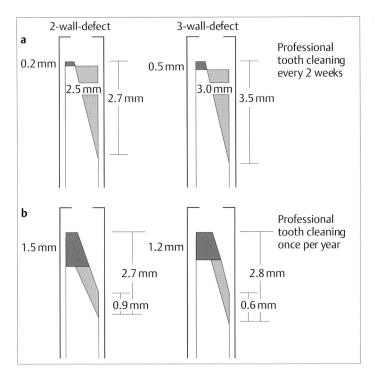

**Fig. 11.18** Bone-fill after flap surgery may be expected mostly in two- and three-wall pockets and in plaque-free dentitions. (After Rosling et al.[14])

**a** After 12 months only slight loss of crestal bone but large fill-in of the bony defect (▨) was observed in individuals with extremely careful plaque control who underwent professional tooth cleaning every two weeks.

**b** In those who underwent yearly check-ups only, virtually no bone-fill was observed, while crestal bone was resorbed (■).

2-wall-defect  3-wall-defect

**a**
0.2 mm  0.5 mm  Professional tooth cleaning every 2 weeks
2.5 mm  3.0 mm
2.7 mm  3.5 mm

**b**
1.5 mm  1.2 mm  Professional tooth cleaning once per year
2.7 mm  2.8 mm
0.9 mm  0.6 mm

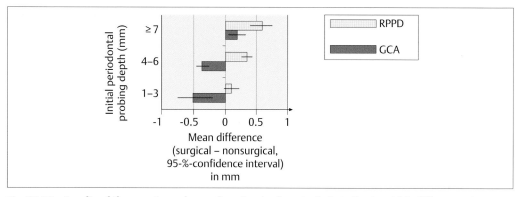

**Fig. 11.19   Results of three meta-analyses of randomized controlled studies in which differences between clinical outcomes of surgical and nonsurgical periodontal therapy were compared.** Mean differences between surgical and nonsurgical periodontal therapy as well as 95% confidence intervals are given. (After Heitz-Mayfield.[15]) Surgical periodontal therapy resulted in greater reduction of periodontal probing depths (RPPD) in moderately deep (4–6 mm) and deep pockets (≥ 7 mm). Greater gains in clinical attachment (GCA) can only be expected in deep pockets of 7 mm or more. After surgery more attachment loss is seen initially in shallow and moderately deep pockets.

An analysis of three systematic reviews on the effects of surgical as compared to nonsurgical debridement of root surfaces by Heitz-Mayfield[15] revealed the following (quality of evidence: moderate):

➤ After 12 months, in general, greater reduction of periodontal probing depth can be expected after periodontal surgery. Quality of evidence: high.
➤ As regards clinical attachment gain, scaling and root planing performs better in shallow and moderately deep pockets, while somewhat greater attachment gain after periodontal surgery may be observed in deep pockets (≥ 7 mm) (**Fig. 11.19**). Quality of evidence: high.

## ■ Periodontal Wound Healing

Until about 30 years ago, the main focus of periodontal therapy was the control of periodontal infection. The major aims of periodontal surgery were to provide *access* to the heavily colonized root surface and to drastically change the *ecology* of the area in such a way as to inhibit bacterial recolonization.

Periodontal lesions treated in that way usually heal with preservation of the anatomical defect, which was caused by the inflammation. Nevertheless, clinical and radiologic alterations are frequently quite impressive and include reduction of periodontal probing depth, gain of clinical attachment, and even some bone-fill in infrabony lesions.

Whether true periodontal *regeneration* has actually occurred can only be assessed *histologically* after biopsy. In humans, this is generally admissible only under experimental conditions and strict observance of ethical principles.

Biological and functional periodontal regeneration means:

➤ Formation of new root cementum (basically acellular extrinsic fiber cementum, see Chapter 1) on a formerly bacterially colonized root surface
➤ Newly formed alveolar bone
➤ Insertion of principal fibers of a new periodontal ligament in either new bone or new cementum

It is well understood that important prerequisites for periodontal regeneration must include the following:

➤ Presence of multipotent progenitor cells
➤ A biocompatible root surface, which has to be re-established
➤ Exclusion of epithelium during wound healing
➤ Stabilization of the wound area

### Presence of Progenitor Cells

Periodontal regeneration requires specific cell activities of progenitor cells (determined stem cells) which have to proliferate, migrate into the wound area, differentiate, and eventually synthesize extracellular matrix components.

Progenitor cells colonizing the periodontal defect should have specific capabilities to form cementum, bone, and periodontal ligament fibers. They are supposed to reside in the remaining periodontal ligament, in the adjacent alveolar bone, and in blood.[16]

### Re-establishment of a Biocompatible Root Surface

An exposed root surface has undergone numerous *pathological alterations* including destruction of Sharpey's fibers which anchor in root cementum, hypermineralization of cementum and/or dentin, and penetration of cementum and, in particular, dentin by toxins or even bacteria. To make a contaminated root surface again biologically acceptable for the organism, certain modifications are necessary:
➤ Scaling and root planing remove bacteria and toxins.
➤ A thorough removal of the smear layer resulting after instrumentation may be achieved by treatment with citric acid, saturated tetracycline solution, or ethylenediaminetetraacetic acid (EDTA).

In **meta-analyses** of 13 and 15 clinical trials by Mariotti[17] in which the effects of chemical root surface modifiers citric acid, tetracycline, or EDTA on periodontal pocket reduction and gain of clinical attachment, respectively, were assessed in patients with chronic periodontitis, no additional pocket reduction or clinical attachment gain could be found. Quality of evidence: low.

### Exclusion of Epithelium

Gingival epithelium is the periodontal tissue with the highest proliferation rate:
➤ Proliferation starts in the initial phase of wound healing along the inner surface of the flap in the apical direction. After about one week the original bottom of the lesion may be reached.
➤ Epithelial cells adhere to the tooth surface by a common epithelial attachment mechanism via hemidesmosomes (see Chapter 1).

➤ *Note*: Epithelium prevents contact between connective tissue and the root surface which may otherwise lead to root resorption.

As has been demonstrated in animal experiments, the various connective tissues of the periodontium exhibit quite different regenerative potentials[18]:
➤ Contact between *gingival connective tissue* and the root surface usually results in *root resorption.*
➤ If *bone tissue* comes into contact with the root surface, *ankylosis* may be the result.
➤ It is assumed that the *periodontal ligament* contains cells which may initiate both cementogenesis and formation of desmodontal fibers.

These observations have ultimately led to the discovery of the biological principle of *guided tissue regeneration*:
➤ Accordingly, the result of any wound healing mainly depends on the kinds of cells which populate the wound area.
➤ For that reason, exclusion of epithelium—for example, by using mechanical barriers such as membranes (see below)—may allow cells from the periodontal ligament to proliferate coronally onto the root surface.

### Wound Stabilization

Healing of an incision wound is a precisely predictable process. Its early (hours) and medium-term (days) events are known in great detail:
➤ Wound healing commences with the immigration of chemotactically attracted cells, which start to clean the wound of any injured and necrotic tissue, foreign material, and microorganisms.
➤ It ends with the production and maturation of extracellular matrix, which bridges the wound margins, supports cells and vessels, and restores resistance to functional strain.
➤ Epithelial cells rapidly bridge the maturing fibrin clot.

Three overlapping wound healing phases may be distinguished (**Fig. 11.20**)[19]:
➤ Early and late *inflammatory phase*:
  – Immigration of neutrophil granulocytes and monocytes which clean the wound from bacteria and traumatized tissues.
  – Macrophages start repair.

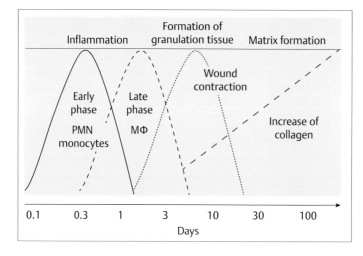

**Fig. 11.20  Three phases characterize wound healing after injury.** In the early inflammatory phase, polymorphonuclear granulocytes (PMNs) and monocytes determine the events, which are subsequently replaced by macrophages (MΦ). Under the influence of growth factors and cytokines, granulation tissue develops which later contracts. Finally, further accumulation of collagen results in tissue maturation and scar formation. (Modified after Kiritsy et al,[19] courtesy of SAGE Publications.)

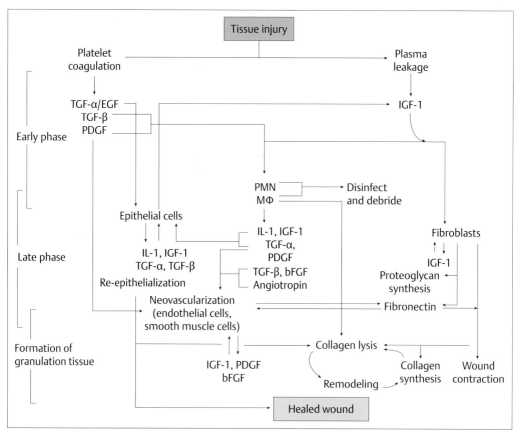

**Fig. 11.21  Interaction between different growth factors and cytokines, which eventually results in wound healing after tissue injury.** (Modified after Kiritsy et al,[19] courtesy of SAGE Publications.) Phases correspond to respective phases in **Fig. 11.20**.

| | | | |
|---|---|---|---|
| TGF | transforming growth factor | MΦ | Macrophage |
| EGF | epidermal growth factor | IL | Interleukin |
| IGF | insulin-like growth factor | PDGF | platelet-derived growth factor |
| PMN | polymorphonuclear granulocyte | bFGF | basic fibroblast growth factor |

➤ Formation of granulation tissue:
  – Mediators released by macrophages (growth factors, cytokines, **Fig. 11.21**) initiate angiogenesis and cell proliferation in the wound area, which result in the formation of granulation tissue.
  – Proliferating cells migrate within the fibrin network and deposit a loose extracellular matrix of collagen, fibronectin, and proteoglycans.
  – The matrix contracts under the influence of cell–cell and cell–matrix contacts.
  – Epithelialization of the wound starts, within hours after injury, from the wound margins. Basal epithelial cells migrate through the fibrin clot.
➤ *Maturation and remodeling* of granulation tissue lead to increasing resistance to functional strain. This phase may last weeks if not several months.

Stabilization of the wound area is the most critical point during initial wound healing after surgery, since the blood clot beneath the flap is rather sensitive to mechanical forces. Disruption of the fibrin clot would lead to apical proliferation of the epithelium.

Wound healing of the periodontium is complicated by several factors:
➤ The mucogingival flap is repositioned against a nonvascular, hypermineralized, firm root surface.
➤ This leads commonly to tear-off of the fibrin clot, usually after a very short period of time.
➤ Subsequent apical proliferation of epithelium prevents regeneration of root cementum and periodontal ligament.

In essence, two complementary concepts govern all therapeutic measures intended to promote periodontal regeneration:
➤ Prevention of apical proliferation of epithelium:
  – Historically, this has been attempted by repeat curettage during wound healing or by excision of gingiva with or without placement of a connective tissue graft. *Note:* The principle has been extended in recent years by Nd:YAG laser application (so-called laser-assisted new attachment procedure, LANAP) with some histological proof of periodontal regeneration.[20,21]

**Table 11.3** Bone and bone replacement grafts

| Graft material | |
| --- | --- |
| Human | • Autogenous grafts<br>  – Extraoral source<br>  – Intraoral source<br>• Allogeneic grafts<br>  – Freeze-dried bone allografts<br>  – Demineralized freeze-dried bone |
| Bone substitutes | • Xenogeneic grafts<br>  – Bovine hydroxyapatite<br>  – Coral calcium carbonate<br>• Alloplastic grafts<br>  – Polymers<br>  – Ceramics<br>• β-tricalcium phosphate<br>• Hydroxyapatite<br>• Bioactive glass |

  – Nowadays, mechanical barriers such as membranes are commonly used.
➤ Stabilization of the fibrin clot:
  – Root conditioning with citric acid, tetracycline, or EDTA (see above).
  – Application of enamel matrix protein (see below).
  – Nonresorbable or resorbable membranes.
  – Autogeneous bone or bone substitutes (**Table 11.3**).
  – Coronal repositioning and fixation of the mucoperiosteal flap.

In future, the principles of *tissue engineering* (**Fig. 11.22**) will be further applied in periodontal regeneration, which may include:
➤ Development of more suitable scaffolds (collagen, bone, bone substitutes)
➤ Addition of desired cells (cell seeding) (e. g., osteoblasts, fibroblasts, cementoblasts, stem cells)
➤ Addition of specific signal molecules such as growth factors, morphogens, and adhesins (see below).

## Bone and Bone Substitutes

Autogeneous bone and bone replacement grafts may have various properties:
➤ *Osteogenesis*: New bone formation by viable osteoblasts contained in the transplanted graft itself.
➤ *Osteoinduction*: Resident progenitor cells in surrounding tissue are induced to form new bone.

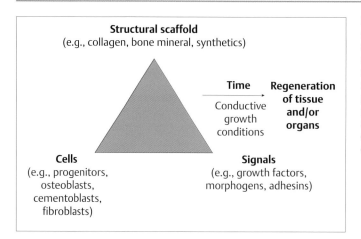

**Structural scaffold**
(e.g., collagen, bone mineral, synthetics)

Time    Regeneration
Conductive    **of tissue**
growth    **and/or**
conditions    **organs**

**Cells**
(e.g., progenitors,
osteoblasts,
cementoblasts,
fibroblasts)

**Signals**
(e.g., growth factors,
morphogens, adhesins)

**Fig. 11.22  Prerequisites for tissue regeneration** are basically suitable scaffolds, as well as the desired cell populations and corresponding signal molecules, for instance PDGF (platelet derived growth factor) or BMPs (bone morphogenetic proteins), in suitable amounts and in correct time succession. (Modified after Lynch,[22] courtesy Quintessence Publishing.)

➤ *Osteoconduction*: Bone formation of already committed cells close to the filling material, which is basically inert and essentially functions as a scaffold.

*Autogeneous bone* (autograft) is mainly osteoconductive and osteoinductive.
➤ However, if vital osteoblasts/bone marrow were transplanted, osteogenesis may be expected.
➤ Autografts are safe; in particular, there is no risk of transmission of infectious disease.
➤ A disadvantage is additional morbidity due to the second extra- or intraoral surgical site.

*Allogeneic graft* (allograft), for example, mineralized/demineralized freeze-dried bone allograft (FDBA, DFDBA), is provided by certified bone banks:
➤ Materials are mainly osteoconductive.
➤ They may also induce bone and cementum formation by differentiation factors in the graft, such as bone morphogenetic proteins (BMPs). Note that the osteoinductive activity of DFDBAs may differ considerably among various bone banks.
➤ *Caution*: Albeit very small, a certain risk of HIV infection and Creutzfeld–Jacob disease may persist. Also, undesired immune reactions cannot entirely be ruled out.

*Alloplastic graft* (alloplasts):
➤ Synthetic materials:
  – Hydroxyapatite (e.g., Ostim, Heraeus Kulzer, Hanau, Germany).

  – β-Tricalcium phosphate (e.g., Cerasorb Dental M, Riemser Dental, Kleinostheim, Germany).
  – Bioactive glasses: amorphous particles of surface reactive glass–ceramic biomaterials containing silicon dioxide, sodium oxide, calcium oxide, and phosphorus pentoxide (e.g., PerioGlas, NovaBone, Jacksonville, Florida, USA). It is claimed that osteoblasts colonize the surface of the particles and replace the slowly resorbing material with bone.
➤ Xenogeneic materials (xenografts):
  – Chemically treated, completely inorganic bovine bone (e.g., Bio-Oss, Geistlich Pharma, Wolhusen, Switzerland). For bone augmentation in combination with resorbable membranes (GBR, guided bone regeneration)
  – Coralline calcium carbonate
➤ *Note:* Alloplastic materials are only osteoconductive. Bone or cementum formation is not induced. They may be used as an inert filler for infrabony lesions. Concerns have been raised that proliferating cells from the periodontal ligament may be blocked. Moreover, difficulties may arise in properly diagnosing persisting periodontal infections.

**Growth and Differentiation Factors**

*Growth factors* are mitogenic polypeptides which locally or systemically influence *growth* and *function* of different cells:
➤ *Autocrine effects*: Growth-factor-secreting cells are themselves stimulated.

> *Paracrine effects*: The numbers of certain target cells and, thus, of their products, are controlled.

*Differentiation factors* control the *phenotype* of certain cells:
> Progenitor cells develop under the influence of differentiation factors into functioning, mature cells.
> For instance, in the presence of BMPs, mesenchymal precursor cells develop into osteoblasts.
> BMPs are members of the TGF-β (transforming growth factor-β) super family: BMP-2, -3, -4, -6 and -7 may induce bone and/or cartilage formation.

Neither growth factors nor BMPs (**Table 11.4**) have so far been approved for periodontal therapy. Currently, genetically engineered human recombinant rhBMP-2 and rhBMP-7 may have an indication in complicated orthopaedic cases. In all likelihood, the structural and functional complexity of periodontal tissues would require high dosages of BMPs owing to diminished responsiveness of tissues in elderly patients and to compensate for rapid clearance from the tissues.

*Platelet-rich plasma* (PRP):
> High concentrations of PDGF (platelet-derived growth factor) and TGF-β may stimulate regeneration of bone and periodontal tissues.
> Both growth factors may be enriched in autologous blood with a cell separator (e.g., ATR Curasan Set, Curasan, Kleinostheim, Germany).
> A **meta-analysis** by Del Fabbro et al[24] concluded that, based on 10 randomized controlled trials in which PRP was used during periodontal surgery including various bone substitutes, PRP resulted in greater gain of clinical attachment in infrabony lesions. Quality of evidence: moderate. The additional application of membranes (see below) was not of advantage. Quality of evidence: high.

## Root Surface Conditioning with Enamel Matrix Proteins

During tooth development, cells of Hertwig's epithelial root sheath (see Chapter 1) secrete enamel matrix proteins (amelogenins). This is one of the basic prerequisites for the formation of acellular extrinsic fiber cementum. A therapeutic approach is to imitate these biological events during development as a means of stimulating periodontal regeneration.[25]

**Table 11.4** Activity of growth and differentiation factors. ++: greatly increased; +: increased; −: no or negative effect. (After Cochran and Wozney[23])

| | Fibroblast proliferation | Pre-osteoblast/ osteoblast proliferation | Extracellular matrix synthesis | Mesenchymal cell differentiation | Vascularization |
|---|---|---|---|---|---|
| Platelet-derived growth factor (PDGF) | ++ | ++ | − | − | + (indirectly) |
| Insulin-like growth factor (IGF) | + | ++ | ++ | − | − |
| Bone morphogenetic proteins (BMPs) | − | +/− | +/− | ++ | ++ (indirectly) |
| Transforming growth factor-β (TGF-β) | +/− | +/− | ++ | − | + (indirectly) |
| Fibroblast growth factor (FGF) | ++ | ++ | − | − | − |

Commercially available enamel matrix proteins for periodontal regeneration are obtained from tooth germs from pigs (Emdogain, Straumann, Basel, Switzerland):

➤ Emdogain is pharmacologically safe and, especially, not immunogenic.
➤ After thorough root debridement during periodontal surgery and removal of the smear layer with a 24% EDTA gel (PrefGel, Straumann), Emdogain is applied to the root surface.

Animal experiments, human biopsies, and controlled clinical studies have produced some promising results[26]:

➤ Formation of cementum on conditioned root surfaces which mostly resembled cellular intrinsic fiber cementum (see Chapter 1).
➤ In clinical experiments, clinical attachment gain was more pronounced after Emdogain application than after conventional flap surgery and may be comparable to results after guided tissue regeneration (**Box 11.1**). Emdogain may have broad indications—for example, infrabony periodontal lesions, furcation involvement, and surgical root coverage.

➤ Emdogain may be combined with synthetic bone substitutes (BoneCeramic, Straumann) for additional tissue support (Emdogain PLUS).
➤ Long-term results point to the stability of the achieved gain of periodontal attachment and bone.

*Caution:* Due to the unclear composition of Emdogain and, in particular, manifold in in vitro studies observed regulatory effects on malignant cells and various factors which are related to carcinogenesis, Emdogain is not recommended in patients with premalignant or malignant oral mucosal lesions.[28]

---

**Box 11.1   Does root conditioning with enamel matrix derivative (Emdogain) during flap surgery in periodontal infrabony defects have any benefits? Do clinical results compare favorably to those after guided tissue regeneration (GTR)?**

Based on meta-analyses of nine randomized controlled trials, Esposito et al[27] concluded:

➤ After 1 year (5-year results were at that time lacking), application of Emdogain resulted in significantly better reduction of periodontal probing depth (average 0.9 mm, 95% confidence interval [CI] 0.44; 1.31) and greater gain of clinical attachment (1.1 mm, 95% CI 0.6; 1.55) than simple flap surgery or in combination with a placebo.
➤ In order to get an idea of the clinical relevance of average values derived from randomized clinical studies, the number of lesions may be calculated which need to be treated to yield one additional clinically relevant treatment outcome (number needed to treat, NNT). If a 2-mm attachment gain is considered clinically relevant, the meta-analysis revealed that nine defects had to be treated with Emdogain to yield one additional attachment gain of 2 mm (NNT = 9).

➤ Because of design issues and large heterogeneity of studies, these results must be interpreted with caution. No data are available as to whether overall tooth prognosis could be improved by the treatment. Quality of evidence: low.
➤ In six studies, application of Emdogain during flap surgery had been compared with technically more demanding GTR. Complications were more often seen when GTR was applied where, in addition, significantly greater recession was observed (average 0.4 mm, 95% CI 0.15; 0.66). Quality of evidence: moderate. However, reduction of probing depth and gain of clinical attachment did not differ. Quality of evidence: low.

When applying minimally invasive surgical techniques, a recent 12-month randomized controlled trial[10] reported excellent clinical results (mean gain of clinical attachment of about 4 mm) regardless whether adjunctive Emdogain was applied or a combination of Emdogain and a bone mineral-derived xenograft.

## ■ Guided Tissue Regeneration

Certain technical tricks have been used to stabilize the wound area and exclude the epithelium during wound healing after periodontal surgery **(Fig. 11.23)**.[29] The procedure is called guided tissue regeneration (GTR), and may employ both nonresorbable and resorbable (biodegradable) membranes (**Table 11.5**).

## Membranes

First generation membranes consisted of expanded polytetrafluoroethylene (ePTFE, Gore-Tex Periodontal Material, Gore, Flagstaff, Arizona, USA) and have long been regarded as the standard for regenerative periodontal therapy by certain practitioners:

➤ They have to be removed in a second surgical operation after 4 to 6 weeks, increasing patients' morbidity.

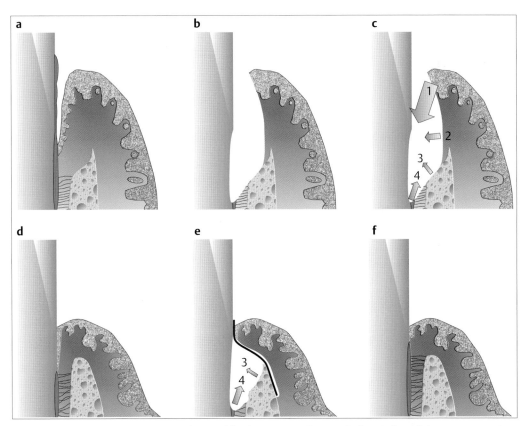

**Fig. 11.23  Current understanding of wound healing events after guided periodontal tissue regeneration.**
**a** Preoperative situation with a bony pocket.
**b** After flap mobilization, granulation tissue is removed and root surface debrided.
**c** Epithelium (1) has the greatest proliferation rate, followed by gingival connective tissue (2).
**d** Therefore, undisturbed wound healing results in a long epithelial attachment, which protects the root surface from contact with cells of the periodontal ligament or bone. Nevertheless, at least in part, bone-fill may take place.
**e** After placement of a mechanical barrier (membrane), cells of alveolar bone (3) and fibroblasts of the periodontal ligament (4) get a chance to colonize the wound area, which is simultaneously protected from tensile forces.
**f** Guided tissue regeneration may thus lead to the formation of new root cementum and functional fiber apparatus of a new periodontal ligament.

**Table 11.5** Requirements of optimum barriers for guided tissue regeneration

| Requirements | Notes |
|---|---|
| Safety | Approval of responsible authorities (US Food and Drug Administration, other national or international administration agencies) |
| Biocompatibility | The material must not be toxic. It must not trigger immunological or inflammatory reactions |
| Tight cervical occlusion | Sutures should be incorporated in the membrane |
| Adaptation to the alveolar bone | |
| Space-making ability | The membrane should not collapse into the defect. Its stiffness should adequately stabilize the wound area |
| Tissue integration | Connective tissue should be able to grow into the structured outer surface of the membrane |
| Permeability | Tissue fluids and growth factors should reach the root surface |
| Functional period | At least 6 weeks. Longer resorption time may be advantageous |
| Easy handling | Suitable configuration and pre-cuts |

➤ If exposed to the oral cavity, the membrane was rapidly colonized by bacteria which considerably increased the risk for infection.
➤ The membrane tended to collapse into the defect. Titanium-reinforced membranes facilitated better space-keeping and might even have allowed regeneration of horizontal bone loss.
➤ While the previous main distributor of transgingival and submerged membranes for guided tissue and bone regeneration (Gore Medical) has meanwhile terminated production and marketing, similar alternatives have become available again (e. g., Cytoplast, Osteogenics, Lubbock, Texas, USA).

Resorbable membranes make a second operation for removal unnecessary. Clinical results obtained with resorbable membranes were very similar to those achieved with nonresorbable membranes (see below). Currently, membranes from natural products as well as synthetic material are available:
➤ Xenogeneic membranes (e. g., Bio-Gide, Geistlich Pharma, or Ossix, OraPharma, Warminster, Pennsylvania, USA) which consist of collagen from porcine tendons (xenograft). Cross-linking technology may lead to functional integrity for about 4 to 6 months.
➤ Polyglycolide, polylactide, and copolymers of these aliphatic polyesters. The Guidor Matrix Barrier (Sunstar, Chicago, Illinois, USA)

consists of biocompatible and safe bioresorbable polylactic acid blended with a citric acid ester. A special design facilitates sufficient stiffness of the membrane and allows tissue integration and fluid flow. Adequate function has been documented for up to 6 months.

**Indications**

Guided tissue regeneration is intended to lead to considerable alteration of the local morphology of certain periodontal defects. As an overall result, both function and prognosis of the tooth should be improved as well. Outcome after GTR largely depends on operator skills and strict adherence to possible indications. As regards attachment gain, certain periodontal lesions may respond considerably better to GTR than to conventional treatment modalities, for example:
➤ Two- and three-wall bony pockets, at least 4 mm deep[30]
➤ Buccal and lingual degree II furcation involvement of mandibular molars
➤ Discrete buccal (possibly mesial) degree II furcation involvement of maxillary molars
➤ Bony defects after surgical removal of impacted wisdom teeth
➤ Deep Miller class I or II gingival recessions

## Contraindications

General contraindications include:
➤ Systemic diseases that make operative risk unjustifiably high
➤ Insufficient oral hygiene
➤ Excessive smoking

Specific contraindications relate to unfavorable defect morphology:
➤ Horizontal bone loss and one-wall bony lesions
➤ Various osseous lesions around multirooted teeth (see below):
  – Incipient (degree I) furcation involvement
  – Through-and-through (degree III) furcation involvement
  – Degree II involvement of distal furcations of maxillary molars
  – Furcation involvement of premolars and wisdom teeth (there might be reasonable exceptions)
➤ Miller class III or IV gingival recession
➤ Periodontally diseased teeth with a hopeless prognosis:
  – Teeth which lack remaining periodontal ligament for desired proliferation (note that there might be reasonable exceptions[31])
  – Teeth with excessive tooth mobility which might interfere with wound healing
  – Teeth without clinical relevance

## Procedure

*Note:* Whenever regenerative periodontal and mucogingival surgical measures (see below) are planned, microsurgical instruments (**Fig. 11.24** and **Table 11.6**) and scalpel blades, special suture material (ePTFE, Gore Medical; or monofilament suture material of sizes 6-0 or 7-0) as well as magnifying loupes and, if necessary, an operative microscope (**Fig. 11.25**) are recommended. The surgeon should strive for maximum soft tissue preservation for complete membrane coverage:
➤ Disinfection
➤ Local anesthesia
➤ Incision:
  – Strictly intracrevicular incision
  – Depending on the available interdental space, preparation of a modified (**Fig. 11.26**) or simplified papilla preservation flap (**Fig. 11.27**)
  – Vertical releasing incision should be avoided. If needed, only one releasing incision about one tooth-width lateral to the defect is placed.
➤ Mobilization of a full-thickness, mucoperiosteal flap. Complete disclosure of the defect.
➤ Removal of any granulation tissue.
➤ Thorough scaling and root planing. If applicable, root conditioning with citric acid, saturated tetracycline solution, or EDTA.

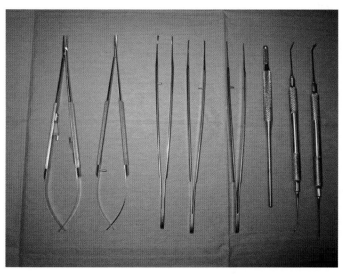

**Fig. 11.24 Microsurgical instruments.** From *left* to *right*: Microsurgical needle holder, scissors, three microsurgical pliers, micro scalpel holder, papilla elevator, dissector (see **Table 11.6**).

**Table 11.6** Microsurgical instruments for guided tissue regeneration or surgical root coverage

| Instruments | Description | Article no., manufacturer |
|---|---|---|
| Scalpel holder for micro blades | For mounting micro blades, e.g.,<br>• lancet<br>• curved<br>• round | 871MH/6, Carl Martin<br>• 871MB/65<br>• 871MB/67<br>• 871MB/71 |
| Papilla elevator | For atraumatically raising the papilla while preserving its anatomy | 1031, Carl Martin |
| Periodontal dissector | Atraumatic dissection of tissue layers<br>• Soft tissue preparation<br>• Harvesting connective tissue grafts | 1121, Carl Martin |
| Microsurgical tissue pliers | • Curved surgical micro-tweezer, 0.8 mm wide, 18 cm long<br>• Straight surgical micro-tweezer, 0.8 mm wide, 18 cm long<br>• Straight anatomical micro-tweezer, 0.8 mm wide, 18 cm long | • 787A/18, Carl Martin<br><br>• 787/18, Carl Martin<br><br>• 781/18, Carl Martin |
| Microsurgical scissors | • Micro tissue scissors, 18 cm<br>• Micro suture scissors, 18 cm | • 855A/18, Carl Martin<br>• 855/18, Carl Martin |
| Needle holder | • Micro needle holder, diamond coated, 18 cm | • 1171DI/18, Carl Martin |
| Suturing material holder | • Micro suturing material holder, 18 cm | • 1171/18, Carl Martin |

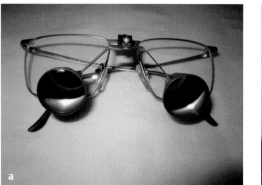
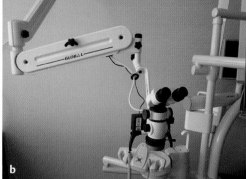

**Fig. 11.25   Magnifying aids.**
**a** Magnification loupes with Galilean ocular lenses and 2.5 times magnification. The working distance is 30 to 50 cm and the visual field 10 to 13 cm. Despite the possible advantages of higher magnification, limited visual field and shallow depth of field have to be considered.
**b** Operative microscope. When selecting a suitable microscope, maneuverability has to be taken into account so that, for example, posterior regions can be properly seen as well.

➤ Selection of an appropriate membrane, which is trimmed according to the bony defect. The membrane should completely cover the defect and overlap the bone margins by about 2 mm (**Fig. 11.28**). The membrane is tightly fixed at neighboring teeth with sling sutures.

➤ The flap is coronally advanced after careful dissection of the periosteum at its base.
➤ Primary closure of the interdental space and tension-free fixation of the flap over the membrane by using horizontal and vertical mattress sutures (**Figs. 11.26** and **11.27**).

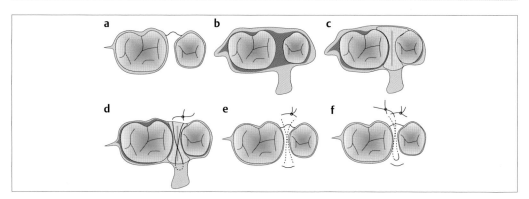

**Fig. 11.26   Modified papilla preservation technique.**[8]
**a** Semilunar incision to preserve the palatal papilla.
**b** Lingual mobilization of the papilla.
**c** A titanium-reinforced membrane is trimmed and placed over the defect. Subsequently, the buccal periosteum is dissected at the base of the buccal flap to allow its tension-free advancement.
**d** A horizontal, internal crossed mattress suture is first placed beneath the mucoperiosteal flap between the base of the palatal papilla and the buccal flap.
**e, f** The interproximal tissue can then be fixed, without any tension, with a second, vertical mattress suture.

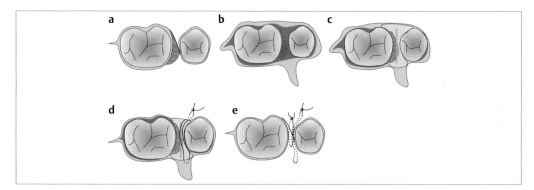

**Fig. 11.27   The simplified papilla preservation flap**[9] is particularly recommended in cases where interdental space is narrow (e.g., at anterior teeth) and where there is an intrabony lesion at one tooth only.
**a** An oblique incision starts at the buccal line angle of the involved tooth to reach the mid-interproximal portion of the papilla of the adjacent tooth.
**b** A full-thickness flap is raised.
**c** The membrane is trimmed and placed over the defect. The buccal periosteum is dissected at the base of the buccal flap to allow its tension-free advancement.
**d** An offset internal horizontal mattress suture is positioned running from the base of the keratinized tissue at the midbuccal aspect of the noninvolved tooth to a symmetrical location at the base of the lingual/palatal flap. The suture rubs against the interproximal root surface, hangs on the residual interproximal bone crest, and is anchored to the lingual/palatal flap.
**e** Primary closure is obtained by one or two interrupted sutures or vertical mattress suture, depending on available space.

Note that sutures have to be left in place for an extended period.
➤ Additional interrupted sutures with finer suturing material (6-0) are used to approximate wound margins.

*Note:* In general, GTR has successfully been combined with autogenous bone grafts or bone allografts.

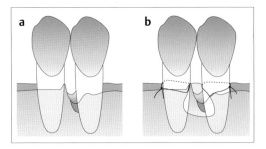

**Fig. 11.28   A trimmed membrane is placed over a combined one-, two-, and three-wall bony lesion and fixed to the neighboring teeth.**

## Postoperative Care

The patient has to be briefed about the delicate wound healing processes. The usual postoperative infection control measures apply:

➤ Mouth rinses twice daily with a 0.1 to 0.2% chlorhexidine solution for about 4 to 6 weeks. Toothbrushing must be avoided in the surgically treated area.

➤ During the first 2 weeks, wound healing should be checked every second or third day. If necessary, supragingival plaque at the gingival margin is carefully removed.

➤ If the membrane is exposed, the patient should apply a 1% chlorhexidine gel twice daily. *Note*: Secondary surgical coverage should never be performed.

➤ Antibiotics are not routinely prescribed.

Sutures should be removed after 4 to 6 weeks. If a nonresorbable membrane had been implanted, it has to be surgically removed after 4 to 6 weeks:

➤ Intracrevicular incision after local anesthesia and mobilization of a small mucoperiosteal flap

➤ Cutting of the sling suture and removal of the membrane with tissue tweezers

➤ Careful removal of granulation tissue at the inner surface of the flap with a universal curette

➤ Repositioning and fixation of the flap with interdental sutures

➤ If complete coverage is not possible, placement of a free gingival graft should be considered to protect the regenerated tissue.

## Critical Assessment

The dentist should take care not to foster unrealistically high expectations on the part of the patient. Guided tissue regeneration is generally not intended to save "hopeless" teeth. Currently, the role of GTR in daily practice is rather limited:

➤ The technique is quite complicated.

➤ Postoperative results depend very much on operator skills.

➤ The range of indications is very limited. For example, infrabony lesions should have a minimum depth of about 4 mm in order to show advantage as compared to conventional flap surgery.[30] Treatment of furcations is largely confined to mandibular molars with degree II involvement.

From a biological point of view, wound healing processes, mostly reparative, are initiated that are not really predictable. In many cases, cellular intrinsic fiber cementum (see Chapter 1) without functional importance is formed. Moreover, newly formed cementum may be loosely deposited and insufficiently attached to the root surface.

Nevertheless, favorable results have been reported in numerous case reports (**Fig. 11.29**) and clinical investigations (**Fig. 11.30**).

*Note:* With resorbable membranes, basically the same clinical results can be achieved as with nonresorbable membranes.

Based on **meta-analyses** of randomized controlled trials,[33] additional gains of clinical attachment, which may have been expected after GTR, were rather low, on average about 1.2 mm (**Box 11.2**).

➤ To achieve maximum effects in an individual case, the following guidelines should be strictly observed:
  – Careful patient selection.
  – Only suitable periodontal defects should be considered; for example, three- or two-wall bony lesions, certain lesions in furcations
  – Employment of magnifying aids (see above)
  – Improved surgical techniques; for example, modified or simplified papilla preservation techniques

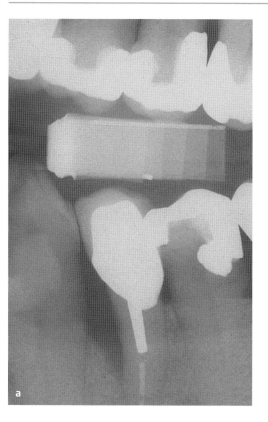

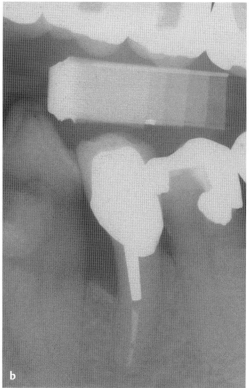

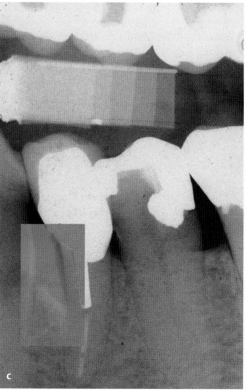

**Fig. 11.29   Result after regenerative periodontal therapy.**

**a** Three-wall infrabony ("intrabony") lesion at tooth 34. Guided tissue regeneration was performed using a nonresorbable ePTFE membrane.

**b** Situation 3 years after surgery. Bone-fill of about 70%.

**c** Subtraction radiography (see **Figs. 6.17** and **6.18**).

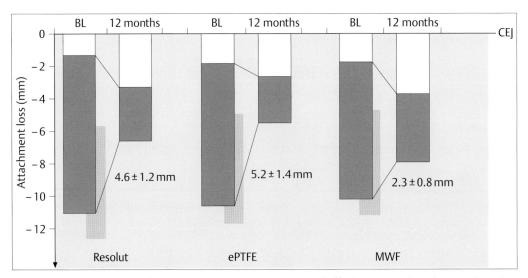

**Fig. 11.30 Controlled clinical trial comparing postoperative results**[32] after 12 months in bony pockets after using synthetic resorbable (Resolut) and nonresorbable membranes (ePTFE) for guided tissue regeneration (GTR) and conventional access flap operations (modified Widman flap, MWF). Excellent comparable attachment gain of up to about 5 mm was observed after GTR, particularly in bony pockets (■). Considerably less favorable results of slightly more than 2 mm attachment gain were calculated, on average, after conventional flap surgery. ePTFE membranes resulted in somewhat less recession (□). ■: Periodontal probing depth.

– *Note:* While microsurgical principles have been suggested, covering a membrane after periosteal dissection basically contradicts these principles.

Meaningful long-term results of randomized controlled trials on GTR, which should include patient-tangible variables like undesired side effects, cost–benefit ratio, and esthetic results, are largely missing. Due to the increased unavailability of patients for follow-up over an extended period, often no definitive conclusions can be drawn. Therefore, it is still not clear whether the prognosis for keeping a certain tooth in the oral cavity can actually be improved by GTR.

*Note:* Evidence from numerous clinical studies (**Box 11.2**) have had a rather negative impact on GTR as a routine measure in periodontal practice. Notably, the main provider of transgingival and submerged membranes for GTR (Gore Medical) has ceased manufacture and distribution after 25 years.

**Box 11.2   Does guided tissue regeneration (GTR) have any benefits as compared to conventional flap surgery in the treatment of periodontal infrabony defects?**

When assessing the efficacy of GTR in the treatment of periodontal infrabony defects as compared to conventional access flap surgery in terms of clinical, radiographic, and patient-centered outcomes after at least 1 year follow-up, Needleman et al[33] identified 16 randomized controlled trials in which GTR was tested alone and two studies in which the combination of GTR and bone substitutes were applied. The authors concluded the following:

➤ Regardless of whether bone substitutes were additionally applied or not, the mean difference in clinical attachment gain between GTR and access flap was 1.22 mm (95 % confidence interval [CI] 0.80; 1.64). Quality of evidence: low.

➤ Likewise, regardless of whether bone substitutes were additionally applied, greater mean reduction of periodontal probing depth of 1.21 mm (95 % CI 0.53; 1.88) was observed in defects treated with GTR. Quality of evidence: low.

➤ Moreover, GTR resulted in significantly less recession (mean 0.26 mm, 95 % CI 0.08; 0.43). Quality of evidence: moderate.

➤ As compared to conventional access flap, eight patients need to be treated with GTR to achieve one additional site with a clinically relevant attachment gain of 2 mm (NNT = 8). Quality of evidence: moderate.

➤ In some studies, hard tissue probing at surgical re-entry operations were done, which unanimously confirmed favorable results after GTR with or without bone substitutes.

➤ Except for increased treatment time with GTR, adverse effects were generally minor. Reasons for considerable variability of results in certain studies are not clear. Whether GTR improves long-term prognosis of diseased teeth has not been studied in any trial.

## ■ Minimally Invasive Surgical Techniques

Minimally invasive surgical techniques (MIST) for periodontal regeneration have become increasingly popular during the past decade.[34] In particular, after a long period of implanting membranes for GTR, for which extensive mucoperiosteal flaps had to be elevated and the periosteum dissected for achieving tight wound closure, it was realized that minimal flap elevation and gentler handling of soft and hard tissue might be important aspects of primary wound closure and blood clot protection; perhaps as important as exclusion of epithelial downgrowth and wound stabilization by mechanical means. A pivotal step in the development of minimally invasive periodontal surgery has been the description of modified and simplified papilla preservation flap designs (MPPF, SPPF; **Figs. 11.26** and **11.27**).

➤ Minimally invasive surgical techniques require magnifying aids as loupes or operative microscopes, microsurgical instruments, and mini-curettes as well as suture material of sizes 6-0 to 8-0.

➤ Despite the description of various closely related flap designs and treatment procedures under slightly different names, as a general rule flaps should be elevated only as required by defect morphology and intended treatment approach; for example, root conditioning with enamel matrix proteins and/ or placement of bone grafts.

➤ This may mean, in certain cases, elevation of just a tiny triangular buccal flap (modified MIST) if access to an interproximal infrabony lesion would be facilitated through that buccal "window."[35] Note that the lesion is not accessed from the lingual/palatal aspect.

– Any granulation tissue filling the defect is sharply dissected from the interdental supracrestal connective tissue of the interdental papilla, which is still in place.

– The root surface is debrided with mini-curettes.

– Emdogain can be applied to the root surfaces and the defect may be filled with bone or bone substitutes (see above).
– An internal horizontal mattress suture (**Fig. 11.26**) secures the buccal flap. Further sutures may be applied if needed.

Based on a **systematic review** of clinical studies employing various minimally invasive periodontal surgical approaches, Cortellini[34] made the following recommendations:
➤ Surgical access to the interdental papilla associated with the infrabony defects:
  – MPPF (**Fig. 11.26**) is chosen whenever the width of the interdental space is greater than 2 mm.
  – SPPF (**Fig. 11.27**) is used if the interdental space is less than 2 mm.
➤ Flap design:
  – Modified MIST is suggested whenever a defect involves one or two sides of a root only and can be debrided from a tiny buccal window.
  – If the interproximal infrabony defect cannot be debrided from a buccal window, an ordinary MIST approach should be performed.
  – If the bony defect involves three or four sides of a root, an extended papilla preservation flap extending to the neighboring teeth is raised and, if needed, periosteal dissection for coronal advancement is done.
➤ Regenerative material to be applied:
  – In case of a modified MIST approach, no regenerative material or Emdogain may be applied.
  – In a MIST approach, in mainly three-wall defects, only Emdogain may be applied, while in one- to two-wall defects, Emdogain may be combined with bone substitutes.
➤ Suturing approach:
  – When MIST or modified MIST is applied, a single internal horizontal mattress suture should suffice to secure the tiny buccal flap.
  – To secure extended MPPF and SPPF, an internal horizontal mattress suture is applied followed by a vertical mattress suture or circular suture to secure the papilla (**Figs. 11.26** and **11.27**).

*Critical remark:* Neither Emdogain alone[36] nor bone substitutes seem to yield additional effects. So, as regards clinical attachment gain in minimally invasive periodontal surgery,[35] miniature flaps of modified MIST, in particular at single-rooted teeth, may be postponed since the lesions are usually accessible for scaling and root planing. Preferably, before planning further regenerative treatment, the therapist should wait for final healing results including bone-fill after thorough nonsurgical therapy of infrabony lesions (see **Fig. 10.9**).

## ■ Treatment of Furcation-Involved Teeth

Because of difficulties in accessing the furcation area, with its bizarre and often unforeseeable structures, treatment of furcation-involved teeth has always been a challenge. Furcation involvement indeed drastically impairs the prognosis of a multirooted tooth.

Dependent on tooth type, the degree of furcation involvement, and several patient factors such as course/expression of periodontal disease, patient's age, and condition of health, compliance, as well as preferences and values, different treatment modalities may be indicated:
➤ *Conservative treatment*, that is, mechanical instrumentation of bacterially colonized root surfaces with or without osteoplasty.
➤ *Resective procedures* such as root amputation, hemisection, premolarization, or tunnel procedures
➤ *Periodontal regeneration*

### Fundamental Morphological Terms

The *anatomic root complex* (**Fig. 11.31**)[37] is that part of a tooth which is located apical to the cementoenamel junction.
➤ The *root cone* is a constant morphological unit. At a given level, a root is classified as either *not separated*, meaning connected to one or more other root cones; or *separated* from one or more other root cones.
➤ The root complex of maxillary molars consists of three *root components* while that of mandibular molars is composed of two.

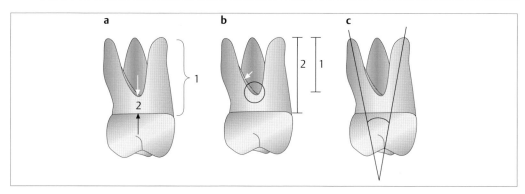

**Fig. 11.31　Anatomic root complex.**
**a** The root complex (1) is that part of the tooth which is located apical to the cementoenamel junction. The root trunk (2) is the part of the root complex that extends from the cementoenamel junction to the furcation entrance.
**b** Degree of separation: The maximum furcoapical extension (1) in relation to the maximum cervicoapical extension (2) of the root complex. Complete separation of the roots (○) by furcation; incomplete separation (*arrow*) by a root groove.
**c** Degree of divergence.

*Note:* Each root component is composed of two or a maximum of three root cones. The *root trunk* is that part of the root complex which is located coronal to the furcation (**Fig. 11.31a**).

➤ Complete (furcation) and incomplete (root groove) *separation structures* may be differentiated. The transitional area between the mainly vertical and the mainly horizontal part of the furcation is called the *furcation entrance.* The furcation's roof is called the *fornix.*

➤ The *separation degree* between two roots or root cones is the maximum furcal–apical extent in relation to the maximum cervical–apical extent of the root complex (**Fig. 11.31b**).

➤ The *degree of divergence* is the angle formed by the cervical half of the long axes of two root cones or roots (**Fig. 11.31c**).

## Structures within the Furcation

As a product of separated enamel organs derived from Hertwig's epithelial root sheet, paraplastic enamel formation may have occurred in the area of the furcation entrance during tooth development, which may promote bacterial proliferation and should therefore be removed:

➤ Enamel projections, which may be classified according to length:
  – Class I: small extensions not extending beyond the root trunk

  – Class II: medium-sized spurs extending up to the furcation entrance
  – Class III: lancetlike projections extending into the furcation
➤ Enamel islands, drops, and pearls

*Cellular mixed stratified cementum* (CMSC) is the common cementum variety (see Chapter 1) in the furcation area. A variably high ridge of CMSC may be seen in the furcation of two-rooted premolars. In the furcation of mandibular molars a central, mesiodistal cementum bulge is found, while at maxillary molars, the cementum bulge is T-shaped.

The bizarre microrelief in the furcation with its depressions and niches, accessory pulp channels, and blind openings may promote bacterial proliferation.

## Conservative Furcation Therapy

Instrumentation of root surfaces in the furcation area is often performed during flap operations. The following instruments may be used:

➤ Curettes (e. g., Columbia 4 R/4 L, or Langer 17/18)
➤ Special furcation curettes (e. g., SQMD 16, SQBL 16, Hu Friedy; **Fig. 11.32**)
➤ In certain cases Hirschfeld periodontal files
➤ Ultrasonic and sonic scalers

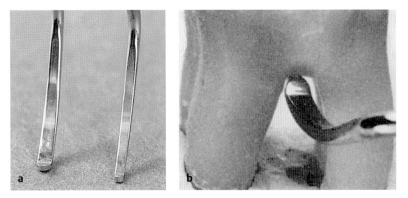

**Fig. 11.32 Special furcation curettes after Quétin.**
**a** 1.3 mm (SQBL 26) and 0.9 mm wide (SQBL 16, Hu-Friedy)
**b** Instrumentation of the furcation fornix. For mesial and distal root surfaces in the furcation, respective furcation curettes (SQMD 26 and SQMD 16) are available as well.

Indication:

➤ Degree I or incipient degree II furcation involvement.
➤ In case of enamel projections or pearls, odontoplasty with fine (40 µm) and extra-fine (15 µm) diamond-coated rotating burs (Perio-Set, Intensiv, Montagnola, Switzerland, see Chapter 10). *Caution:* Use of diamond-coated burs in the furcation may lead to undesired and uncontrolled damage of the root surface and should not be used for routine root debridement.

*Note*: In any case of advanced furcation involvement (degrees II and III), conservative measures may only result in transient improvement of the situation. In particular, horizontal attachment gain should not be expected after conventional (conservative) treatment because of poor access to the furcation area and rapid bacterial recolonization.

**Root Amputation and Hemisection**

Resective measures such as root amputation and hemisection are mainly performed to preserve a strategically important molar. Definitions:

➤ *Root amputation:* The removal of one or several roots while preserving most parts of the crown. It is mainly confined to maxillary molars.
➤ *Hemisection:* The removal of a root together with the corresponding crown portion. It is usually done in mandibular molars.

The range of *indications* is wide and not limited to periodontal disease:

➤ *Periodontal indications:* Degree II and III furcation involvement, particularly of first and second molars.
➤ *Endodontic indications:*
  – Obstructed root canal inaccessible to instrumentation
  – Post and core which cannot be removed
➤ *Iatrogenic indications:*
  – Fractured endodontic instrument which cannot be removed from the root canal
  – Class IV root perforation; that is, perforation into the furcation area
  – Class II root perforation; that is, intra-alveolar perforation within the middle root third.
➤ *Other indications* include intractable root caries in the furcation area and, in rare cases, fractional extraction during orthodontic treatment.

Careful *treatment planning* is mandatory. Resective measures should never be conducted ad hoc. Proper endodontic treatment should be performed in due time before the planned resection. Roots which are to be kept should definitively be root-filled. The root which is to be removed may receive a temporary root filling with $Ca(OH)_2$. In order to avoid leakage, the coronal part of the temporary filling in the root to be removed should be replaced by composite resin. When the root is later removed, the cut is made within the composite (see below).

Procedure for *root amputation* (**Fig. 11.33**):

➤ Disinfection
➤ Local anesthesia

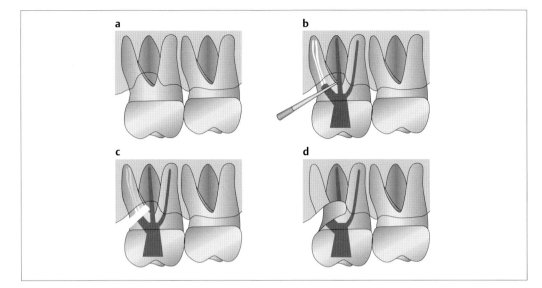

**Fig. 11.33   Root amputation.**
**a** Advanced buccal–mesial furcation involvement of a maxillary first molar. The mesial root is to be removed.
**b, c** Definitive endodontic treatment of the distal and palatal root canal; temporary filling with Ca(OH)$_2$ in both mesial canals. Composite resin should be placed in the coronal part of the mesial root. After flap mobilization and removal of the granulation tissue, the mesial root is separated with a needle-shaped diamond bur from the remaining tooth within the composite to avoid leakage. Cooling with sterile saline is mandatory.
**d** After careful osteotomy the root can easily be removed with a small luxating elevator or root pliers. The amputation area should be smoothened.

➤ Mobilization of a mucoperiosteal flap to disclose the whole furcation area
➤ Removal of all granulation tissue
➤ Separation of the root with a needle-shaped diamond-coated bur:
  – Continuous cooling with saline. Note: the root complex that is intended to be kept and neighboring teeth must not be damaged.
  – The definitive separation of the root from the remaining root complex is usually done with a periosteal or thin luxating elevator. The patient should be informed in advance about the cracking sound.
➤ Removal of the root with luxating elevator or root pliers.
➤ If required, osteoplasty with Schluger's bone file or universal curette.
➤ Smoothing of the amputation area with fine (40 µm) and extrafine (15 µm) diamond-coated burs under continuous cooling.
➤ Careful scaling and root planing of the now largely visible furcation area.

➤ The flap is then repositioned. If necessary, it may slightly be advanced after dissecting the periosteum at its base. Flap margins are approximated and secured with interrupted sutures.
➤ In any case, a periodontal dressing (CoePak) is placed.

The usual postoperative care is provided and chemical plaque control established (e.g., twice-daily mouth rinses with 0.1–0.2% chlorhexidine solution).

After proper healing, restorative treatment is scheduled. Depending on the amount and shape of the remaining tooth substance, in most cases a full or partial crown is indicated. If the tooth was caries-free, a small occlusal restoration may suffice.

Procedure for *hemisection* of mandibular molars (**Fig. 11.34**):
➤ Disinfection
➤ Local anesthesia
➤ Immediately before flap mobilization, the crown portion of the tooth should be sepa-

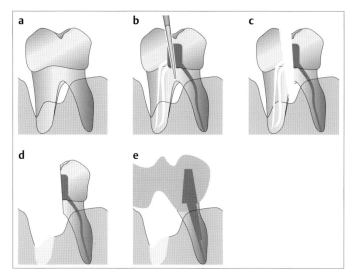

**Fig. 11.34 Hemisection of a mandibular molar.**
**a** Advanced furcation involvement of a mandibular first molar. The mesial root is to be removed.
**b** Root canal therapy. Temporary root canal filling of the mesial canals with $Ca(OH)_2$. Before mobilization of a mucoperiosteal flap, the crown portion of the tooth has to be separated as far as the floor of the pulp chamber.
**c** Final separation of the tooth (at the expense of the part to be extracted).
**d** The root is removed with root pliers.
**e** A fixed dental prosthesis is incorporated.

rated with a needle-shaped diamond bur as far as the floor of the pulp chamber. Carry out generous separation at the expense of the root to be extracted. The cutting direction may be indicated by a straight periodontal probe inserted into the furcation.
➤ A mucoperiosteal flap is mobilized.
➤ Further separation of the tooth with the diamond-coated bur:
  – Continuous and sufficient cooling with saline.
  – Definitive separation of the root from the remainder of the tooth is accomplished with a periosteal or small luxation elevator. Again, the patient should be informed in advance about the cracking sound.
➤ The root and the corresponding part of the crown can now be extracted with root pliers.
➤ All granulation tissue is removed and root surfaces are thoroughly scaled and root-planed.
➤ The cut tooth surface is smoothed with fine (40 µm) and extrafine (15 µm) diamond-coated burs under continuous cooling with saline.
➤ Flap margins are secured with interrupted sutures.
➤ A periodontal pack (CoePak) is placed.

The usual postoperative care is provided and chemical plaque control established (e. g., twice-daily mouth rinses with 0.1–0.2 % chlorhexidine solution).

Restorative treatment may be scheduled after about three months. Depending on the remaining crown substance, the distal root might need post and core. A fixed dental prosthesis with the hemisectioned tooth as abutment may be incorporated. In some cases, the remainder of the tooth may serve as abutment for a single crown.

Critical assessment:
➤ Resective measures do not improve the prognosis of the tooth per se.
➤ Technical problems, which may often emerge during restorative treatment, do affect the long-term prognosis of a root-resected tooth. Examples are:
  – Errors in endodontic treatment with immediate loss of the tooth (e. g., root fracture, perforation)
  – Endodontic errors that carry a risk of late complications (e. g., insufficient instrumentation, insufficient quality of root canal filling)
  – Loss of retention of the restoration
➤ *Note*: The individual risks of each treatment step multiply. The total failure risk may largely increase with the number of procedures. Long-term tooth preservation can only be expected if each treatment step has been performed correctly.

## Premolarization

Premolarization can only be performed—and then rarely—in mandibular molars.

Indications:
➤ Degree II or III furcation involvement of mandibular first molars in which proximal bone has largely been preserved.
➤ Important prerequisites are root divergence of more than 30° and a separation degree of three-quarters or more (**Fig. 11.31**).

Procedure:
➤ After successful root canal treatment, the tooth is separated with a needle-shaped diamond-coated bur.
➤ If required, post and core is fabricated for the distal root. Thereafter single crowns are incorporated on either root.
➤ If the tooth is the most posterior tooth and the space between the roots is narrow, a small fixed partial denture may be incorporated after further orthodontic distalizing the distal root.

## Tunnel Preparation

The furcation entrance may be surgically opened to enable the patient to perform daily toothbrushing of the area. Prerequisites are:
➤ Excellent oral hygiene.
➤ Low caries susceptibility. It may make sense to assess oral load of mutans streptococci and lactobacilli as well as salivary flow rate and buffering capacity with appropriate chairside tests (e.g., CRT, Ivoclar Vivadent, Schaan, Liechtenstein) before scheduling the patient for tunnel preparation.
➤ Periodical recall and excellent compliance.

Indications:
➤ Advanced degree II or III furcation involvement of mandibular first molars.
➤ Divergence of more than 30° and separation degree of more than three-quarters.

Contraindications:
➤ Low degrees of either divergence or separation.
➤ High caries susceptibility. *Caution*: If root caries occurs in the furcation area, the tooth is usually doomed and should be extracted.

➤ Any doubt about compliance of the patient.

Procedure for tunnel preparation on mandibular molars (**Fig. 11.35**):
➤ Disinfection
➤ Local anesthesia
➤ Incisions:
  – Intracrevicular incision on the buccal aspect. Two vertical releasing incisions may demarcate the surgical site at a distance of about half of a tooth's width mesial and distal to the treated tooth.
  – Lingually, a 0.5 mm paramarginal incision is made but vertical incisions are avoided in order not to injure the lingual nerve.
➤ Elevation of a mucoperiosteal flap. Buccally, the flap is mobilized beyond the mucogingival border, lingually up to the bone crest.
➤ All granulation tissue in the furcation area is removed. To widen the furcation entrance for interdental brushes, often some bone has to be removed (ostectomy), preferably with bone files (**Fig. 11.36**):
  – Smaller Sugarman files (FS 1/26) are used in the beginning, followed by larger Schluger files (FS 9/10S 6, Hu-Friedy).
  – Bone may also be removed by rose head burs in a reducing hand piece. Sufficient cooling with saline is mandatory.
➤ Scaling and root planing:
  – Careful removal of any bacterial deposits
  – Complete removal of all supra-alveolar desmodontal fibers and root cementum to prevent reattachment of connective tissue
➤ The flaps are apically repositioned (see above) and secured with single periosteal sutures (**Fig. 11.37**). The lingual flap can also be slightly shortened in order to expose the furcation. Interrupted sutures are used for releasing incisions.
➤ A periodontal dressing (CoePak) is applied to secure the flap position and to keep the furcation area open.
➤ The usual postoperative care is provided and chemical plaque control established (e.g., twice-daily mouth rinses with 0.1–0.2% chlorhexidine solution).

Critical assessment:
➤ Tunnel preparation alters the unfavorable morphology of the furcation area and en-

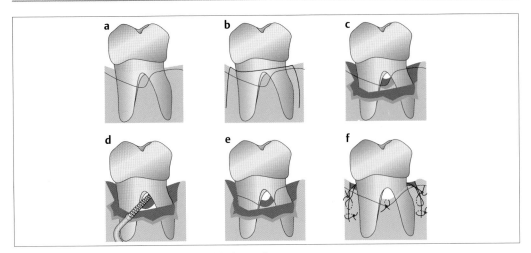

**Fig. 11.35   Tunnel preparation on a mandibular molar.**
**a** Through-and-through furcation in a mandibular first molar. Proximal bone is largely preserved.
**b** Intracrevicular incision, vertical releasing incisions demarcate the surgical area laterally.
**c** A mucoperiosteal flap is mobilized and granulation tissue removed.
**d** Osteoplasty with a Sugarman bone file (see **Fig. 11.36b**).
**e** Following widening of the furcation area, all desmodontal fibers and root cementum is to be removed to prevent reattachment.
**f** Periosteal sutures (see **Fig. 11.11**) for apical repositioning of the flap, interradicular suture, and interrupted sutures for releasing incisions.

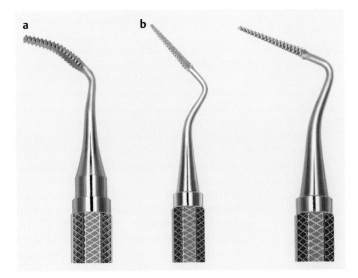

**Fig. 11.36**   Bone files: (**a**) after Schluger, (**b**) after Sugarman.

ables the patient to clean the furcation on a daily basis (**Fig. 11.38**).

➤ The patient has to be trained in brushing the furcation with small interdental brushes (see **Fig 10.5**). In the evening, 1% fluoride gel (Elmex Gelée, GABA, Basel, Switzerland) should be applied; in the morning, 1% chlor-

hexidine gel (Corsodyl, GlaxoSmithKline, Brentford, UK) is applied.

➤ The patient has also to be informed about the possibility of pulpitis-like sensations.
  – Since cementum was completely removed from the entire furcation area to prevent reattachment, dentinal tubules have been

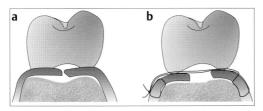

**Fig. 11.37** A full mucoperiosteal flap (**a**) is to be repositioned in an apical position by use of periosteal sutures (**b**).

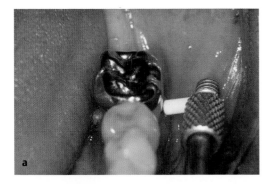

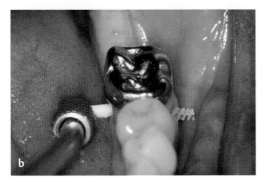

**Fig. 11.38** In order to keep the furcation open, to remove any bacterial plaque, and to apply fluoride and chlorhexidine gels, a molar with a tunnel must be cleaned with interproximal brushes on a daily basis, if necessary from both the buccal and the lingual entrance.

opened across a wide area. In addition, accessory channels (see above) may connect the furcation with the pulp chamber.
- If hypersensitivity persists, the tooth may require root canal treatment.
- Note that long-lasting dentinal hypersensitivity may interfere with the patient's compliance. Consequently, there is a high risk of new soft tissue closure requiring

repeated surgical intervention. Developing root caries in the furcation area is usually an indication for extraction.

**Regenerative Procedures**

Indications:
➤ Mostly mandibular molars with moderately advanced (degree II) buccal and/or lingual furcation involvement.
➤ In some cases, maxillary molars with an isolated buccal (or mesial) degree II furcation involvement.

Contraindications:
➤ General, patient-related contraindications are severe systemic disease possibly interfering with surgical procedures, poor compliance, and excessive smoking.
➤ Local contraindications:
  - Degree I furcation involvement, except in combination with a deep intrabony pocket
  - Through-and-through (degree III) involvement
  - Complicated furcation involvement of maxillary molars without any chance of sufficient debridement (e. g., degree II involvement of a distopalatal furcation)
  - Combinations with advanced proximal bone loss

Procedure (**Fig. 11.39**):
➤ Disinfection
➤ Local anesthesia
➤ Incisions should be made seeking preservation of soft tissue as far as possible:
  - Buccal and lingual/palatal intracrevicular incisions.
  - Two vertical releasing incisions may demarcate the surgical site at a distance of about half of a tooth's width mesial and distal to the treated tooth.
➤ Mobilization of a full mucoperiosteal flap beyond the mucogingival border.
➤ Complete removal of all granulation tissue:
  - Disclosure of the entire furcation defect and surrounding bony pockets.
  - If the defect morphology is unfavorable (communicating furcations, proximal bone loss extending to a level apical to the furcation entrance, deep bony pockets), alternative treatment modalities must be chosen—for example, tunnel pre-

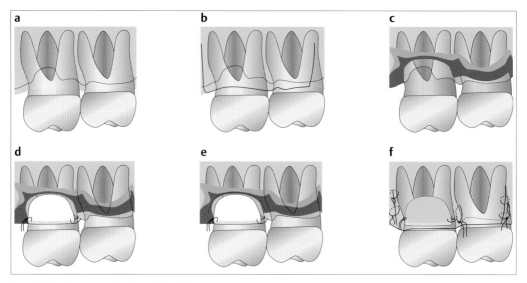

**Fig. 11.39   Regenerative furcation therapy.**
**a** Buccal degree II furcation involvement of a maxillary first molar. Favorable situation for guided tissue regeneration: No proximal bone loss; mesial and distal furcations are not affected.
**b** Intracrevicular incision. Two vertical releasing incisions are made laterally.
**c** A mucoperiosteal flap is mobilized and the granulation tissue removed, with thorough scaling and root planing.
**d** A suitable membrane is trimmed and fixed to the tooth with a sling suture. The membrane should overlap the bone margin by about 2 to 3 mm.
**e** Dissection of the periosteum at the base of the flap and sharp preparation of a split flap for flap advancement.
**f** The flap can now be coronally displaced without any tension. Tight suturing with vertical mattress sutures and fine interrupted sutures to further approximate the wound margins in the proximal region; interrupted sutures for vertical incisions.

paration or hemisection (see above); in certain cases even extraction.
➤ Scaling and root planing:
– This is the critical step which basically determines success or failure of the operation. *Note*: Special operative tricks are meaningless unless the bacterial infection has been controlled.
– If necessary, the furcation entrance should be widened by osteoplasty (see above) to gain better access to the root surfaces in the furcation area.
– The fornix of the furcation is debrided with universal curettes (e.g., Columbia 4 R/4 L, Langer 17/18 or special furcation curettes SQBL 1, SQMD 1; see **Fig. 11.26**). Sonic scalers in combination with extra-fine diamond-coated burs (15 μm) may be used as well.

➤ The membrane is then selected and carefully trimmed. It should overlap the bone margins by about 2 to 3 mm and has to be tightly fixed with a sling suture. The knot should be placed interproximally.
➤ The mucoperiosteal flap should cover the membrane completely without any tension. Therefore, the periosteum has to be dissected at its base. Further sharp preparation of a split flap allows tension-free coronal advancement.
➤ The flap is then tightly sutured. Interdentally, vertical mattress sutures are placed (**Figs. 11.11** and **11.37**) with additional interrupted sutures for further wound margin approximation. Finally, vertical releasing incisions are secured with interrupted sutures.
➤ No periodontal dressing should be applied.

Postoperative care:
➤ Antibiotics are not routinely prescribed.
➤ During the first two weeks, postoperative follow-up sessions should be scheduled every second or third day. If necessary, supragingival bacterial deposits in the surgical area are carefully removed.
➤ Postoperative infection control:
  – While toothbrushing in the surgical site should be avoided for about 4 to 6 weeks, chemical plaque control has to be established (i.e., mouth rinses twice daily with a 0.1–0.2% chlorhexidine solution).
  – If the membrane was exposed after some days or weeks, the patient should apply 1% chlorhexidine gel with a cotton swab twice daily. Secondary surgical coverage should never be performed.
➤ A nonresorbable membrane has to be surgically removed after 4 to 6 weeks.

Critical assessment:
➤ Guided tissue regeneration (GTR) can markedly improve the clinical periodontal situation of furcation-involved teeth if indications are strictly observed (**Fig. 11.40, Box 11.3**).

➤ In clinical studies, in which GTR was compared with access flaps, better healing results were achieved in the following situations:
  – Buccal and/or lingual degree II involvement of mandibular molars
  – Isolated buccal or mesial degree II involvement of maxillary molars
  – Best results may be expected in keyhole-like furcations with a small furcation width and height.
➤ Results obtained with resorbable and nonresorbable membranes were largely comparable. Exclusive or additional use of bone substitutes (e.g., demineralized freeze-dried bone allografts), or root conditioning with citric acid, for example, did not lead to better results.
➤ *Note*: The conversion of moderately advanced furcation involvement (degree II) into a slight involvement (degree I) may be regarded as a success. Slight involvements can then be managed during supportive periodontal therapy (see Chapter 12).

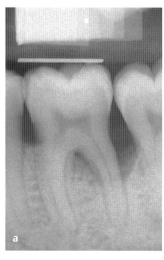 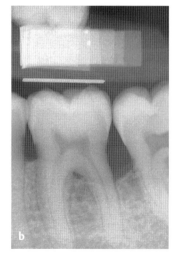

**Fig. 11.40 Result after guided tissue regeneration** of a combined infrabony and furcation lesion in a lower molar.
**a** Intrasurgically confirmed degree II furcation involvement and three-wall intrabony pocket at the lower first molar. Regenerative treatment was accomplished with a synthetic, biologically degradable membrane.
**b** Considerable bone-fill in the furcation and the intrabony pocket, 12 months after therapy.

**Box 11.3    Does guided tissue regeneration (GTR) have any benefits as compared to conventional flap surgery in the treatment of furcation-involved multirooted teeth?**

For well-known reasons, clinical assessment of furcation involvement is rather problematic. The true extent and severity of furcation involvement has to be reassessed during surgery. Therefore, particularly in scientific research, an assessment of whether reduction of horizontal attachment loss has occurred after therapy should only be done during an explorative re-entry operation.

In meta-analyses by Jepsen et al,[38] Murphy and Gunsolley,[39] and Kinaia et al[40] basically randomized controlled studies of at least 6 months duration were considered in which efficacy of GTR for furcation-involved teeth had been studied. All three meta-analyses reported significant heterogeneity of results in single studies, most of which aroused considerable design and execution concerns. Explorative surgery after at least 6 months revealed the following:

➤ In buccal or lingual degree II furcations of mandibular molars, GTR led to a greater mean gain of horizontal attachment of about 1.5 mm as compared to conventional access flap surgery. Quality of evidence: low.

➤ At maxillary molars with degree II furcation involvement, the mean difference was about 1 mm. There is some evidence that GTR yielded somewhat better results than conventional access flap surgery in buccal and mesial degree II furcations of maxillary molars. Quality of evidence: low.

➤ Results achieved with bioresorbable membranes were somewhat better than those achieved with nonresorbable membranes. Quality of evidence: low.

➤ When GTR was combined with bone substitutes, considerably greater horizontal attachment gain could be achieved when compared to GTR alone. Quality of evidence: very low.

➤ Whether complete closure of a degree II furcation after GTR occurs is not foreseeable. A closure of a through-and-through furcation (degree III) has so far not been observed.

## Possible Treatment Strategies

The decision for one treatment modality or another is essentially influenced by the following factors (**Fig. 11.41**):

➤ Tooth type and site of involvement
➤ Degree of furcation involvement
➤ Strategic importance of the tooth
➤ Patient's willingness and ability to cooperate
➤ The question as to whether extensive restorative treatment is planned

In individual cases several further factors have to be considered:

➤ General factors:
  – Patient's age and health condition
  – Form or expression of periodontitis
  – Patient's preferences and values
➤ Local factors:
  – Amount of the remaining periodontal supportive apparatus at individual roots
  – Mobility of individual roots (which cannot be determined preoperatively)
  – Anatomic-topographic relationship between roots
  – Dental caries and endodontic situation

Effective treatment of furcation-involved *premolars* is largely limited. The separation degree of the root complex is usually low, and very conical roots exhibit considerably increased tooth mobility. On the other hand, maxillary premolars, especially, often have high strategic importance. For that reason, palliative measures, such as repeat scaling and root planing, may be indicated to avoid extensive restorative treatment. Furcation-involved *wisdom teeth* are usually of low strategic importance and should be extracted in an early phase of the treatment. There might be reasonable exceptions.

A **systematic review** by Huynh-Ba et al[41] of studies, which have addressed the survival rate of multirooted teeth with furcation involvement, allowed relatively promising conclusions for various therapeutic interventions:

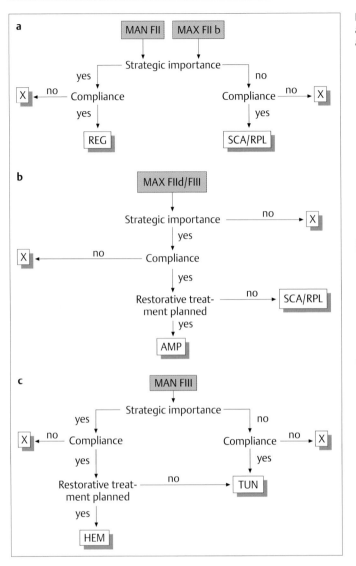

**Fig. 11.41 Decision diagrams for advanced furcation involvement.**
**a** Degree II furcation involvement (F II) of mandibular molars (MAND) and isolated buccal or mesial degree II involvement (F IIb/m) of maxillary molars (MAX). If the tooth has strategic importance and compliance is excellent, regenerative treatment (REG) might be considered. Otherwise, repeated palliative scaling and root planing (SCA/RPL) may improve the prognosis of the tooth. If compliance is poor, the tooth should be extracted in an early treatment phase.
**b** Distal degree II furcation involvement (F IId) or through-and-through involvement(F III) of maxillary molars. If the morphological and topographical situation is favorable, compliance excellent and restorative treatment planned, root amputation may be considered.
**c** Through-and-through furcation involvement (F III) of mandibular molars. If no local factors interfering with the treatment are present, restorative measures planned and patient's compliance is excellent, hemisection (HEM) might be a treatment option. A hemisectioned tooth may be incorporated in a fixed dental prosthesis. If the dentition is largely plaque-free, tunnel preparation (TUN) may be an alternative treatment, especially if restorative treatment can be avoided.

➤ 43 to 96% of furcation-involved teeth treated with conventional flap surgery had been retained during observation periods of between 5 and 53 years.
➤ 62 to 100% of furcation-involved teeth, in which one or more roots had been resected, were still in place after 5 to 13 years.
➤ Reported survival rates of molars in which a tunnel procedure had been done were between 43% and 93% after 5 to 8 years.

➤ Incipient furcation involvement (degree I) may be controlled by nonsurgical periodontal therapy. More than 90% of teeth were still in place after observation periods of between 5 and 9 years.
➤ Survival rates after regenerative treatment were 83 to 100% after 5 to 12 years of observation.
➤ The most frequent complications after furcation therapy were vertical root fracture and endodontic failure after resective measures.

# ■ Mucogingival Surgery

Functional or esthetic mucogingival disorders include, in particular, an aberrant (i.e., marginal insertion of) lip, cheek, or tongue frenula, decreased vestibular depth, and localized or generalized gingival recessions.

Mucogingival surgery in the strict sense refers to certain operative techniques for plastic surgical correction of tooth-surrounding soft tissue, which includes morphology, position, and amount of tissue.

The aim of so-called *plastic periodontal surgery* is the correction of anatomical, developmental, traumatic, or disease-derived defects of gingiva, alveolar mucosa, and alveolar bone; for example:

➤ Surgical widening of the zone of attached and keratinized gingiva.
➤ Correction of soft tissue defects of the mucogingival region and the alveolar process.
➤ In a wider sense, pocket elimination by an apically repositioned flap (see above), which preserves the amount of keratinized gingiva, may belong to the field of plastic periodontal surgery as well.

## Widening of the Zone of Keratinized Tissue with a Free Gingival Graft

Large differences in gingival width are manifest between and within individuals. A minimal width of less than 3 mm on average is commonly found at vestibular aspects of canines and premolars of the mandible.

A narrow band or even absence of attached gingiva may be either a normal variant or due to gingival recession. *Note*: If oral hygiene is optimal, the gingival margin may be kept inflammation-free and stable, even when there is a very narrow band of keratinized tissue. Narrow or unattached gingiva is not in itself an indication for surgical widening of the vestibule or zone of keratinized tissue. In some cases, however, this condition may render oral hygiene procedures more difficult.

Possible indications for a free gingival graft:

➤ Shallow vestibule in combination with marginal insertion of a lip or cheek frenulum
➤ Before surgical root coverage by coronally repositioned flap (see below)
➤ Pre-prosthetically in case of a subgingival preparation line and thin gingiva; likewise, before placing a dental implant when keratinized mucosa is largely lacking
➤ Before or during orthodontic treatment, when anterior teeth are to be moved through the alveolar bone and the attached gingiva is thin or even absent

Procedure (**Fig. 11.42**):

➤ Disinfection
➤ Local anesthesia
➤ Preparation of a periosteal wound bed for a free gingival graft:
  – Supraperiosteal incision with a no. 15 scalpel blade at the mucogingival border, about one tooth-width mesial and distal to the tooth to be treated.

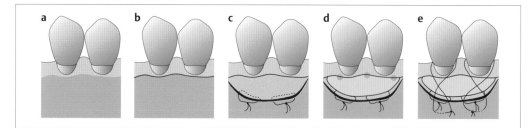

**Fig. 11.42  Free gingival graft.**
**a** Narrow band of gingiva and decreased vestibular depth.
**b** Supraperiosteal incision at the mucogingival border.
**c** Supragingival preparation of a recipient site for the graft. The mucosal flap is fixed with two mattress sutures to the periosteum with resorbable suture material.
**d** The trimmed graft is compressed with a gauze tampon for 2 minutes and subsequently glued at two or three spots on the coronal margin with tissue glue (Histoacryl).
**e** Alternatively, the graft may be fixed with two crossed suspensory sutures, so-called basket sutures.

– Supraperiosteal sharp preparation of a mucoperiosteal flap. *Caution*: The mental nerve in the region of mandibular premolars must not be injured.
– Removal of any remaining muscle fibers with LaGrange gingival scissors.
– Apical fixation of the mucosa with a horizontal mattress suture (resorbable suture material, 5-0).
– A template corresponding to the size and shape of the wound bed may be cut from the sterile suture's wrapping material.

➤ Local anesthesia of the greater palatine nerve.
➤ A gingival graft is harvested from the masticatory mucosa either between the second premolar and the second molar or the tuberosity. The region of the palatal rugae should rather be avoided:
– The template is placed on the palatal mucosa about 2 mm central to the gingival margin.
– It is circumcised by a 1.5 mm deep incision. The template is then removed and a graft of 1 to 1.5 mm thickness is harvested with the scalpel.
– *Caution:* The palatal blood vessels must not be injured. They are usually located more centrally and run deeper in the submucosa. If the procedure is carried out correctly, injury can virtually be ruled out.
➤ The palatal wound is covered with a periodontal dressing (CoePak), which is fixed interdentally.
➤ The connective tissue side of the graft is trimmed with gingival scissors or a scalpel. Any fatty tissue is removed and the level of the graft adjusted for even thickness. Size and shape are adjusted according to the wound bed. *Note*: In the region of the vestibular fold about 1 mm of the wound should not be covered by the graft.
➤ The graft is compressed with a saline-soaked gauze tampon for 2 minutes to avoid hematoma formation.
➤ It is then fixed at the gingival margin with two spots of tissue sealant (e. g., Histoacryl, B. Braun, Melsungen, Germany). Alternatively, the graft may be secured with a so-called basket suture (**Fig. 11.42e**). *Note*: The graft should not be sutured with interrupted sutures.

➤ No periodontal dressing should be applied at the grafted site since this might result in dislocation of the graft.

The usual postoperative care is provided and chemical plaque control established. Toothbrushing of the surgical site is suspended for two to three weeks while the patient rinses his or her mouth twice daily with 0.1 to 0.2 % chlorhexidine solution.

Wound healing and epithelial differentiation has been described to pass through three distinct phases[42]:
➤ *Initial phase* (days 1–3):
– Plasma circulation facilitates graft vitality.
– Wound transudate enters the graft by capillary action.
– The epithelium degenerates and is desquamated.
➤ *Revascularization* (days 2–11):
– Capillaries proliferate from the wound margins.
– Formation of anastomoses which re-establish blood circulation.
– Metabolism within the graft increases.
– Amoeboid migration of epithelial cells, which originate from the surrounding tissues, onto the vital graft surface.
➤ *Maturation* (up to the end of the sixth week and thereafter):
– The number of blood vessels within the graft decreases
– The epithelium matures, a keratinized layer forms.

*Note:* Epithelial differentiation is influenced by the connective tissue beneath (which stems from the hard palate). Therefore, the epithelium will likely be orthokeratinized (see Chapter 1).

Critical assessment:
➤ A graft of sufficient dimensions should be harvested. Grafts that are too thin (e. g., less than 0.7 mm) have a strong tendency to shrink. An even and defined thickness may be achieved with a special machine-driven mucotome (Nouvag, Goldach, Switzerland). Apart from considerable costs, a disadvantage is that the grafts are rectangular and trimming them to the size and shape of the wound bed involves considerable tissue waste.

➤ Generally, free gingival grafts have a high success rate. In some cases, "creeping attachment," that is, coronal proliferation of the gingiva onto a corresponding root recession site, may be observed after the elimination of muscle pulls.
➤ The palatal wound may cause some discomfort.
➤ Due to orthokeratinization of palatal mucosa (see Chapter 1), grafts harvested from the hard palate are usually of a different color than the surrounding tissues.

A free gingival graft may also be used to cover a shallow recession of not more than 1 mm. Procedure:
➤ De-epithelialization of the tissue which surrounds the recession.
➤ A fairly thick gingival graft (1.5–2 mm) is harvested.
➤ After thorough scaling of the root surface, the graft is placed supramarginally, and compressed for several minutes with saline-soaked gauze.
➤ It is then secured with a basket suture (**Fig. 11.42e**).

Vestibular extensions without free gingival grafts (e. g., the Edlan-Mejchar surgical technique) are nowadays rarely performed. There might be pre-prosthetic indications to improve the situation for a removable dental prosthesis.

## Gingival Recessions

Recessions have a multifactorial etiology. *Primary causes* are frequent trauma to the gingival margin and inflammation. Numerous *predisposing factors* have been identified, for example:
➤ Prominent position of a tooth in the dental arch
➤ Dehiscence or fenestration of the alveolar bone
➤ Orthodontic tooth movement in a labial direction through the alveolar bone

To treat gingival recessions, oral hygiene practices must be checked first. There is often a discrepancy between the frequency and intensity of toothbrushing and its effectiveness. An optimal oral hygiene must be established first. The patient should be trained in removing bacterial deposits from the tooth surfaces effectively with appropriate effort but without injuring gingival tissues.

Following this hygienic phase, the situation should be carefully documented:
➤ Intraoral photographs should be taken.
➤ Stone model casts are made which document frenula and their position, the vestibular fold, and any gingival recessions.
➤ A recession chart (see **Fig. 6.12**) is filled in.

In certain cases, corrective mucogingival surgery may then be planned.

## Lateral Sliding Flap

Indications for a lateral sliding flap as described by Grupe and Warren[43]:
➤ Localized, shallow (≤2 mm) Miller class I or II recessions with adequately wide gingiva lateral to the tooth to be treated
➤ Especially, at anterior teeth in the maxilla where the vestibule is rather deep

Contraindications:
➤ Miller class III or IV recessions
➤ Several neighboring teeth with recessions
➤ Generally shallow gingiva
➤ Shallow vestibule, especially when recessions in the mandible are to be treated

Procedure (**Fig. 11.43**):
➤ Disinfection
➤ Local anesthesia
➤ Thorough scaling and root planing to remove any microbial deposits from the root surface that has been exposed to the oral environment
➤ To remove the smear layer and demineralize the dentin surface to disclose its collagen matrix, the root surface may be conditioned with citric acid (pH 1) or saturated tetracycline solution. *Note*: In comparative clinical studies, no superiority were observed after root conditioning (see above).
➤ Incision:
  – Intracrevicular incision in the area of the recession to remove the junctional epithelium.
  – Horizontal incision within the attached gingiva lateral (usually distal) to the tooth to be treated.

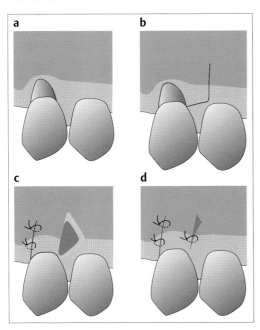

**Fig. 11.43 Lateral sliding flap.**

**a** Localized recession with sufficiently wide gingiva lateral to the neighboring tooth.

**b** Thorough scaling of the root surface which has been exposed to the oral environment. If necessary, it may be conditioned with citric acid (pH 1) or saturated tetracycline solution. An intracrevicular incision is made at the tooth to be treated, a horizontal incision in the area of the attached gingiva, and a vertical, slightly oblique incision into the vestibule.

**c** A mucoperiosteal flap is prepared. The periosteum is dissected at the base of the flap and the flap is rotated without tension to cover the recession. The wound margins around the exposed bone are carefully undermined.

**d** Virtually complete wound closure can be achieved.

- Vertical, slightly oblique incision into the alveolar mucosa. Care should be taken to ensure a wide base of the flap.
➤ A mucoperiosteal flap is mobilized beyond the mucogingival border. The periosteum at the flap base is dissected and a split thickness flap prepared. The flap is rotated tension-free coronally and laterally to cover the recession.
➤ The flap is secured with interrupted sutures. The tissues close to the exposed bone surface are carefully undermined, which will in most cases allow wound closure even in the area of the vertical incision.

➤ No periodontal dressing is placed and postoperative care is provided and the usual infection control measures are established.

## Coronally Advanced Flap after Vestibular Extension with Free Gingival Graft

Indications for a coronally advanced flap as described by Bernimoulin et al[44]:
➤ Localized or several neighboring, moderately deep or deep ($\geq 2$ mm) Miller class II recessions in combination with a shallow vestibule.
➤ *Note*: For root coverage of Miller class I recessions, deepening of the vestibule is not necessary.

Contraindications include Miller class III or IV recessions.

In a first operation, vestibular extension is carried out and a free gingival graft placed (**Fig. 11.42**). The possibility of slight creeping attachment after removing muscle pulls should be taken into account. Three months later, root coverage may be done by a coronally repositioned flap.

Procedure (**Fig. 11.44**):
➤ Disinfection
➤ Local anesthesia
➤ Thorough instrumentation and, if considered necessary, chemical conditioning of the root surface
➤ The location of the new tip of the papilla is identified as follows:
  - The recession depth is determined with a periodontal probe.
  - The respective distance is then subtracted from the present tip of the papilla at the surgical site.
➤ Incisions:
  - Intracrevicular incision in the area of the recession to remove the junctional epithelium
  - Interdentally, horizontal incisions which circumcise the new papillary tips
  - Two vertical, slightly diverging incisions into the alveolar mucosa confine the surgical site
➤ Preparation of a mucoperiosteal flap:
  - The flap is mobilized beyond the mucogingival border.

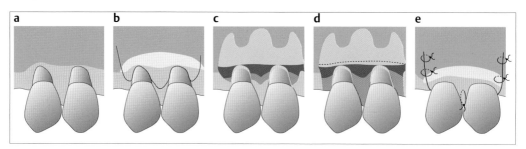

**Fig. 11.44   Coronally advanced flap.**
**a** Two neighboring recessions with narrow gingiva and decreased vestibular depth.
**b** Situation about three months after vestibular extension with a free gingival graft (**Fig. 11.42**). Incision lines for mobilization of a trapezoidal flap. A new papillary tip is defined according to the depth of the recession. Vertical incisions into the vestibule confine the flap laterally.
**c** A mucoperiosteal flap is mobilized and the papillae de-epithelialized to create a suitable wound bed.
**d** The periosteum is dissected at the base of the flap and the flap advanced without tension for root coverage.
**e** The wound is closed with interrupted sutures for vertical incisions and a vertical mattress suture interdentally.

- The periosteum is dissected at the base of the flap and a split-thickness flap prepared.
- The papillae are de-epithelialized to create a suitable wound bed.
- The flap is advanced coronally tension-free to cover the recession(s) and compressed for about 2 minutes with a gauze tampon soaked in saline.
➤ Careful wound closure:
  - Interrupted sutures for lateral incisions
  - Interdental vertical mattress suture (**Fig. 11.11**)

No periodontal dressing should be placed. The usual postoperative care is provided and infection control measures are established.

Note that the adjunct application of enamel matrix proteins (Emdogain) may lead to considerably better results; in particular, a higher rate of complete root coverage is obtained in the coronally advanced flap procedure. On the other hand, application of platelet rich plasma (PRP, see above) did not influence postoperative results after surgical root coverage with coronally advanced flaps.

**Coronally Advanced Flap with Connective Tissue Graft**

Indications for a coronally advanced flap as described by Langer and Langer[45] are localized deep Miller class I or II recessions, especially in case of thin gingiva. Contraindications include Miller class III or IV recessions.

The procedure is similar to that of the coronally advanced flap[44] but without the preceding surgical deepening of the vestibule.

Sufficiently thick connective tissue grafts may be harvested from three areas of the masticatory mucosa of the hard palate (**Fig. 11.45**): the premolar area, the area of the second molar, and the tuberosity.

*Note*: The rather thin mucosa covering the palatal root of the first molar is not suitable for graft harvesting. An anatomical barrier separates the part of the hard palate containing minor salivary glands (extends up to the soft palate) from the part containing adipose tissue (in the premolar region).[46]

Procedure for harvesting a palatal connective tissue graft:
➤ Disinfection
➤ Local anesthesia of the greater palatine nerve
➤ Incisions:
  - Perpendicular to the alveolar bone, an incision is made about 2 mm from the palatal gingival margin, the length of which depends on the desired size of the graft.
  - A semilunar undermining incision dissects the main part of the lamina propria/submucosa from a thin layer of connective tissue covered by epithelium.[47] Alternatively, two vertical incisions confine the area for harvesting the connective tis-

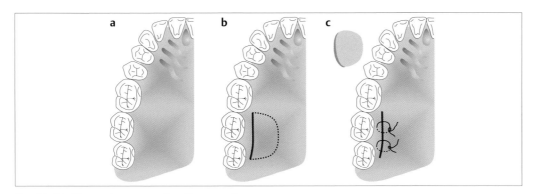

**Fig. 11.45  Harvesting connective tissue grafts.**
**a** Topography of the hard palatal mucosa. Suitably thick mucosa is found in the premolar region and in the region of the second and third molars. A barrier in the region of the palatal root of the first molar usually prevents harvesting connective tissue of sufficient thickness.
**b** Harvesting the connective tissue graft from a more distal area. The first incision is made perpendicular to tooth axis up to the surface of the alveolar bone. A second, undermining, incision is made parallel to the bone surface. After mobilization the circumcised graft is carefully removed.
**c** Closure with interrupted sutures.

sue graft, the so-called trap door flap. *Caution:* Care must be taken not to injure the major blood vessels.
- Incisions made with a special double-blade scalpel[48] yield evenly thick connective tissue grafts with a small epithelial collar.
➤ The largely circumcised graft is mobilized with a small periosteal elevator and removed with tissue pliers.

After thorough root instrumentation and, if considered necessary, chemical conditioning, the trimmed graft is secured with resorbable sling sutures. The mucoperiosteal flap is coronally advanced and secured tension-free with vertical mattress sutures (see above). The palatal wound is closed with interrupted sutures.

No periodontal dressing is placed. The usual postoperative care is provided and infection control measures are established.

## Semilunar Coronally Repositioned Flap

Indications for a semilunar coronally repositioned flap[49] are localized, shallow (less than 3 mm) Miller class I recessions, especially at maxillary teeth. Contraindications include Miller class II, III, or IV recessions.

Procedure (**Fig. 11.46**):
➤ Disinfection
➤ Local anesthesia
➤ Thorough instrumentation and, if considered necessary, chemical conditioning of the root surface
➤ Incisions:
  - Intracrevicular incision in the area of the recession to remove the junctional epithelium.
  - Semilunar incision apically to the recession within the alveolar mucosa. The distance between the incision and the soft tissue margin should correspond to the depth of the recession plus a further 2 to 3 mm.
  - Undermining incision to dissect a split-thickness flap.
➤ The semilunar split flap is coronally advanced tension-free and compressed for 2 to 3 minutes with gauze soaked in saline.
➤ The apical wound is not sutured. A periodontal dressing (CoePak) might be applied.

The usual postoperative care is provided and infection control measures are established.

## Envelope Technique

Indications for the envelope technique[50] are localized, rather shallow Miller class I or II recessions, especially when the gingiva is rather thin.

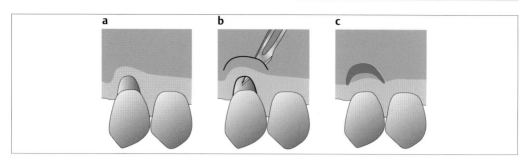

**Fig. 11.46  Semilunar coronally repositioned flap.**
**a** Localized Miller class I recession. The exposed root surface is scaled and, if necessary, conditioned with citric acid (pH 1) or saturated tetracycline solution.
**b** Semilunar incision in the vestibule. The distance between the incision and the gingival margin should exceed the recession depth by 2 to 3 mm. This is followed by sharp preparation of a split-thickness mucosal flap, marginally perforating the gingival sulcus.
**c** Coronal mobilization and compression of the tissue with a soaked gauze tampon for about 3 minutes. The apical wound is not sutured.

Contraindications include deep recession (≥ 3 mm) and Miller class III or IV recessions.
Procedure (**Fig. 11.47**):
➤ Disinfection
➤ Local anesthesia
➤ Thorough instrumentation and, if considered necessary, chemical conditioning of the root surface.
➤ Incisions:
 – Intracrevicular incision to remove junctional epithelium
 – Sharp, undermining preparation of a supraperiosteal pouch around the recession site
 – A further access incision in the alveolar lining mucosa about a tooth's width dis-

tally to the recession has been recommended.
➤ A sufficiently large connective tissue graft is harvested from the hard palate's masticatory mucosa (**Fig. 11.45**), trimmed, and placed into the prepared pouch ("envelope") preferably from the distal access incision.[51] Note that only a small part of the graft covers the root surface while its major parts are located in the pouch to assist survival of the graft.
➤ The graft may be secured with tissue glue (Histoacryl) and a periodontal dressing applied.
➤ The palatal wound is closed with interrupted sutures.

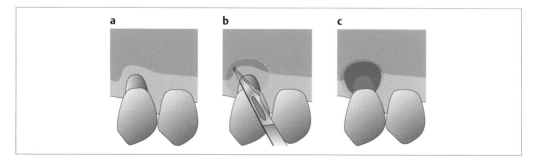

**Fig. 11.47  Envelope technique.**
**a** Localized Miller class I recession. The exposed root surface is scaled and, if necessary, conditioned with citric acid (pH 1) or saturated tetracycline solution.
**b** Intracrevicular incision to remove the junctional epithelium undermining, and supraperiosteal preparation of a pouch ("envelope") for the connective tissue graft.
**c** The major part of the graft, which should be further secured with Histoacryl tissue glue, lies in the pouch.

The usual postoperative care is provided and infection control measures are established.

If several adjacent recessions are to be treated, the closely related *tunnel technique*[52] may be applied. An undermining incision of interdental papillae is done with a special microsurgical dissector to avoid perforation. Note that the technique requires very long connective tissue grafts which can often not be harvested given the anatomical peculiarities of the hard palate (see **Fig. 11.45**). Then, an allogeneic transplant, for example, acellular dermal matrix (Alloderm, BioHorizons, Birmingham, Alabama, USA) is recommended.

## Guided Tissue Regeneration

Specially designed membranes are used to provide and maintain sufficient space for the proliferation of cells originating in the surrounding periodontal ligament:

➤ To avoid collapse of the membrane on the root surface, a special ePTFE membrane is employed which is reinforced with a titanium cross or scaffold. The membrane has to be removed after 4 to 6 weeks in a second operation. Note that the main provider (Gore Medical) has meanwhile ceased manufacture of transgingival and submerged membranes for GTR, but similar alternatives have recently become available again (e.g., Cytoplast, Osteogenics, Lubbock, Texas, USA).

➤ Special resorbable membranes with space-keeping function (e.g., Guidor PPS Biore-sorbable Matrix Barrier, Sunstar, Chicago, Illinois, USA).

Indications:

➤ Localized or neighboring, deep (3 mm or more) Miller class I or II recessions.
➤ Especially, recessions at maxillary canines and premolars.
➤ A shallow Black class V cavity. For exploration, the restoration has to be removed.

Contraindications include shallow recessions, a decreased depth of the vestibule and Miller class III or IV recessions.

Procedure (**Fig. 11.48**):

➤ Disinfection
➤ Local anesthesia
➤ Thorough instrumentation to freshen the root surface and create a concave root surface; for example, using rotating diamond-coated fine (40 μm) and extrafine (15 μm) burs
➤ If considered necessary, chemical conditioning of the root surface with citric acid (pH 1) or saturated tetracycline solution to remove the smear layer and expose dentin collagen fibers
➤ To define the location of the new papilla tips, the rec^ession depth is determined with a periodontal probe. The respective distance is subtracted from the present tip of the papilla at the surgical site (see above).
➤ Incisions:
  – Intracrevicular incision in the area of the recession to remove the junctional epithelium.

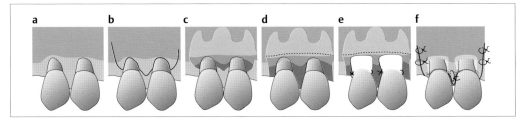

**Fig. 11.48    Root coverage employing guided tissue regeneration.**

**a** Neighboring Miller class I or II recessions. The exposed root surface is scaled and, if necessary, conditioned with citric acid (pH 1) or saturated tetracycline solution.

**b–d** Incisions, flap mobilization, and periosteal dissection as for coronally advanced flap (see **Fig. 11.44**).

**e** Membranes are trimmed and secured with sling sutures.

**f** The flap is coronally advanced and secured in a tension-free manner with a vertical mattress suture (interdentally) as well as interrupted sutures (lateral releasing incisions).

– Interdentally, horizontal incisions are made circumcising the new papilla tips.
– Two vertical, slightly diverging incisions into the alveolar mucosa laterally border the surgical site.
– Intracrevicular incision at the palatal/lingual aspect.
➤ Preparation of a mucoperiosteal flap:
– In the vestibule, the trapezoidal flap is raised beyond the mucogingival border.
– Palatally/lingually, papillae are raised and the flap is slightly elevated up to the bone level.
– The periosteum is dissected at the base of the buccal flap.
– Papillae are de-epithelialized to create a suitable wound bed.
➤ A suitable membrane (e. g., Guidor PPS Bioresorbable Matrix Barrier) is selected. The membrane is trimmed until it overlaps the bony margins apically by about 2 mm, laterally by 1 mm. The membrane is secured with sling sutures (integrated in the Guidor membrane).
➤ The vestibular flap should be coronally advanced without any tension.
➤ Careful wound closure: interdentally, a vertical mattress suture (**Fig. 11.11**) is placed (ePTFE suture material), lateral incisions are secured with interrupted sutures.
➤ No periodontal dressing is placed.

Postoperative infection control:
➤ *Note*: Antibiotics are not prescribed on a routine basis. The patient should rinse his or her mouth twice daily with a 0.1 to 0.2% chlorhexidine solution for 4 to 6 weeks.
➤ During the first two postoperative weeks, wound healing is checked every second or third day. Any plaque present at the gingival margin is carefully removed.
➤ If the membrane is exposed, the patient is advised to apply a 1% chlorhexidine gel twice daily. Secondary surgical coverage should *never* be performed.

If a resorbable membrane was placed, sutures are removed after 2 to 3 weeks.

## Critical Assessment

New methods and modifications for root coverage have been developed, especially since the mid-1980s when recessions were properly classified (see Chapter 6):
➤ Miller class I and II recessions may be covered with different methods including guided tissue regeneration (GTR). Root coverage may vary between 80% and 100%.[53]
➤ On the other hand, suboptimal results are to be expected in cases of Miller class III (interproximal attachment loss) recessions, while class IV recessions (interdental bone loss up to a level apical to the marginal tissue recession) cannot satisfactory be treated yet.
➤ Deep and, especially, wide recessions cannot be covered as successfully as shallow and narrow ones.

Quality of the new dentogingival connection:
➤ When GTR is applied for surgical root coverage, new cementum and a new connective tissue attachment on the previously exposed root surface may be expected.[54]
➤ With all other methods for root coverage, wound healing may essentially result in the formation of a long junctional epithelium. However, due to the fairly large area from which regenerative processes can take place (apical and lateral borders of the recession), some new cementum and new connective tissue attachment may also be expected after coronally advanced flaps with and without connective tissue grafts.

Increasing width and thickness of the gingiva:
➤ After coronally advanced flaps—especially when preceded by widening of the vestibule with a free gingival graft and after placement of connective tissue grafts—both width and thickness of the gingiva may considerably increase.
➤ This may be particularly important in patients with a persistent tendency to injure the gingival tissues during toothbrushing.
➤ *Note:* Widening of the gingiva is not to be expected after GTR. However, the resorbing granulation tissue may lead to reversible thickening of the tissue during the resorption period.[55]

The literature on surgical root coverage is amazingly rich with comparisons (**Box 11.4**), which makes decision-making in individual cases difficult. On the basis of a recent Bayesian network meta-analysis of 29 randomized controlled trials of at least 6 months duration, in which treatment outcomes of Miller class I and II recessions were assessed, Buti et al[56] concluded the following:

➤ The coronally advanced flap in combination with a connective tissue graft was the most effective procedure for surgical root coverage in terms of recession reduction and clinical attachment gain. It might be considered the *gold standard* in the treatment of Miller class I and II gingival recessions. Quality of evidence: moderate.

➤ The coronally advanced flap in combination with Emdogain ranked first for complete root coverage. The odds of achieving complete root coverage were increased fourfold if Emdogain was used in the procedure. Quality of evidence: moderate.

➤ In terms of gain of keratinized tissue, coronally advanced flaps in combination with connective tissue graft or collagen matrix or acellular dermal matrix (see above) yielded quite comparable results. Quality of evidence: low.

---

**Box 11.4   Which method for surgical root coverage of Miller class I and II recessions of at least 3 mm depth may yield best results as regards reduction of recession depth and complete root coverage?**

A systematic review by Chambrone et al[53] considered 12 randomized controlled trials of at least 6 months follow-up. The authors conclude that subepithelial connective tissue grafts, coronally advanced flaps and guided tissue regeneration (GTR) may all be applied to achieve reasonable coverage of recession. A mean coverage of 81% (range 50–97%) was calculated in a meta-analysis. On the other hand, complete root coverage was only achieved in about 47% on average (range 8–92%). In two long-term studies of 2 and 6 years, respectively, mean coverage and percentage complete coverage decreased again. As compared to GTR with resorbable membranes, subepithelial connective grafts yielded superior results as regards reduction of recession depth (quality of evidence: moderate) and keratinized tissue (quality of evidence: low).

A Bayesian network meta-analysis by Buti et al[56] which compared numerous root coverage procedures, had tried to rank efficacy and identify best treatment modalities. The authors considered 29 randomized controlled trials of at least 6 month duration in which treatment outcomes of Miller class I and II recessions were compared. As regards recession reduction and clinical attachment gain, a coronally advanced flap involving connective tissue grafts may be considered the gold standard. Quality of evidence: moderate.

The highest rate of complete root coverage was achieved by a coronally advanced flap in combination with Emdogain. The odds of achieving complete root coverage were increased by a factor of 3.91 (95% confidence interval 1.76; 9.48) if Emdogain was used in the procedure. Quality of evidence: moderate.

Coronally advanced flaps combined with either connective tissue graft or collagen matrix yielded best results as regards the amount of keratinized tissue. In cases where an adequate connective tissue graft cannot be harvested, acellular dermal matrix may be an alternative. Quality of evidence: low.

A further meta-analysis of 13 randomized controlled trials by Cheng et al[57] compared clinical effects of a coronally advanced flap alone or in combination with Emdogain and/or a connective tissue graft. It was confirmed that placement of a connective tissue graft or application of Emdogain led to significantly more keratinized tissue in coronally advanced flap procedures. Quality of evidence: low.

The application of Emdogain may potentially lead to reduced probing pocket depth and might also result in increased keratinized tissue, but not to the effect of placing a connective tissue graft. Quality of evidence: low.

## Frenectomy

For the surgical correction of lip and cheek frenula mainly three procedures have been used, namely V-Y or Z plasty (**Fig. 11.49**), or a free gingival graft (see above).

Indications include:

➤ Distinct labial frenum, which should be surgically corrected before and during orthodontic closure of a diastema

➤ Marginally inserting frenula interfering with effective oral hygiene, or wound healing after periodontal surgery

Procedure for V-Y plasty (**Fig. 11.49b–d**):
➤ Disinfection
➤ Local anesthesia
➤ Incision:
  – V-shaped circumcision of the frenum of the lip
  – Supraperiosteal preparation of a mucosal flap and dissection of muscle pulls
➤ Apical mobilization of the flap and fixation with interrupted sutures

Procedure for Z plasty (**Fig. 11.49e–f**):
➤ Disinfection
➤ Local anesthesia
➤ Z-shaped incision through the frenum
➤ Supraperiosteal preparation of two triangular flaps
➤ Exchange of the position of the flaps
➤ Fixation with interrupted sutures

A periodontal dressing is not necessary for either technique. The usual postoperative care is provided and infection control measures are established.

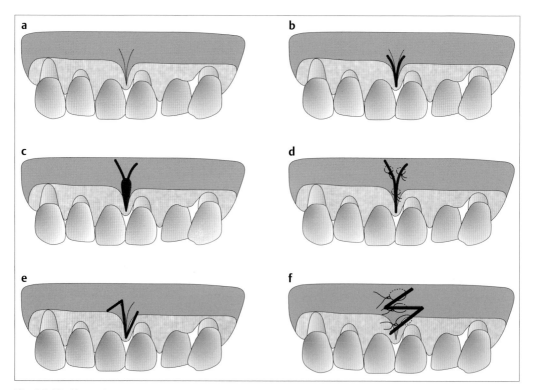

**Fig. 11.49   Frenectomy.**
**a** The marginally inserting, interfering frenum of the lip is supposed to be removed.
**b–d** V-Y plasty: V-shaped circumcision (**b**). Supraperiosteal preparation of a mucosal flap and apical repositioning (**c**). The two resulting sides of the "Y" are apically secured with interrupted sutures (**d**).
**e, f** Z plasty: Z-shaped supraperiosteal incision. Preparation of two triangular mucosal flaps (**e**). Swap position of the flaps, which are secured with interrupted sutures (**f**).

## ■ Occlusal Therapy

Occlusal forces may affect various structures of the stomatognathic system:
➤ Marginal and apical parts of the periodontium
➤ Pulp–dentin complex
➤ Occlusal surfaces of the teeth
➤ Temporomandibular joint
➤ Neuromuscular system

Causes of occlusal trauma, which may occur in combination, include:
➤ *Psychological stress*, frequently resulting in parafunctions such as clenching and bruxism
➤ *Premature occlusal contacts*
➤ Other forms of nonphysiological strain (e. g., an inappropriate dental prosthesis)

Experiments in animals and humans have shown the following[58]:
➤ Occlusal trauma cannot induce inflammatory lesions in the marginal periodontium.
➤ However, excessive jiggling forces may accelerate the progression of existing periodontitis.
➤ Increased tooth mobility may have a negative effect on the ecological conditions in the pocket. Especially, periodontal pathogens may proliferate.

*Note*: Although the pathogenic significance of occlusal trauma for the periodontium has long been considered rather low, new evidence from clinical studies points to considerable negative effects especially on periodontal treatment outcomes.[59,60]

Signs of a periodontal occlusal trauma include:
➤ Marked deviation of the tooth during articulation
➤ Progressively increasing tooth mobility
➤ Widening of the periodontal ligament space at the alveolar crest and, sometimes, around the apex

*Note*: Increasing *tooth mobility* due to occlusal interference is essentially regarded as a sign for *physiological compensation*: A tooth with increased mobility may evade excessive forces during articulation.

The deviation of a tooth crown has historically been measured with Mühlemann's *periodontometer*.[61] Two kinds of tooth mobility may be distinguished:
➤ *Desmodontal (initial) tooth mobility.* Small forces up to 1 N lead to linearly increasing deviation of the crown of between 0.05 mm and 0.1 mm due to displacement of the tooth within the periodontal ligament space.
➤ *Periodontal (secondary) tooth mobility.* Larger forces up to 5 N lead to distortion and compression of the alveolar process. The crown may be displaced by 0.08 to 0.15 mm.
  – Secondary tooth mobility varies among teeth (incisors > canines > premolars > molars).
  – It is greater in children than in adults and greater in women than in men.
  – Furthermore, it increases towards the end of pregnancy.

Elimination of an occlusal trauma as part of periodontal therapy may include:
➤ Minor orthodontic measures
➤ Temporarily wearing an occlusal splint to minimize the influence of potentially harmful parafunctions.
➤ Occlusal adjustment
➤ Semipermanent or permanent splinting of teeth
➤ Stabilization of remaining and replacement of lost teeth by definitive prosthetic treatment

### Occlusal Splint

For short-term relief of parafunctional problems in patients with tense jaw, face, and neck muscles[62]:
➤ Relaxation of the tense muscles
➤ Stabilization of the occlusion in centric relation
➤ *Note*: Before occlusal surfaces are irreversibly altered by selective grinding or extensive restorations, for example, occlusal therapy with appropriate splints should be carried out.

A resin acrylic splint (e. g., Michigan splint) for the maxilla (in the case of Angle class III malocclusion, mandibular splints are also possible) is manufactured as follows:

➤ Axis-orbital mounting of stone model casts in a semi adjustable articulator (see below).
➤ In order to fashion an acceptable splint for the patient, the vertical occlusal dimension should only be slightly increased.
➤ Plane and smooth occlusal surface. Centric stops and canine guidance are waxed up.
➤ Interference-free gliding of the teeth with freedom in centric must be achieved.
➤ The splint is transformed into acrylic resin, trimmed and polished.

The splint should be worn all the time, day and night, during the first three weeks.

## Occlusal Adjustment

Clinical occlusal analysis may sometimes reveal evidence of occlusal trauma:
➤ While the main symptom is progressive tooth mobility (i.e., increasing over time), that can only be assessed longitudinally.
➤ Further hints for occlusal trauma are palpable and visible deviation of a tooth in maximum intercuspidation and, in particular, during articulation.
➤ *Note:* In the case of hypermobile teeth, model cast analysis in a semi-adjustable articulator can hardly provide important information as regards occlusal interferences.

In view of anatomic structures of the periodontium, any tooth mobility is a function of the height of the alveolar bone, the width of the periodontal ligament space, and the morphology of the root complex. Careful differential diagnosis is therefore necessary. *Note:* Teeth which are hypermobile because of advanced bone loss cannot become firm after occlusal adjustment.

Occlusal trauma may be a sequel of advanced periodontitis which may greatly aggravate the situation, as teeth frequently change their position during the course of progressive periodontitis, for example:
➤ Unilateral pressure exerted by granulation tissue in a bony pocket may cause the tooth to move away from the periodontal lesion.
➤ The resulting occlusal interference may lead to periodontal trauma, since the tooth is alternately pushed during function into one or the other direction (jiggling).

Interfering contacts should be removed early during therapy. Selective grinding should be done to eliminate interferences in centric occlusion and, in particular, balancing interferences. Working side contacts should be harmonized. Possible further indications for occlusal adjustments may include:
➤ Prevention or diminishing of excessive parafunctional habits such as clenching and bruxism
➤ Harmonization of the occlusal plane
➤ Corrections after orthodontic and before restorative treatment

*Note*: An "ideal" occlusion created by extensive occlusal adjustment including restorative procedures is not a desirable treatment aim in itself.

## Semipermanent Splinting

Increased tooth mobility as a result of a reduced periodontium is fairly acceptable as long as the occlusion is stable and chewing comfort is not impaired. However, an unfavorable relation between the clinical crown and the total tooth length may result in considerable forces at the alveolar crest and at the apex during function (**Fig. 11.50**), the so-called *secondary occlusal trauma*. In these cases splinting of teeth results in a reduction of the periodontal ligament space, since the detrimental forces are distributed among several teeth.[63]

Indications for semipermanent splinting of, in particular, anterior teeth include:
➤ Significant reduction of the tooth-supporting apparatus
➤ Progressive tooth mobility
➤ Risk of tooth loss during function or treatment

Procedure:
➤ The teeth are meticulously scaled and polished. Rubber dam is applied.
➤ Splinting with composite after etching quite large enamel areas of the tooth to be splinted and its neighboring teeth. If class III cavities or restorations are present, the splint may be reinforced with carbon fiber or dental floss ligatures, or metal or acrylic mesh.
➤ Creation of small, mobile units is of advantage (**Fig. 11.51b**). If more than three teeth

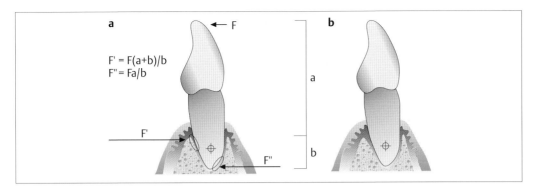

**Fig. 11.50  Secondary occlusal trauma.**
**a** If the relation between the length of the clinical crown (a) and the total length of the tooth (a + b) is unfavorable, considerable forces may arise at the alveolar crest and at the apex during normal function.
**b** If periodontal infection is under control, compensatory bone resorption in the region of the alveolar crest and the tooth's apex mean that in this situation, too, the tooth can evade detrimental forces and attachment loss is not to be expected. Clinically, tooth mobility may be progressive, which may make splinting necessary.

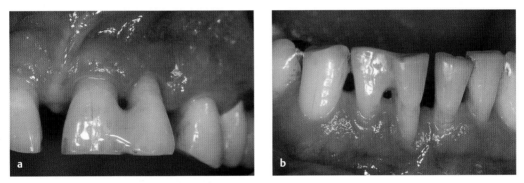

**Fig. 11.51  Semipermanent splinting with composite.**
**a** Esthetically somewhat problematic splinting of hypermobile tooth 22. After periodontal treatment the splint may be removed if the tooth's mobility was consolidated.
**b** Semipermanent splint of teeth 41 and 42. *Note:* A small, still slightly mobile unit is less susceptible to fracture, since teeth are allowed to evade occlusal forces during functional strain. Effective homecare hygienic measures are possible.

are bonded, the risk of fracture (at the firm tooth) increases considerably.
➤ The occlusion must carefully be checked. Especially for anterior teeth in the maxilla, an esthetically somewhat problematic situation may arise (**Fig. 11.51a**).
➤ Periodontal hygiene must not be hampered. Cleaning of embrasures with interdental brushes or dental floss (Superfloss) at home must be possible.

Splints that do not functionally interfere and are esthetically acceptable may remain permanently in place.

### Perio-Prosthetic Aspects

Generalized aggressive and severe chronic forms of periodontitis usually lead to early loss of molars. The remaining teeth frequently exhibit markedly increased tooth mobility.

In addition to the necessary replacement of lost teeth in order to restore chewing function and to improve esthetics, stabilization of the remaining teeth is a major treatment goal of restorative therapy.
➤ In cases of increased tooth mobility, chewing comfort can be improved considerably by permanently splinting teeth in a fixed

dental prosthesis. *Note*: Increased tooth mobility and advanced loss of the tooth-supporting apparatus are not in themselves contraindications for fixed prostheses.

➤ In patients with a reduced number of teeth and increased tooth mobility, fixed dental prostheses have several advantages as compared to removable prostheses:
  – Greater stability of the construction
  – Better distribution of chewing forces

➤ Particularly in patients over 60 years of age, the possibility of a shortened tooth arch (premolar occlusion) should be seriously considered as well.

➤ Occlusal stabilization in patients with unilateral or bilateral shortening of the dental arch[64] may also be achieved by distal cantilevers:
  – if possible as a bilateral fixed dental prosthesis.
  – A unilateral fixed prosthesis needs at least two abutments.
  – Abutments with low retention are contraindications.

➤ To avoid loss of retention, abutments should be prepared with maximum height and minimum taper:
  – The principle of self-retention must be observed.
  – The inclination of the crowns should be opposite to the dislocating force that acts on the cantilever.

➤ In certain cases orthodontic distalizing of a premolar and subsequent insertion of a fixed partial denture may be possible.

➤ Teeth should not be combined with oral implants in fixed restorations.

Restorative treatment may be conducted about 4 to 6 months after completion of periodontal therapy.

Procedure for manufacturing fixed dental prostheses in dentitions with marked tooth mobility:

➤ A two-stage procedure is recommended by which one jaw is restored first (in **Fig. 11.52**, the upper jaw is shown).

➤ Study model casts are mounted in a semiadjustable articulator in maximum intercuspidation.

➤ If required, incisor–canine guidance is recorded.

➤ An acrylic *registration plate* is made in the articulator.

➤ *Preparation of abutment teeth*. The preparation height should amount to more than 4 mm to achieve maximum retention of the crowns:
  – This is usually not a problem in the case of long clinical crowns after periodontal treatment of advanced periodontitis.
  – However, in case of marked divergence of abutment teeth, root canal treatment and incorporation of post and core may be indispensable.
  – The possibility of attachments should be considered in this case.

➤ *Impression taking:*
  – Double-mix impression material (silicone) may be used in a perforated tray.
  – *Caution:* Hydrocolloid impression material should be avoided. Teeth with marked root exposure are at a high risk of irreversible thermal pulp damage. Likewise, very firm, addition silicone or polyether impression material should not be used. Considerable problems may arise during removal of the impression from the oral cavity as well as from the model cast.

➤ An alginate impression is made of the opposite jaw with a rim-lock tray.

➤ The master model and opposite jaw model are manufactured.

➤ *Note*: In the case of very mobile teeth, registration of cusp tips of the dental arch should not be done in situ but must be performed on the registration plate using the master model:
  – Zinc oxide eugenol paste (e. g., Temp-Bond, Kerr Dental, Orange, California, USA) is applied on the registration plate.
  – The watered master model is placed on the registration plate. An impression of the cusps is made with the soft paste.
  – The paste is allowed to set—in a water bath, for example.

➤ After the registration paste has set, impressions that are too deep are trimmed with a scalpel blade. The fit of the impressions in the patient's mouth is checked.

➤ In order to minimize an increased vertical dimension, the registration plate is ground from the mandibular side until a small perforation in centric occlusion is noted.

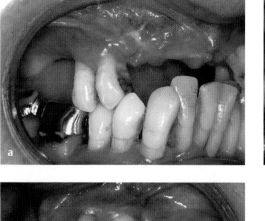
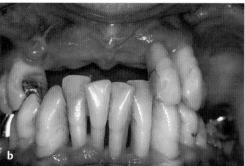
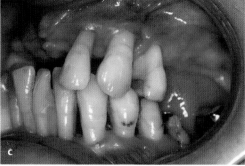

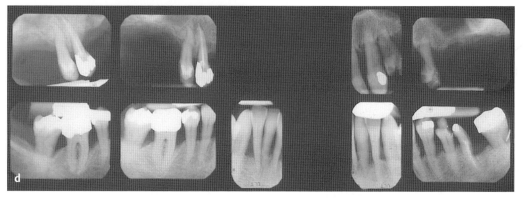

**Fig. 11.52**  Perioprosthetic treatment of a patient with generalized severe chronic periodontitis.
**a–d** After extraction of furcation-involved maxillary molars and periodontal therapy, the patient presents with advanced bone loss of the remaining teeth.

Continued ▶

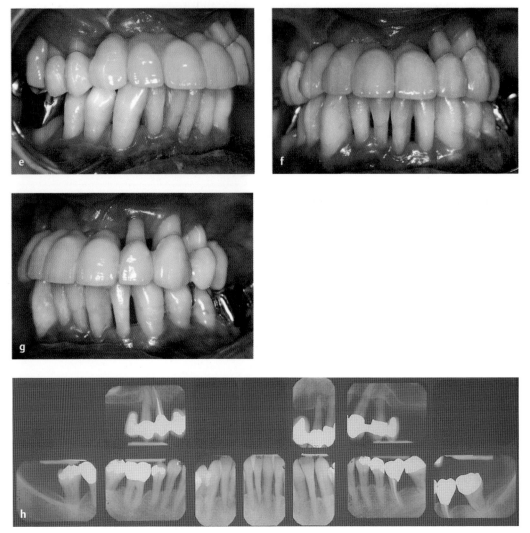

**Fig. 11.52** Continued
**e–h** 10 years of maintenance therapy following permanent splinting of maxillary teeth with a fixed dental prosthesis.

➤ *Centric relation record*:
  – On the mandibular side of the registration plate a small amount of heated thermoplastic impression compound (Kerr Dental) is applied in the region of the central incisors.
  – The mandible is guided in centric relation towards the inserted registration plate. The frontal stop within the thermoplastic

material should just prevent contact of the posterior teeth to the plate.
  – It should be repeatedly checked that the patient can easily find the frontal stop in the centric occlusion.
  – Zinc oxide eugenol paste is applied to the mandibular side of the registration plate in the region of the posterior teeth. The maxillary side of the plate is inserted

into the patient's mouth, and the patient closes in centric occlusion.
- Pressure-free molds of the mandible's posterior teeth cusps are made in the soft registration paste.

➤ After the registration paste has set, the plate is removed from the mouth. The frontal stop is discarded with a scalpel blade. Impressions are shortened to a level where only the tips of the cusps remain visible.
➤ The fit of master and opposite jaw models with the registration plate is checked.
➤ Model casts are then mounted in a semiadjustable articulator. The upper jaw model is mounted using a face-bow. The lower jaw model is mounted using the centric relation record. The mounting is checked with the patient's clinical situation.

When manufacturing the dental prosthesis in the dental laboratory, the risk of fracture of the fixed partial denture must be taken into account:
➤ Bridgework should be of proper dimensions and possess the necessary rigidity. It must also allow adequate interdental hygiene.
➤ Fixed partial dentures should not be soldered. Instead, sliding attachments should be inserted which function as stress breakers.
➤ Although in principle feasible, cantilever bridges should be avoided whenever possible because of an increased risk of failure due to loss of crown retention, fracture of the metal frame, or even tooth fracture.
➤ Combinations with implants are often a better alternative (see below).

*Note*: Subgingival crown margins are largely incompatible with gingival health.
➤ In all areas not exposed to view, supragingival crown margins should be placed, if necessary, after surgical crown lengthening.
➤ In esthetically demanding areas, some compromise has to be sought:
- Slightly subgingival (about 0.5 mm), technically perfect (marginal imperfections of not more than 50 µm) crown margins are tolerable.
- The *biological width* must be taken into account. There should be a distance of 2.5 to 3 mm between the alveolar crest and the margin of the restoration. *Note*:

The biological width is smaller in individuals with narrow and thin gingiva.
- If the biological width is disregarded, attachment loss, or recurrent and frequently proliferating inflammation of the gingiva, is to be expected.

Failure after incorporation of fixed dental prostheses for stabilization of periodontally impaired dentitions is frequently due to technical and biophysical factors:
➤ Loss of retention of the crown
➤ Fracture of the metallic frame
➤ Root fracture after incorporation of post and core
➤ *Note*: As a basic principle, the most important prerequisite for long-term success is the control of periodontal infection.

In a **systematic review** of nine studies by Ong et al[64] in which survival and success rates of implants in patients with previous periodontitis were compared with those in patients without periodontitis, the following trends were revealed (quality of evidence: very low):
➤ In four out of five identified studies of patients with 4 to 14 years follow up, survival rates of implants in those with previous periodontitis were significantly lower.
➤ Likewise, in four out of five studies considerably more unfavorable success rates were reported in patients with previous periodontitis.
➤ In all three studies in which incidence of peri-implantitis had been assessed, this was considerably greater in patients who had previously been treated for periodontitis.

Insertion of dental implants for restoring patients with largely mutilated dentitions due to generalized aggressive or severe chronic periodontitis has to be planned thoughtfully. Broad application of possible indications may in fact lead to increased loss rates in patients with previous periodontitis. Likewise, implants in heavy smokers have an increased risk for failure or loss. If resorption of the alveolar process is considerable, bone augmentation is often inevitable.[66] Further routinely applied measures include:
➤ Guided bone regeneration (GBR) using membranes in combination with autoge-

nous bone and/or bone substitutes (xeno-grafts, allografts, or synthetics; see above).
➤ Onlay graft, that is, a block of autogenous bone.
➤ Sinus floor elevation.[67]
➤ Distraction osteogenesis, which has a comparably high rate of complications.

A **systematic review** by Telleman et al[68] concluded that short implants (< 10 mm) may be of advantage when trying to avoid possible complications due to bone augmentation and sinus floor elevation. Unsurprisingly, the survival rate of implants increased with their length. Quality of evidence: low.

## ■ Treatment of Peri-implant Infections

*Early dental implant failures* are caused by lack of or insufficient osseointegration and are usually the result of improper implant bed preparation, bacterial contamination and wound healing complications, lack of primary stability and/or premature loading. If osseointegration was not accomplished, the implant has to be explanted.

*Late failures* that occurred after primary osseointegration has been achieved are usually the result of bacterial infection (peri-implant mucositis, peri-implantitis) and/or excessive load.

To manage peri-implant infections in practice, depending on severity, increasingly invasive interventions are recommended (cumulative interceptive supportive therapy, CIST)[69]:
➤ *Peri-implant mucositis* (increased probing depth with bleeding on probing but no bone loss; **Fig. 11.53**):
  – Remotivation for effective oral hygiene.
  – Supra- and subgingival scaling with special graphite or plastic scalers (Perio Soft-Scaler, Kerr Dental). *Note:* The titanium surface of the implant may easily be destroyed by metal instruments.
  – Topical application of a 1% chlorhexidine gel, mouth rinsing with 0.1 to 0.2% chlorhexidine mouthwash, twice daily.
  – If required, surgical correction of unfavorable soft tissue morphology.
➤ *Peri-implantitis* (increased probing depth with bleeding on probing and also bone loss; **Fig. 11.53**):
  – As in case of peri-implant mucositis, effective oral hygiene has to be re-established. Supra- and subgingival scaling and application of chlorhexidine preparations.
  – If applicable, topical application of antibiotics with controlled or sustained release—for example, Ligosan (doxycycline,

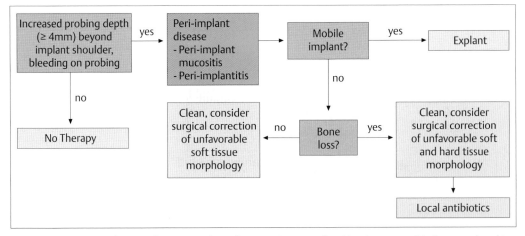

**Fig. 11.53 Decision diagram for peri-implant diseases.** In cases of peri-implant mucositis (increased probing depth without marginal bone loss but with bleeding on probing) the dental implant should be cleaned with special graphite or plastic scalers. Surgical correction of unfavorable soft tissue morphology may be considered as well. In the case of peri-implantitis (with bone loss), the dental implant has to be explanted, if mobile. In all other cases surgical correction of soft and hard tissue morphology is indicated. Topical application of an antibiotic (preferably with controlled or sustained release) should be considered as well.

Heraeus Kulzer, Hanau, Germany) or Chlo-Site (chlorhexidine, Zantomed, Duisburg, Germany), see Chapter 13.
- After resolution of acute inflammation, surgical correction of both soft and hard tissue morphology. Basically resective or, if applicable, regenerative measures apply. *Note:* While radiographs after about one year may reveal partial fill-in of osseous defects (**Fig. 11.54**), re-osseointegration should not be expected.
- If the implant is mobile, it has to be explanted.

In a systematic review, Esposito et al[70] identified nine studies in which the results of numerous different treatment modalities for peri-implantitis, both nonsurgical (mechanical and machine-driven debridement, topical antibiotics, laser therapy) and surgical (access flap, GTR, bone augmentation), were reported. The authors concluded that reliable evidence of efficacy is currently lacking:

➤ A single small trial at unclear risk of bias revealed that the use of topical antibiotics in addition to subgingival debridement yielded a statistically significant additional 0.6 mm mean reduction of probing attachment level (PAL) and pocket depth (PPD) over a 4-month period in patients with severe peri-implantitis. Another small trial at high risk of bias indicated that, after 4 years, improved PAL and PPD of about 1.4 mm, on average, were obtained when a xenograft bone substitute with a resorbable membrane was compared to nanocrystalline hydroxyapatite in peri-implant infrabony defects. (Quality of evidence: moderate.)
➤ There is no evidence from four trials that more complex and expensive therapies were superior to control treatments, which basically consisted of subgingival mechanical debridement.
➤ Follow-ups longer than one year suggested recurrence of peri-implantitis in up to 100% of treated cases for some of the tested interventions.

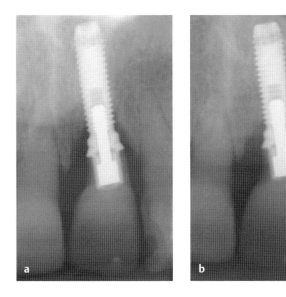

**Fig. 11.54 Treatment of peri-implantitis.**
**a** Radiographically discernable bone loss at a dental implant in the region of 021. Clinically, probing depths of 9 mm were measured and profuse bleeding on probing and emanation of pus recorded. During surgical treatment the implant surfaces were cleaned with graphite scalers and a saturated solution of tetracycline (content of a capsule dissolved in saline) applied with cotton pellets. Systemic amoxicillin (1.5 g/d) and metronidazole (1.2 g/d) was prescribed for 7 days (see Chapter 13).
**b** Ten months after therapy, radiographically discernable partial bone-fill had occurred. Clinically, probing depths were 4 mm and mucosa did not bleed after probing.

# 12 Phase III—Supportive Periodontal Therapy

## ■ Risk Assessment, Risk Communication, Risk Management

Immediately after periodontal surgery, the progress of healing should be followed up weekly or every other week. After two to three months, the periodontal situation is re-evaluated. Thereafter, *supportive periodontal therapy* (SPT), which is phase III of periodontal therapy, commences.[1]

In patients susceptible to periodontal disease, a high risk of recurrent infection with periodontal pathogens has to been assumed. Therefore, after completion of corrective therapy, lifelong supportive care should be organized on an individual basis.

Risk assessment, its communication to the patient, and risk management are cornerstones of supportive care. The goals of this third treatment phase, which has also been termed maintenance therapy, are:
➤ Risk-related medical and dental history-taking and clinical examination.
➤ Remotivation of the patient and providing continuous medical support.
➤ Timely and appropriate intervention in any case of recurrent periodontitis.
➤ Avoidance of any under- or overtreatment.

*Note*: Long-term success of any periodontal therapy depends less on particular surgical measures or devices, but more on the quality of supportive periodontal care.

### Risk Assessment

If possible, reduction of deleterious influences of established risk factors is nowadays regarded as a central treatment aspect of any complex, multifactorial, chronic disease. This applies to periodontal diseases as well, since both onset and progression of periodontitis are largely determined by individual risks:
➤ Risk factors are either part of the *causal chain* or they *expose* the individual to disease.

➤ *Note*: Once disease has broken out, elimination of the risk factor does not necessarily lead to healing.

Risk assessment for recurring periodontitis is usually performed at three levels[2]:
➤ Local risk assessment
➤ Dentition-related risk assessment
➤ Systemic risk assessment.

### Local Risk Factors

*Redness* and *swelling* of the gingiva are cardinal symptoms of inflammation and should be carefully assessed in any periodontal examination. They are visible signs of inflammatory reactions, especially to supragingival plaque. Because of very low sensitivity, they are not a suitable diagnostic for periodontal activity.[3]

*Bleeding on probing* to the bottom of the sulcus or pocket (**Fig. 12.1**) can easily be checked by local examination. Especially if a pressure-controlled probe is used with a force of about 0.25 N (e.g., ClickProbe, KerrHawe, Bioggio, Switzerland), it gives a fairly reliable impression of local inflammation within the sulcus or pocket:
➤ Bleeding on probing has been used as a *diagnostic test* for attachment loss during supportive periodontal care. *Frequent bleeding on probing* has low sensitivity (many false-negative findings) but quite high specificity (few false-positive findings) in detecting active periodontal disease.
➤ If a site bleeds whenever the patient attends the office for periodontal maintenance, the risk for attachment loss at that particular site may be increased about two- to three-fold. Absence of or infrequent bleeding on probing, on the other hand, signifies a stable periodontal condition.[3]

*Purulent exudate* had in the past been a name-giving symptom of the disease, *pyorrhea alveolaris*. It is nowadays rarely observed, in particular not during supportive periodontal care:

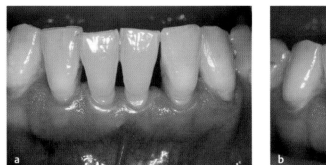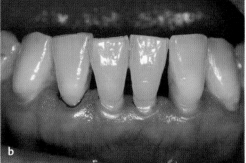

**Fig. 12.1 Bleeding on probing.**
**a** Clinically, the periodontal situation shows no signs of inflammation.
**b** Profuse bleeding after probing at the distal aspect of the right lateral incisor. Small bleeding spots are seen distal to the right and mesial to the left central incisor. Frequent bleeding after probing has been shown to be rather insensitive but relatively specific for periodontal activity after therapy.

➤ Because it lacks sensitivity (many false-negative findings), purulent exudate is not a prognostic indicator.
➤ If present, it should always prompt therapeutic measures.

*Increased probing depth*: Periodontal probing depths of more than 3 mm are frequently noted after periodontal therapy. Basically two differential diagnoses are possible:
➤ Increased probing depth due to a long junctional epithelium after periodontal surgery. In that case, there is no inflammation and, in particular, no bleeding on probing (see Chapter 11).
➤ Increased probing depth because of presence of a periodontal pocket. The inflammatory response in the tissue then results in bleeding on probing.

In residual periodontal pockets that bleed after probing, there is high risk of further attachment loss.[3] For this reason, *combined findings* should be recorded: For instance, bleeding on probing may be documented in the periodontal chart (see **Fig. 6.8**) by underlining (in red) the periodontal probing depth.
*Furcation involvement* may drastically impair the prognosis of the affected tooth.[4,5] The risk for extraction of a tooth with insufficiently treated furcation involvement may be increased by a factor of 2. Likewise, persisting *bony pockets* have a slightly increased risk, by about 30%, for further attachment loss.[6]

Local presence of *periodontal pathogens* (e.g., cell numbers $> 10^4$ for *Aggregatibacter actinomycetemcomitans* and $> 10^5$ for *Porphyromonas gingivalis*), have been shown to drastically increase the risk of local attachment loss. Microbiological tests of plaque from individual tooth surfaces are very expensive and therefore not suitable as a diagnostic tool (see Chapter 6 and below).

## Dentition-Related Risk Factors

The proportion of *tooth surfaces covered by supragingival plaque* (after disclosing) and the proportion of *gingival units bleeding after probing* may be used for remotivating a patient who is under supportive periodontal care. During supportive periodontal care, excellent oral hygiene is required.
➤ In plaque-infected dentitions, further progression of periodontal disease has to be expected.[7]
➤ The proportion of gingival units that bleed after probing corresponds well with the overall inflammatory condition of the tissues.
➤ The *relation between both parameters*, namely the percentage of plaque-covered surfaces and gingival units bleeding on probing (e.g., the plaque-bleeding ratio, or the site-specific association), may better relate to the risk of future attachment loss:
  – Supposedly, a low proportion of tooth surfaces covered by plaque but a high propor-

tion of sites bleeding on probing might signal a higher risk.

– High proportions of plaque, but rather lower proportions of sites that bleed on probing—that is, a weaker association—have been observed in IL-1 genotype positive individuals (see Chapter 8) with plaque-induced gingivitis.[8]

– Likewise, smokers usually have comparable amounts of plaque and slightly more calculus than nonsmokers (see Chapter 8). Bleeding tendency after probing may, on the other hand, be reduced. *Note:* This masking effect of smoking may lead to risk miscalculation.

Both the number of *residual pockets* and the number of *open furcations* considerably expand the habitat for obligately anaerobic periodontal pathogens. As a consequence, numerous residual periodontal pockets of, say, 5 mm or more and open, inappropriately treated, furcations raise the periodontitis risk for the whole dentition.

The intraoral load of selected periodontal pathogens such as *A. actinomycetemcomitans*, *P. gingivalis*, *Prevotella intermedia*, *Tannerella forsythia*, and *Treponema denticola* may be assessed in a pooled sample of, for instance, the four deepest pockets. This may provide valuable information, particularly in aggressive forms of periodontitis and cases refractory to periodontal therapy (see Chapters 6 and 13). In either case, persistent periodontal infection with *A. actinomycetemcomitans* may have some prognostic value. *Note:* Microbiological tests should not be performed on a routine basis. Any possible gain in information must always be set against the considerable expenses involved.

*Tooth loss* due to periodontitis may signal increased susceptibility for periodontal disease. The risk of further tooth loss may be higher if numerous teeth had already been extracted due to periodontal disease. Since the decision for or against an extraction is not always entirely based on the periodontal prognosis of the particular tooth, other reasons for previous extractions need to be taken into account.

*Bone loss* in relation to age: advanced, generalized bone loss at a young age signifies high risk of further attachment loss. On the other hand, mild or moderate bone loss in middle or old age usually indicates low risk.

*Complex restorative treatment* entails numerous risks (see Chapter 11) which have to be assessed on a regular basis. They include:

➤ Occlusal instability leading to increasing tooth mobility
➤ Possible fracture of the construction or loss of retention
➤ Tooth fracture
➤ Endodontic problems
➤ Possible oral hygiene impediment

### General Risk Factors

Due to likely *genetic predisposition* (see **Tables 3.4** and **3.5**) and possible *persistent infection* with periodontal pathogens that are difficult to eradicate, such as *A. actinomycetemcomitans*, patients with aggressive and early-onset periodontitis generally need more intensive supportive care than patients with more chronic forms of the disease.

Some *systemic diseases* are important risk factors for periodontitis. Therefore, periodical updating of medical history is mandatory, especially in older patients. In the context of supportive periodontal care, close cooperation with medical specialists may be necessary: for example, diagnosis and metabolic control of patients with diabetes mellitus; management and prevention of menopausal osteoporosis; or for patients with HIV infection.

The most important risk factor for periodontitis is *tobacco consumption*,[9] and quitting smoking is an important aim during all phases of periodontal therapy. Smoking status can be assessed and documented in a suitable questionnaire (see **Table 8.4**). Although smoking is causing a plethora of serious and life-threatening diseases, the dentist may be a natural first contact person for medical counseling and assistance in quitting smoking.

### Communication

Established and presumed risks for onset and progression of periodontal disease (**Table 12.1**) may be graphically displayed in multidimensional risk diagrams (**Fig. 12.2**). Visualization of the individual risk may considerably improve communication with the patient and allow joint planning of how to proceed. Important aspects are renewed improvement of oral hygiene; in smokers, alteration of smoking habits;

**Table 12.1** Known and presumed risks for development and progression of periodontal disease

| Risk | Examples | Relative risks |
|---|---|---|
| Etiological factors | • Poor oral hygiene<br>• Periodontal pathogens<br>  – A. actinomycetemcomitans<br>  – P. gingivalis<br>  – T. forsythia<br>  – T. denticola | 2<br>2–3; possibly much higher (~17) in periodontal infections with highly leukotoxic clone of A. actinomycetemcomitans, JP2 |
| Genetic susceptibility | • Allele 2 (C→T) of IL1A(−889) and IL1B (+3954) | ~2 in Caucasians |
| Drugs | • Immune suppressive agents<br>  – cyclosporin A<br>  – tacrolimus<br>• Ca²⁺ antagonists | |
| Behavior | Coping with emotional stress | 1.5–2 |
| Background variables | • Age<br>• Gender<br>• Race | Increases with age<br>Males > females<br>Blacks > Asians > Caucasians |
| Systemic diseases | • Diabetes mellitus<br><br>• Osteopenia/osteoporosis | 2.8–3.4; may be much higher in poorly controlled diabetics |
| External exposition | Smoking | 2.5–6; may be much higher in young populations |
| Socioeconomic factors | • Education<br>• Poverty | |

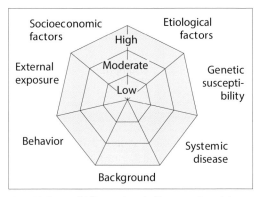

**Fig. 12.2 Multidimensional diagram for risk assessment of complex diseases.** The different sectors represent clusters of different factors (**Table 12.1**). Polygonals connect comparably low, moderate, and high risks. This allows the risk in a given case to be more easily visualized. Note that dentition-related and (superordinate) general risks should be presented in separate risk diagrams. (Adapted from Tonetti.[9])

and facilitating overall cooperation with the patient's physician.[10,11]

For long-lasting compliance the patient should be able to fully comprehend the suggested therapeutic measures.

### Risk Management

Supportive periodontal therapy may be carried out during a one-hour appointment:
➤ *Examination* (about 15 minutes):
  – Update of medical/dental history
  – Intraoral, especially periodontal, examination (see **Figs. 6.8** and **6.13**)
  – Risk assessment
➤ Detailed counseling (about 15 minutes):
  – If required, motivation to improve oral hygiene
  – If required, medical support in quitting smoking
  – Discussion of further procedure
➤ Active measures (about 30 minutes):
  – Supragingival scaling.
  – Subgingival scaling only at sites with periodontal probing depths of ≥4 mm which have bled upon probing. *Note:* Subgingival scaling in shallow pockets of up to 3 mm

leads to attachment loss (see Chapter 10). Frequent removal of root substance may also result in hypersensitive teeth.

– In particular, open furcations must be carefully debrided with hand instruments and/or ultrasonic or sonic scalers.
– Polishing with polishing paste. Local fluoridation with high-dose fluoride gel.

If any surgical procedures would be necessary— for example, if more than four bleeding sites with a periodontal probing depth of 5 mm or more were found—a separate session should be arranged.

Recall intervals should basically depend on individual risks:

➤ For patients at *high risk* (combined systemic and behavioral risks, complex and prolonged perio-prosthetic treatment, or uncertainty about recurrence of periodontitis), the next SPT session should be scheduled after two or three months. *Note*: The proportion of these patients should not exceed 10% in a specialized periodontal practice.
➤ For patients at *moderate risk* who have certain, easy-to-control risks, recall intervals of about four to six months are appropriate. In a specialized periodontal practice, these patients amount to about 60%.
➤ For patients at *low risk*, yearly sessions are sufficient. *Note*: Any overtreatment and leaving patients in uncertainty about the course of the disease should be avoided.

# 13 Medication and Supplements

## ◼ Antibiotic and Antimycotic Therapy

### Systemically Administered Antibiotics

Adjunct antibiotic therapy may be justified because of the infectious character of most periodontal diseases, which may be caused by a limited number of bacteria.

A distinction has to be made between specific, *microbiologically oriented* chemotherapy following the detection of specific pathogens; and *empirically oriented* chemotherapy in acute cases, which demand immediate treatment. In the wake of a surge of new information on the complexity of the oral microbiota (see Chapter 2) and results from randomized controlled trials,[1] microbiologically oriented antibiotic therapy has recently lost some ground and the value of microbiological diagnosis has been put into perspective (see Chapter 6).

Concerns about increasing antibiotic resistance (e.g., methicillin-resistant *Staphylococcus aureus*, multidrug-resistant tuberculosis, antibiotic resistance of bacteria causing common infections of the urinary tract, pneumonia, or bloodstream infections), which jeopardizes effective prevention and treatment of life-threatening infections, should be taken seriously when considering adjunct antibiotic therapy of periodontal diseases. After all, periodontal infections are not life-threatening diseases and can usually be controlled without adjunctive antibiotics.

➤ *Note*: Apart from generalized severe cases, chronic periodontitis should not be treated in the first place with adjunct systemic antibiotics.

➤ In cases of aggressive or refractory periodontitis, microbiological diagnosis (see Chapter 6) may allow the targeting of specific pathogens such as *Aggregatibacter actinomycetemcomitans* and *Porphyromonas gingivalis*. Responsible use of antibiotics takes into account the possible development of bacterial *resistance*, antibiotic *toxicity*, and the risk of *sensitizing*.

Some basic characteristics of various types of infections,[2] that is, acute, chronic, delayed, or biofilm-induced, should be carefully considered (**Table 13.1**):

➤ Not life-threatening *acute bacterial infections* usually do not require antibiotics. Supportive treatment measures such as bed rest, supply of liquids and minerals, and fever-reducing drugs suffice in most cases. A typical example of an oral infection in this group is acute necrotizing ulcerative gingivitis (ANUG, see Chapter 9).

➤ Development of *chronic disease* signals problems of the host to properly cope with the infection. Chronic necrotizing ulcerative periodontitis is a typical oral example. In this case, adjunct antibiotic therapy may be of considerable advantage.

➤ In many *delayed infections*, causative agents have long been mysterious (e.g., the role of *Helicobacter pylori* in the pathogenesis of peptic ulcer). Once the cause has been identified, antibiotic treatment may be straightforward.

➤ In contrast, *biofilm infections* which are caused by members of the resident microflora (see Chapter 2) require a completely different approach, namely mechanical disruption of the highly organized biofilm. As outlined in Chapter 2, alterations in the ecosystem may also have considerable therapeutic effects. In addition, antiseptics are successfully applied as well (see Chapter 10).

Before any administration of adjunctive systemic antibiotics, the dentogingival biofilm has to be disrupted by thorough scaling and root planing:

➤ Structured plaque within the pocket may be as thick as 400 µm (see Chapter 2). It is unlikely that an antibiotic can penetrate these bacterial masses which are colonizing the root surface.

➤ Moreover, because of the extremely high number of bacteria in the pocket, the antibiotic appearing in gingival exudate is rapidly depleted.

**Table 13.1** Some characteristics of bacterial infections. (Modified and supplemented after Socransky and Haffajee[2])

| | Acute infection | Chronic infection | Delayed infection | Biofilm-induced infection |
|---|---|---|---|---|
| **Examples** | • Upper respiratory tract<br>• Gastrointestinal tract<br>• Local abscess<br>• Acute necrotizing ulcerative gingivitis | • Tuberculosis<br>• Leprosy<br>• Necrotizing ulcerative periodontitis | • Rheumatic fever<br>• Syphilis<br>• Peptic ulcer<br>• Lyme disease | • Dental caries<br>• Periodontitis/ peri-implant diseases<br>• Denture stomatitis<br>• Conjunctivitis in patients wearing contact lenses |
| **Onset after colonization** | Rapid | Slow | Delayed | Delayed |
| **Course** | Days, weeks | Months, years | Years | Years |
| **Causative agent(s)** | Exogenous | Exogenous, also endogenous | Exogenous | Endogenous |
| **Source of infection** | Often unknown | Sometimes unknown | Often unknown | Unknown |
| **Characteristics** | After entry into the body, rapid resolution | After entry into the body, failure of host to cope | Inauspicious onset, later new form of the disease | • Biofilm<br>• Pathogens reside basically outside the body |
| **Treatment** | • **Supportive**<br>• *Antibiotics* | • **Antibiotics**<br>• *supportive* | • **Antibiotics**<br>• **?** | • **Mechanic disruption**<br>• **Ecological**<br>• Antiseptic<br>• *Antibiotics?* |

➤ Bacterial metabolism and proliferation rate are much decreased in biofilms. Minimum inhibitory concentrations of antibiotics for bacteria residing in biofilms may therefore be 100 to 1,000 times higher than concentrations effective in planktonic cultures (see Chapter 6).

➤ The risk for resistance development is therefore particularly high.

Adjunctive systemic antibiotic therapy basically aims at the reduction or eradication[3] of specific periodontal pathogens, while the physiological flora is preferably not affected. Superinfection with resistant microorganisms should be avoided.

Possible indications for the use of adjunctive antibiotics include[4–6]:

➤ Aggressive (**Fig. 13.1**), especially early-onset, periodontitis.

➤ Refractory chronic periodontitis (**Fig. 13.2**).

➤ Severe forms of generalized periodontitis in patients with systemic disease, for example:

– Diabetes mellitus
– Low numbers or dysfunction of polymorphonuclear granulocytes
– HIV infection and < 200/mm³ CD4 cells

➤ Necrotizing ulcerative periodontitis and periodontal abscess (**Fig. 13.3**), especially if general symptoms, fever, and/or lymphadenitis are present.

➤ For indications for antibiotic prophylaxis, see Chapter 8.

In cases of moderate or localized severe, chronic periodontitis the first step should always be a vigorous attempt to control the periodontal infection by conventional means (see Chapters 10 and 11), namely scaling and root planing and, after re-evaluation, access flap surgery if required. Only if that strategy has apparently failed, should a critical analysis be done as to the following questions:

➤ Is the oral hygiene of the patient sufficient?

➤ Have teeth with furcation involvement and infrabony defects been treated properly?

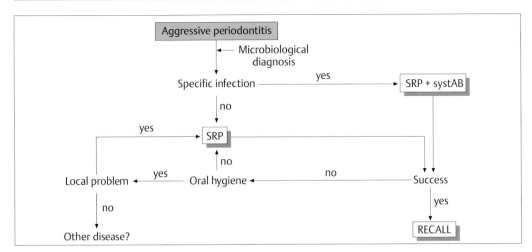

**Fig. 13.1   Flow chart for decision-making regarding adjunctive systemic antibiotics (systAB) in cases of aggressive periodontitis.** A microbiological test for presence of pathogens, such as *Aggregatibacter actinomycetemcomitans* and/or *Porphyromonas gingivalis*, should be done at the very outset of the therapy, not least for forensic reasons. Possible differential diagnoses of other diseases (e.g., malignancy, Langerhans' cell histiocytosis, mucocutaneous disorders, inflammatory alterations associated with corrosion phenomena) should be taken into account, as well. SRP: scaling and root planing; after reevaluation, if required, also in combination with flap surgery.

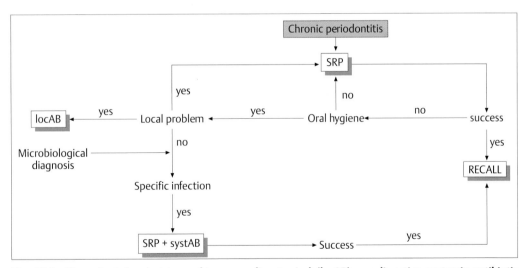

**Fig. 13.2   Flow chart for decision-making regarding topical (locAB) or adjunctive systemic antibiotic treatment (systAB) in cases of chronic periodontitis.** Note that microbiological tests should be arranged only after conventional therapy has failed. SRP: scaling and root planing which, after re-evaluation, may be combined, if required, with flap surgery.

➤ Is the patient a heavy smoker?
➤ Could there be any underlying systemic disease?

Before prescribing systemic antibiotics, the existing problems in the patient need to be properly addressed. *Note:* Reducing the need for periodontal surgery by adjunct antibiotics may be short-sighted. Anatomical defects such as

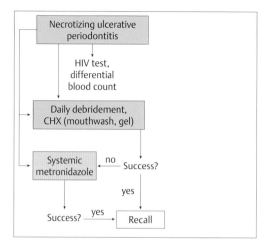

**Fig. 13.3   Flow chart for decision-making in necrotizing ulcerative periodontitis.** In order to rule out respective infections or blood diseases, an HIV test and differential blood count should be arranged. If general symptoms of fever and lymphadenitis are present, daily debridement should be supplemented by systemic metronidazole treatment.

furcation involvement and infrabony lesions, which are the main indications for periodontal surgery (see Chapter 11), will not resolve after subgingival scaling and adjunct antibiotic treatment. In light of the global problem of antibiotic resistance, any recommendation for repeat courses of antibiotic therapy to reduce the need for minor surgical intervention in a not life-threatening disease should be considered inappropriate.

Within the framework of comprehensive periodontal therapy, an adjunct antibiotic agent should have the following properties:
➤ *Specificity*: Antibiotics of great importance in general medicine that are reserved for life-threatening conditions should not be used to fight periodontal infections.
➤ *Effectiveness*: Microbial diagnosis (e. g., culture) may be combined with susceptibility testing. Antibiotics should be bactericidal rather than merely bacteriostatic.
➤ *Substantivity*: The appropriate antibiotic should appear at sufficient concentration at the site of action (i.e., the periodontal pocket). *Note:* Since periodontal pathogens can be found on all mucous membranes of the oral cavity and may even invade epithelial cells, an antibiotic should appear in effective concentrations in the saliva as well (**Table 13.2**).
➤ *Safety*: Low toxicity and low risk of sensitization.
➤ Possibility of *oral administration*: Parenteral or intramuscular applications are usually not suitable in dental practice.

The following antibiotics have been used as an adjunct to conventional periodontal therapy (**Table 13.3**). Note that relevant contraindications have to be observed in each case:
➤ *Penicillins*:
  – Interfere with bacterial cell wall synthesis.
  – Exhibit in-vitro antibacterial activity against most periodontal pathogens.

**Table 13.2** Concentrations of antibiotics in serum, gingival exudate, and saliva after oral administration of standard doses

| | Dosage (mg) | Serum concentration (µg/mL) | Concentration in gingival exudate (µg/mL) | Concentration in saliva (µg/mL) |
|---|---|---|---|---|
| Penicillin | 500 | 3 | ~0 | ~0 |
| Amoxicillin | 500 | 8 | 3–4 | ~0 |
| Doxycycline | 200 | 2–3 | 2–8 | 0.5 |
| Tetracycline | 500 | 3–4 | 5–12 | 0.1–0.3 |
| Azithromycine | 500 | 0.3–0.4 | 3.3–6.5* | 2 |
| Clindamycin | 150 | 2–3 | 1–2 | 0.2–0.3 |
| Metronidazole | 500 | 6–12 | 8–10 | 6–12 |
| Ciprofloxacin | 500 | 1–2.5 | 2.5 | 1.3 |

* Concentration in gingival tissue.

**Table 13.3** Recommended dosages for adjunctive systemic antibiotic therapy

| Antibiotic | Dosage for adults (70 kg) | Duration of medication |
|---|---|---|
| Tetracycline<br>• Tetracycline-HCl<br>• Doxycycline-HCl<br><br>• Minocycline-HCl | <br>• 4 × 250 mg/day<br>• 1 × 200 mg/day,<br>  afterwards 1 × 100 mg/day<br>• 1 × 200 mg/day | <br>• 14–21 days<br>• 1 day, 13–20 days<br><br>• 14–21 days |
| Metronidazole | 3 × 400 mg/day | 7–10 days |
| Amoxicillin/clavulanic acid (Augmentin) | 3 × 500 mg/day | 7–10 days |
| Ciprofloxacin | 2 × 500 mg/day | 7–10 days |
| Clindamycin | 4 × 300 mg/day | 7 days |
| Azithromycin | 2 × 250 mg/day | 3 days |
| Combinations<br>• Metronidazole/<br>  amoxicillin<br>• Metronidazole/<br>  ciprofloxacin | <br>• 3 × 400 mg/day<br>• 3 × 500 mg/day<br>• 2 × 500 mg/day<br>• 2 × 500 mg/day | <br>7–10 days<br><br>7–10 days |

– However, pocket exudate generally contains sufficient amounts of β-lactamase (penicillinase), which cleaves the β-lactam ring of the penicillin and nullifies any antimicrobial effect. β-lactamases may be produced by certain periodontal pathogens.

– *Note:* If penicillin without β-lactamase inhibitor was prescribed, untreated periodontitis may even exacerbate. Multiple periodontal abscesses may develop (see Chapter 9).

➤ *Penicillins with β-lactamase inhibitors:* Broad-spectrum penicillin amoxicillin may be combined with clavulanic acid (Augmentin) or sulbactam (Sultamicillin), which both carry the β-lactam ring. They have basically no antimicrobial activity but high affinity to β-lactamases which are irreversibly blocked.

➤ *Tetracyclines:*
– Bacteriostatic antibiotics with a broad spectrum of antimicrobial action. Tetracyclines interfere with protein synthesis of bacteria.

– Considerable substantivity: Systemically administered tetracyclines bind to root surfaces within the pocket and may be released even after intake has ceased. This may lead to higher concentrations of tetracycline (**Fig. 13.4**), doxycycline, and minocycline in gingival exudate than in serum.[8]

– On the other hand, tetracyclines are rarely secreted into the saliva (**Table 13.2**),

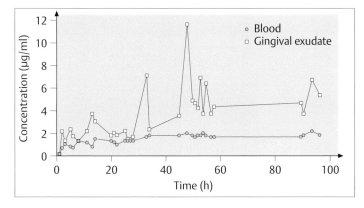

Fig. 13.4 **Compared to achievable blood levels, concentrations of tetracycline may become two to four times higher in gingival exudate.** Oral dosage: 250 mg every 6 hours. (Adapted from Gordon et al.[7])

which might be the main reason for their failure to eradicate infections, such as due to oral *A. actinomycetemcomitans*,[4] when administered as an adjunct to subgingival scaling.

– Irrespective of their antimicrobial effect, tetracyclines inhibit tissue collagenase (see below).

➤ *Nitroimidazole derivatives* (metronidazole, ornidazole):

– Inhibit nucleic acid synthesis by disrupting the DNA of microbial cells.

– Small spectrum of activity against protozoa (e.g., trichomonads) and obligate anaerobes.

– After administration of therapeutic doses, similar concentrations are found in gingival crevice fluid and serum. Metronidazole is also secreted into the saliva.

– Metronidazole is the antibiotic of first choice for necrotizing ulcerative periodontitis, aggressive periodontitis, and refractory periodontal infections with obligately anaerobic periodontal pathogens.

– In laboratory animal experiments mutagenicity and carcinogenicity have been observed.

– *Note:* Metronidazole, and possibly ornidazole, may cause severe nausea and vomiting if taken in adjunction with alcohol (disulfiram reaction).

➤ *Clindamycin:*

– Interferes with bacterial protein synthesis.

– Is especially active against gram-negative, obligately anaerobic bacteria.

– Is virtually not secreted into saliva.

– It may be applied as an adjunct antibiotic in refractory cases not associated with *Eikenella corrodens* (which is resistant to clindamycin).

– *Caution*: Pseudomembranous colitis after superinfection of the gut with *Clostridium difficile,* which is resistant to clindamycin. Clindamycin should therefore only be administered if other antibiotics are contraindicated.

➤ *Azalides*, a new generation of macrolides, in particular azithromycin:

– Displays antimicrobial activity against anaerobic and gram-negative bacteria.

– High concentrations can be achieved in the saliva and gingival tissues.

➤ *Quinolones* (e.g., ciprofloxacin, ofloxacin, moxifloxacin):

– Quinolones, which inhibit DNA gyrase, have excellent activity against numerous facultatively anaerobic, gram-negative bacteria, including nosocomials like *Pseudomonas aeruginosa.*

– In particular, moxifloxacin has favorable pharmacokinetic properties (high saliva concentration, penetration of neutrophil granulocytes and epithelial cells) and excellent activity against *A. actinomycetemcomitans.*[9]

– *Note*: Quinolones should not routinely be used in dentistry owing to its excellent activity in serious nosocomial infections and high risk for resistance development.

➤ Combinations:

– Metronidazole and amoxicillin have widely been used in combination, especially in periodontal infections, with *A. actinomycetemcomitans* and/or *P. gingivalis.*

– In patients who are allergic to penicillins, as an exception ciprofloxacin may be combined with metronidazole.

In **systematic reviews** by Herrera et al[10] and Haffajee et al[11] adjunct systemic antibiotic therapy of periodontitis has been critically assessed. **Meta-analyses** of studies in which patients with chronic or aggressive periodontitis had been treated revealed the following:

➤ If subgingival scaling was supplemented by systemic antibiotics, greater gain of clinical attachment, particularly in deep periodontal pockets, was reported. A great number of different antibiotics including tetracyclines, metronidazole, spiramycin and, notably, combinations of amoxicillin and metronidazole, all showed similar effects in this regard. Quality of evidence: moderate.

➤ In particular, patients with aggressive or active periodontitis may benefit from adjunct systemic antibiotics.

In another **systematic review** of 19 randomized controlled trials by Zandbergen et al,[12] clinical effects of nonsurgical periodontal therapy were compared to systemic administration of combined metronidazole and amoxicillin as adjunct. The additional pocket reduction after 6 months averaged 1.50 mm (95% confidence interval [CI] 1.46; 1.54) while additional clinical attachment gain was 0.98 mm, on average (95% CI 0.93; 1.03). Quality of evidence: moderate.

Whether the choice of a suitable antibiotic should be based on the predominant pathogens or presence of resistant bacteria had been a matter of dispute. In particular the combination of amoxicillin and metronidazole appears to result in a considerable improvement of periodontal conditions, as regards pocket depth reduction and clinical attachment gain, in the majority of cases with aggressive and refractory chronic periodontitis. Moreover, at least for a short period, a reduced surgical treatment need was reported.[13]

Microbiological testing may in fact be helpful when selecting a suitable antibiotic in therapy-resistant cases of chronic periodontitis (see Chapter 2). Not least for forensic reasons they are recommended after a thorough analysis of possible reasons for the present partial failure of conventional periodontal therapy (**Fig. 13.2**).

*Note:* Due to known and in part considerable adverse effects, any decisions about adjunct antibiotic therapy of periodontal diseases should be made with caution.

## Topical Administration of Antimicrobial Substances

For the use of antiseptics in mouth rinses and toothpastes see Chapter 10.

Periodontal disease tends to occur locally. Consequently, topical application of antimicrobial agents may be a reasonable treatment approach. In order to be pharmacologically effective, topically applied drugs have to fulfill the following criteria[14]:

➤ The drug must reach the site of action—in this case, the bottom of the periodontal pocket.
➤ It must remain there for sufficient time.
➤ It must be effective at concentrations that can be achieved.

Clinical and microbiological effects of pocket irrigation as well as application of preparations with sustained and controlled delivery (**Fig. 13.5**) of various drugs have been tested in numerous studies:

➤ *Pocket irrigation* with a blunt cannula or special irrigators: for example, povidone–iodine (Betadine), 3% $H_2O_2$, or chlorhexidine

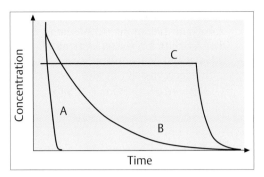

**Fig. 13.5 Clearance of intracrevicularly administered antimicrobial drugs.**
**a** Pocket irrigation.
**b** Drug delivery device with sustained release.
**c** Controlled delivery of the drug. (Adapted from Tonetti.[14])

solution. In the case of a periodontal abscess (see Chapter 9):
– Since the bottom of the pocket is not reliably reached by the active agent and the time for which it remains in the pocket at effective concentrations is too short, pocket irrigation basically exerts only minor effects.
– The adjunct subgingival irrigation with chlorhexidine or hydrogen peroxide had no additional clinical effect.[15]

➤ Preparations with *sustained drug delivery* may exert bactericidal action for extended periods[16–18]:
– 1.5% chlorhexidine in a gel which contains 2.5% xanthan gum (ChloSite, Zantomed, Duisburg, Germany) may be applied in periodontal and peri-implant pockets with a rounded-down cannula. The gel may stay up to 3 weeks in the pocket while chlorhexidine is consistently released.
– 25% metronidazole benzoate gel consisting of glyceryl monooleate and sesame oil (Elyzol, Dentalgel, Colgate-Palmolive, New York, USA). The gel, which sets under the influence of gingival exudate or saliva, is applied with a rounded-down cannula in two sessions, one week apart.
– 14% doxycycline hyclate in a biologically degradable slow-release gel formulation (Ligosan Slow Release, Haereus Kulzer, Hanau, Germany).

- Adhesive film solution of piperacillin/tazobactam (Periofilm T, Medirel, Agno, Switzerland) for the treatment of periodontal and peri-implant pockets.
- 2% minocycline-HCl in an ointment containing hydroxymethyl cellulose, aminoalkyl methacrylate, triacetin, and glycerin (Periocline, Sunstar, Chicago, Illinois, USA).
➤ Preparations with *controlled drug delivery*[19,20]:
  - A gelatin chip with 2.5 mg chlorhexidine (PerioChip, Dexcel Pharma, Or Akiva, Israel). This biologically degradable chip is 5 mm long, 5 mm wide, and about 1 mm thick. It is trimmed to fit the pocket morphology. The chlorhexidine concentration in gingival exudate may reach 125 μg/mL for about 1 week.
  - Minocycline in biodegradable microglobuli (Arestin, OraPharma, Plainview, NY, USA). Concentrations in gingival exudate of up to 340 μg/mL may be maintained for 2 weeks.
  - Within the framework of guided tissue regeneration (see Chapter 11), freely applied resorbable gel barrier containing 4% doxycycline (Atrisorb D FreeFlow, Tolmar, Fort Collins, Colorado, USA).

In **meta-analyses**[21,22] of randomized controlled trials of 6 months duration (±3 months) on the efficacy of adjunct local antibiotic/antiseptic therapy with various active agents (tetracycline, minocycline, doxycycline, metronidazole, chlorhexidine chip) the following was concluded:
➤ As compared to sole scaling and root planing, the combined treatment with topical application of antimicrobial agents resulted in significantly lower periodontal probing depths (average 0.2 to <0.5 mm). Additional clinical attachment gains were even smaller and not always significant. Quality of evidence: low.
➤ *Note:* Additional mean pocket depth reduction or clinical attachment gain in the range of fractions of a millimeter must be considered clinically irrelevant.

According to **meta-analyses**,[23–25] the sole application of topical antibiotics as compared to scaling and root planing may lead to similar results as regards pocket depth reduction and gain of clinical attachment. Quality of evidence: low.

*Critical assessment:* Preparations with controlled drug delivery may be employed in certain cases as an alternative to mechanical debridement, for example:
➤ During supportive periodontal care in the case of marked dentin hypersensitivity
➤ After considerable loss of tooth substance due to repeat scaling
➤ *Note:* Combination therapy (scaling and root planing plus local antimicrobial therapy) had in most cases no additional effect. Possible exceptions may include deep periodontal pockets which have not sufficiently responded to mechanical debridement—for example, open furcations or deep infrabony pockets, and in particular peri-implantitis (see Chapter 11).

As a matter of fact, periodontal pathogens do not only colonize periodontal pockets. Most pathogens are widely distributed within the oral cavity and topical application of antimicrobial agents would hardly affect other habitats. Especially in cases of periodontal infection in which invasive[26] and difficult-to-eradicate bacteria are involved (e.g., *A. actinomycetemcomitans* in aggressive periodontitis), topical antibiotic therapy is therefore not indicated.

## Local Antimycotic Therapy

Diagnosis of oral candidosis:
➤ Clinically, white coatings or patches of pseudomembranous slough (so-called thrush) predominate, which leave a red, bleeding surface if removed. In other cases erythematous areas emerge. *Note:* Angular cheilitis of the corner of the mouth is often a co-infection of *Candida albicans* and *Staphylococcus aureus*.
➤ Swab samples may be directly streaked onto an elective medium (Nickerson) and cultivated at room temperature. Suspect colonies of *Candida* spp. may be assessed after 24 to 48 hours.
➤ Cytology of swab samples and proof of mycelium, in some cases hyphae which have invaded epithelial cells. In chronic cases biopsy and serology are recommended.

Therapy involves improvement of oral and, if applicable, denture hygiene, supplemented with adjunctive use of chlorhexidine mouthwash/gel. In refractory cases topical antimycotic therapy (lozenges, mouth rinsing, chewing gum, gel, ointment, denture varnish) with nystatin, amphotericin B or miconazole, or systemic therapy (fluconazole) may be necessary.

In immune-suppressed patients antimycotic prophylaxis of oral candidiasis is indicated. *Note*: Re-infection of the oral cavity is likely if the intestinal tract is not treated concomitantly.

## ■ Modulation of the Host Response

### Inhibitors of Tissue Collagenase

To exploit the inhibitory effect of tetracyclines on matrix metalloproteinases released by, in particular, polymorphonuclear granulocytes, peri- and post-therapeutic medication of low-dose tetracycline derivatives as an adjunct to mechanical periodontal therapy has long been considered. A low-dose doxycycline hyclate preparation (Periostat, Alliance Pharma, Chippenham, UK) has been approved for host modulation as an adjunct to scaling and root planing in patients with periodontitis. The drug is systemically administered at a nonantimicrobial dosage of 20 mg/day twice daily for up to 9 months.

In a **systematic review** by Reddy et al[27] the efficacy of host modulating low-dose doxycycline as a sole measure or in combination with conventional nonsurgical periodontal therapy was assessed. It was concluded:

➤ Long-term application of subantimicrobial doses of doxycycline in combination with subgingival scaling and root planing does result in statistically significant greater clinical improvement of the periodontal conditions.
➤ **Meta-analyses** of five, respectively six, randomized controlled trials revealed slightly more clinical attachment gain (0.4–0.45 mm) and reduced probing depths (about 0.45 mm) in moderately deep (4–6 mm) or deep (≥ 7 mm) periodontal pockets. Quality of evidence: moderate.

*Note:* At least in theory, there might be an increased risk for the development of bacterial resistance. Tetracycline derivatives have been developed that strongly inhibit tissue collagenases but do not have any antimicrobial action. They have not yet been approved by national or international agencies and are therefore not available.

### Modulation of Bone Metabolism

Bisphosphonates (e. g., allendronate, etidronate) may be prescribed for patients at increased risk for osteoporosis/osteopenia.

➤ *Caution:* Long-term administration increases the risk for osteonecrosis in particular after tooth extraction.
➤ Adjunct administration of bisphosphonates in chronic periodontitis for modulation of bone metabolism is therefore strongly discouraged.

### Omega-3 Polyunsaturated Fatty Acids

Omega-3 polyunsaturated fatty acids are substrates for enzymatic conversion of bioactive lipid mediators (lipoxins, or their more stable aspirin-triggered form, resolvins, and protectins), with protective and inflammation-resolving properties. Production of proinflammatory molecules, such as eicosanoids, proinflammatory cytokines and reactive oxygen species, may be reduced.[28]

There is some evidence for therapeutic effects for a number of inflammatory diseases, such as rheumatoid arthritis, cystic fibrosis, ulcerative colitis, asthma, as well as atherosclerosis and cardiovascular diseases.

Preliminary clinical results suggest positive effects of adjunct, long-term administration of omega-3 polyunsaturated fatty acids in combination with low-dose acetylsalicylic acid during nonsurgical therapy of chronic periodontitis.[29]

## ■ Anti-inflammatory Drugs

### Nonsteroidal Anti-inflammatory Drugs

Metabolites of arachidonic acid are strongly associated with the development of inflammatory periodontal lesions as well as modulation and regulation of inflammatory cells:

➤ Nonsteroidal anti-inflammatory drugs (NSAIDs) interfere with the cyclooxygenase

(COX) pathway and thus prostaglandin production (see **Fig. 3.2**).

➤ Prostaglandin inhibitors largely suppress destructive processes during acute inflammation.

Limited additional effects of systemically administered NSAIDs, such as ibuprofen, naproxen or flurbiprofen, on periodontal treatment results have been reported. In a **systematic review** Reddy et al[27] assessed the efficacy of anti-inflammatory therapy of periodontally diseased patients when combined with conventional treatment:

➤ In six studies in which alterations of alveolar bone levels were reported, a significant benefit of anti-inflammatory therapy was observed. Quality of evidence: low.

➤ On the other hand, in nine studies in which primarily clinical attachment levels were considered, no significant benefit of anti-inflammatory therapy was reported. Likewise, in 8 out of 10 studies in which effects on periodontal probing depths or further secondary variables, such as gingival inflammation, were reported, adjunct anti-inflammatory therapy did not yield benefits as regards respective outcomes. Quality of evidence: low.

Routine prescription is not recommended owing to frequent adverse side effects including:

➤ Gastrointestinal complaints including peptic ulcer.

➤ Impairment of the hematopoietic system.

➤ Note that long-term medication of selective COX-2 inhibitors may lead to an increased risk of cardiovascular events.

If not contraindicated, infrequent postoperative complaints (pain, swelling) after periodontal surgery (see Chapter 11) may be controlled with paracetamol ($3 \times 500$ mg/day) or ibuprofen ($3 \times 400$ mg/day). Acetylsalicylic acid (aspirin) is explicitly not recommended due to increased postoperative bleeding tendency.

### Local Glucocorticoids

Glucocorticosteroids have marked anti-inflammatory and immune suppressive effects. Inhibition of early and late inflammatory reactions includes:

➤ Vasodilation, edema formation, and exudation of neutrophil granulocytes are inhibited.

➤ Capillary proliferation, fibroblast proliferation, and collagen formation are suppressed.

➤ Excessive release of lysosomal enzymes is prevented due to membrane stabilization.

➤ Synthesis of proinflammatory cytokines and mediators, such as IL-1, TNF-$\alpha$, and $PGE_2$, are inhibited.

➤ T cell activity is suppressed.

Short-term local application of, for example, prednisolone in cases of bacterial, acute-inflammatory, painful processes including:

➤ Necrotizing ulcerative gingivitis/periodontitis

➤ Pericoronal abscess

Painful forms of oral lichen planus should be treated with topical glucocorticoids, for example:

➤ 0.1 % betamethasone valerate and 0.5 % vitamin A in a suitable ointment

➤ Application three times per day for the first three weeks, then gradual reduction of the dosage over several weeks

## ■ Nutritional Supplements, Probiotics

### Vitamins

The *vitamin B complex* contains a group of water-soluble, essential vitamins: thiamin ($B_1$), riboflavin ($B_2$), niacin ($B_3$), pantothenic acid ($B_5$), pyridoxine ($B_6$), biotin ($B_7$), folate ($B_9$), cyanocobalamin, and various other cobalamins ($B_{12}$).

➤ Deficiencies are associated with malfunctioning protein, fat, and carbohydrate metabolisms and increased susceptibility to infections.

➤ Supplemental administration of the vitamin B complex may have positive effects on wound healing. In combination with periodontal surgery, superior gain of clinical attachment has been reported as well.[30]

The fat-soluble *vitamin D* plays an important role in calcium metabolism and is essential for bone growth and mineralization. The hormonally active form of vitamin D, calcitriol (1,25 dihydroxyvitamin $D_3$ or 1,25[OH]$_2$D) suppresses the release of proinflammatory cytokines IL-1 and TNF-α, enhances expression of anti-inflammatory IL-10, and induces expression of the IL-10 receptor.

> In the population-based NHANES III study (see Chapter 5), increased serum levels of calcifediol (25-hydroxyvitamin D or 25[OH] D), a marker for a patient's vitamin D status, were associated with a reduced tendency of gingival bleeding after probing (**Fig. 13.6a**) which was dose-dependent and possibly related to vitamin D's anti-inflammatory action.[31]

> In a recent population-based 5-year longitudinal study in Germany, serum 25(OH)D was inversely associated, in a dose-dependent manner, with the incidence of tooth loss.[32]

> Vitamin D deficiency may also negatively influence the postoperative results after periodontal surgery.[33] On the other hand, consistent supportive periodontal care (see Chapter 12) improves the clinical situation independent of vitamin D supplementation.[34]

*Vitamin C* deficiency has long been associated with scurvy, in particular bleeding gums and loosening of teeth due to severe periodontitis. Based on NHANES III data, estimated vitamin C

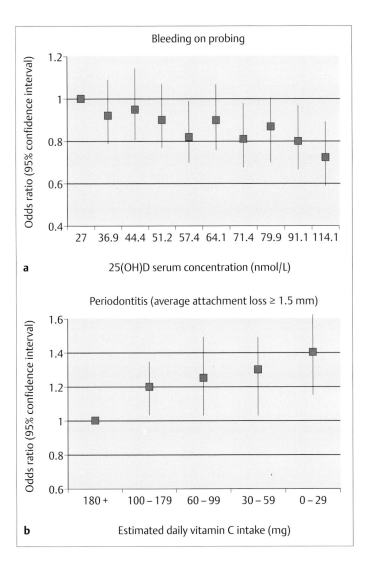

**a** Relationship between serum concentrations of 25-hydroxyvitamin D (25[OH]D) and bleeding on probing. The odds for bleeding on probing were reduced by 30% in the highest decile (114.1 nmol/L) as compared to the lowest decile (27 nmol/L). (After Dietrich et al.[31])

**Fig. 13.6 Vitamins and periodontal diseases in the population-based NHANES III study.**

**a** Relationship between serum concentrations of 25-hydroxyvitamin D (25[OH]D) and bleeding on probing. The odds for bleeding on probing were reduced by 30% in the highest decile (114.1 nmol/L) as compared to the lowest decile (27 nmol/L). (After Dietrich et al.[31])

**b** Relationship between estimated daily intake of vitamin C and periodontitis (as defined by average attachment loss of 1.5 mm). Periodontitis was associated with low vitamin C intake. (After Nishida et al.[35])

intake was negatively associated with periodontal disease (**Fig. 13.6b**).[35] In smokers, insufficient supply seems to increase the risk for periodontitis. Presently no intervention studies are available which might have shown prevention of attachment loss after supply of increased doses of vitamin C.

## Calcium

Based on NHANES III data, insufficient intake of calcium may be associated with periodontitis.[36]

To date, there is insufficient evidence as to whether dietary intake recommendations and guidelines need to be changed in order to promote periodontal health.[37] In particular, properly designed and conducted intervention studies are lacking. Future studies may also focus on overall diet and healthy eating patterns rather than trying to consider individual nutrients in isolation.

## Probiotics

Probiotics are viable microorganisms which may, if supplied in sufficient amounts, exert health promoting effects[38]:

➤ A generally beneficial, but rather ill-defined, influence on the immune system has been claimed.
➤ Moreover, pathogenic microorganisms in the intestinal tract or oral cavity may be replaced by more beneficial bacteria.

➤ There is actually some evidence for beneficial effects of probiotics in cases of acute diarrhea and Crohn's disease.

Replacement of pathogenic bacteria in the oral ecosystem by probiotics is a basically attractive concept for the prevention of dental caries[39] and periodontal disease or, as a further example, halitosis. Probiotic bacteria, including several lactobacilli (*Lactobacillus reuteri, L.brevis, L. bulgaricus*), streptococci (*Streptococcus thermophilus, S. salivarius*), and *Weissella cibaria*, were tested in a number of clinical and microbiological studies. For example, *L. reuteri* releases the bacteriocins reuterin and reutericyclin, which apparently interfere with the proliferation of certain oral pathogens. The bacterium also suppresses secretion of proinflammatory cytokines in the mucosa of the small intestine.

Currently, *L. reuteri* may be administered, for example, in chewing gum (GUM PerioBalance, Sunstar, Chicago, Illinois, USA). Whether clinical effects on gingivitis may be expected is not clear.[40]

*Note:* Whether specific nutritional supplements have a beneficial influence on the development and progression of destructive periodontitis or the clinical outcome after periodontal therapy can only be assessed in randomized controlled trials. So far available results, which are often based on retrospective analyses of epidemiological studies, do not justify definitive recommendations.

# 14 References

## 1 Anatomy and Physiology

1. Berkovitz BKB, Holland GR, Moxham BJ. Oral Anatomy, Histology and Embryology. 4th ed. Edinburgh: Mosby Elsevier; 2009
2. Nancy A. Ten Cate's Oral Histology, Development, Structure and Function. 8th ed. Edinburgh: Mosby Elsevier; 2012
3. Schroeder HE. The periodontium. In: Oksche A, Vollrath L, eds. Handbook of Microscopic Anatomy, vol V/5. Berlin, Heidelberg: Springer; 1986
4. MacNeil RL, Somerman MJ. Development and regeneration of the periodontium: parallels and contrasts. Periodontol 2000 1999;19:8–20
5. Bosshardt DD, Nanci A. Hertwig's epithelial root sheath, enamel matrix proteins, and initiation of cementogenesis in porcine teeth. J Clin Periodontol 2004;31(3):184–192
6. Schroeder HE. Oral Structural Biology. New York: Thieme Medical; 1991
7. Lindhe J, Wennström J, Berglundh T. The mucosa at teeth and implants. In: Lindhe J, Lang NP, eds. Clinical Periodontology and Implant Dentistry. 6th ed. Oxford: Wiley-Blackwell; 2015
8. Schroeder HE. Biological problems of regenerative cementogenesis: synthesis and attachment of collagenous matrices on growing and established root surfaces. Int Rev Cytol 1992;142:1–59

## 2 Periodontal Microbiology

1. Turnbaugh PJ, Ley RE, Hamady M, Fraser-Liggett CM, Knight R, Gordon JI. The human microbiome project. Nature 2007;449(7164):804–810
2. Human Oral Microbiology Database. http://www.homd.org/modules.php?op=modload&name=-HOMD&file=index (Retrieved May 19, 2015)
3. Paster BJ, Boches SK, Galvin JL, et al. Bacterial diversity in human subgingival plaque. J Bacteriol 2001;183 (12):3770–3783
4. Pozhitkov AE, Beikler T, Flemmig T, Noble PA. High-throughput methods for analysis of the human oral microbiome. Periodontol 2000 2011;55(1):70–86
5. Dewhirst FE, Chen T, Izard J, et al. The human oral microbiome. J Bacteriol 2010;192(19):5002–5017
6. Guarner F, Malagelada JR. Gut flora in health and disease. Lancet 2003;361(9356):512–519
7. Leys EJ, Griffen AL, Beall C, Maiden MF. Isolation, classification, and identification of oral microorganisms. In: Lamont RJ, Hajishengallis GN, Jenkinson HF, eds. Oral Microbiology and Immunology. 2nd ed. Washington DC: ASM Press; 2014

8. Paster BJ, Olsen I, Aas JA, Dewhirst FE. The breadth of bacterial diversity in the human periodontal pocket and other oral sites. Periodontol 2000 2006;42:80–87
9. Aas JA, Paster BJ, Stokes LN, Olsen I, Dewhirst FE. Defining the normal bacterial flora of the oral cavity. J Clin Microbiol 2005;43(11):5721–5732
10. Carlsson J. Microbiology of plaque-associated periodontal disease. In: Lindhe J, ed. Textbook of Clinical Periodontology. 2nd ed. Copenhagen: Munksgaard; 1989
11. Stoodley P, Sauer K, Davies DG, Costerton JW. Biofilms as complex differentiated communities. Annu Rev Microbiol 2002;56:187–209
12. Socransky SS, Haffajee AD. Dental biofilms: difficult therapeutic targets. Periodontol 2000 2002;28:12–55
13. Kolenbrander PE, Andersen RN, Blehert DS, Egland PG, Foster JS, Palmer RJ Jr. Communication among oral bacteria. Microbiol Mol Biol Rev 2002;66(3):486–505
14. Brecx M, Theilade J, Attström R. An ultrastructural quantitative study of the significance of microbial multiplication during early dental plaque growth. J Periodontal Res 1983;18(2):177–186
15. Ramberg P, Sekino S, Uzel NG, Socransky S, Lindhe J. Bacterial colonization during de novo plaque formation. J Clin Periodontol 2003;30(11):990–995
16. White DJ. Dental calculus: recent insights into occurrence, formation, prevention, removal and oral health effects of supragingival and subgingival deposits. Eur J Oral Sci 1997;105(5 Pt 2):508–522
17. Socransky SS. Criteria for the infectious agents in dental caries and periodontal disease. J Clin Periodontol 1979;6(7):16–21
18. Haffajee AD, Socransky SS. Microbial etiological agents of destructive periodontal diseases. Periodontol 2000 1994;5:78–111
19. Haffajee AD, Teles RP, Socransky SS. Association of *Eubacterium nodatum* and *Treponema denticola* with human periodontitis lesions. Oral Microbiol Immunol 2006;21(5):269–282
20. Hill AB. The environment and disease: association or causation? Proc R Soc Med 1965;58:295–300
21. Fredricks DN, Relman DA. Sequence-based identification of microbial pathogens: a reconsideration of Koch's postulates. Clin Microbiol Rev 1996;9(1):18–33
22. Socransky SS, Haffajee AD, Cugini MA, Smith C, Kent RL Jr. Microbial complexes in subgingival plaque. J Clin Periodontol 1998;25(2):134–144
23. Colombo APV, Boches SK, Cotton SL, et al. Comparisons of subgingival microbial profiles of refractory periodontitis, severe periodontitis, and periodontal health using the human oral microbe identification microarray. J Periodontol 2009;80(9):1421–1432
24. Holt SC, Kesavalu L, Walker S, Genco CA. Virulence factors of *Porphyromonas gingivalis*. Periodontol 2000 1999;20:168–238

25. Henderson B, Ward JM, Ready D. *Aggregatibacter (Actinobacillus) actinomycetemcomitans:* a triple A* periodontopathogen? Periodontol 2000 2010;54(1):78–105
26. Ishihara K. Virulence factors of *Treponema denticola.* Periodontol 2000 2010;54(1):117–135
27. Sharma A. Virulence mechanisms of *Tannerella forsythia.* Periodontol 2000 2010;54(1):106–116
28. Lally ET, Kieba IR, Golub EE, Lear JD, Tanaka JC. Structure/function aspects of *Actinobacillus actinomycetemcomitans* leukotoxin. J Periodontol 1996;67:298–308
29. Haubek D, Poulsen K, Kilian M. Microevolution and patterns of dissemination of the JP2 clone of *Aggregatibacter (Actinobacillus) actinomycetemcomitans.* Infect Immun 2007;75(6):3080–3088
30. Macheleidt A, Müller HP, Eger T, Putzker M, Fuhrmann A, Zöller L. Absence of an especially toxic clone among isolates of *Actinobacillus actinomycetemcomitans* recovered from army recruits. Clin Oral Investig 1999;3(4):161–167
31. Haubek D, Ennibi OK, Poulsen K, Vaeth M, Poulsen S, Kilian M. Risk of aggressive periodontitis in adolescent carriers of the JP2 clone of *Aggregatibacter (Actinobacillus) actinomycetemcomitans* in Morocco: a prospective longitudinal cohort study. Lancet 2008;371(9608):237–242
32. Socransky SS, Haffajee AD, Dzink JL, Hillman JD. Associations between microbial species in subgingival plaque samples. Oral Microbiol Immunol 1988;3(1):1–7
33. Müller HP, Heinecke A, Borneff M, Knopf A, Kiencke C, Pohl S. Microbial ecology of *Actinobacillus actinomycetemcomitans, Eikenella corrodens* and *Capnocytophaga* spp. in adult periodontitis. J Periodontal Res 1997;32(6):530–542
34. Hammond BF, Lillard SE, Stevens RH. A bacteriocin of *Actinobacillus actinomycetemcomitans.* Infect Immun 1987;55(3):686–691
35. Meurman JH, Stamatova I. Probiotics: contributions to oral health. Oral Dis 2007;13(5):443–451
36. Hritz M, Fisher E, Demuth DR. Differential regulation of the leukotoxin operon in highly leukotoxic and minimally leukotoxic strains of *Actinobacillus actinomycetemcomitans.* Infect Immun 1996;64(7):2724–2729
37. Bramanti TE, Holt SC. Effect of porphyrins and host iron transport proteins on outer membrane protein expression in *Porphyromonas (Bacteroides) gingivalis:* identification of a novel 26 kDa hemin-repressible surface protein. Microb Pathog 1992;13(1):61–73
38. Könönen E, Müller HP. Microbiology of aggressive periodontitis. Periodontol 2000 2014;65(1):46–78
39. Fine DH, Markowitz K, Fairlie K, et al. A consortium of *Aggregatibacter actinomycetemcomitans, Streptococcus parasanguinis,* and *Filifactor alocis* is present in sites prior to bone loss in a longitudinal study of localized aggressive periodontitis. J Clin Microbiol 2013;51(9):2850–2861
40. Köhler B, Andréen I. Mutans streptococci and caries prevalence in children after early maternal caries prevention: a follow-up at 19 years of age. Caries Res 2012;46(5):474–480
41. Dabdoub SM, Tsigarida AA, Kumar PS. Patient-specific analysis of periodontal and peri-implant microbiomes. J Dent Res 2013; 92(12, Suppl)168S–175S
42. Pye AD, Lockhart DE, Dawson MP, Murray CA, Smith AJ. A review of dental implants and infection. J Hosp Infect 2009;72(2):104–110

## 3 Pathogenesis of Biofilm-Induced Periodontal Diseases

1. Seymour GL, Trombelli L, Berglundh T. Pathogenesis of gingivitis. In: Lindhe J, Lang NP, eds. Clinical Periodontology and Implant Dentistry, 6th ed. Oxford: Wiley-Blackwell: 2015
2. Schroeder HE, Listgarten MA. The gingival tissues: the architecture of periodontal protection. Periodontol 2000 1997;13:91–120
3. Page RC, Schroeder HE. Structure and pathogenesis. In: Schluger S, Yuodelis R, Page RC, Johnson RH, eds. Periodontal Diseases. 2nd ed. Philadelphia: Lea & Febiger; 1990
4. Darveau RP, Tanner A, Page RC. The microbial challenge in periodontitis. Periodontol 2000 1997;14:12–32
5. Kornman KS, Page RC, Tonetti MS. The host response to the microbial challenge in periodontitis: assembling the players. Periodontol 2000 1997;14:33–53
6. van de Winkel JG, Capel PJ. Human IgG Fc receptor heterogeneity: molecular aspects and clinical implications. Immunol Today 1993;14(5):215–221
7. Ishikawa I, Nakashima K, Koseki T, et al. Induction of the immune response to periodontopathic bacteria and its role in the pathogenesis of periodontitis. Periodontol 2000 1997;14:79–111
8. Liljenberg B, Lindhe J, Berglundh T, Dahlén G, Jonsson R. Some microbiological, histopathological and immunohistochemical characteristics of progressive periodontal disease. J Clin Periodontol 1994;21(10):720–727
9. Heitz-Mayfield LJ, Lang NP. Comparative biology of chronic and aggressive periodontitis vs. peri-implantitis. Periodontol 2000 2010;53:167–181
10. Gemmell E, Seymour GJ. Immunoregulatory control of Th1/Th2 cytokine profiles in periodontal disease. Periodontol 2000 2004;35:21–41
11. Korn T, Bettelli E, Oukka M, Kuchroo VK. IL-17 and Th17 cells. Annu Rev Immunol 2009;27:485–517
12. Schenkein HA, Koertge TE, Brooks CN, Sabatini R, Purkall DE, Tew JG. IL-17 in sera from patients with aggressive periodontitis. J Dent Res 2010;89(9):943–947
13. Gemmell E, Yamazaki K, Seymour GJ. Destructive periodontitis lesions are determined by the nature of the lymphocytic response. Crit Rev Oral Biol Med 2002;13(1):17–34
14. Dixon DR, Bainbridge BW, Darveau RP. Modulation of the innate immune response within the periodontium. Periodontol 2000 2004;35:53–74

15. Takayanagi H. Inflammatory bone destruction and osteoimmunology. J Periodontal Res 2005;40(4):287–293

16. Hwang AM, Stoupel J, Celenti R, Demmer RT, Papapanou PN. Serum antibody responses to periodontal microbiota in chronic and aggressive periodontitis: a postulate revisited. J Periodontol 2014;85(4):592–600

17. Hajishengallis E, Hajishengallis G. Immunology of the oral cavity. In: Lamont RJ, Hajishengallis GN, Jenkinson HF, eds. Oral Microbiology and Immunology. 2nd ed. Washington DC: ASM Press; 2014

18. Offenbacher S. Periodontal diseases: pathogenesis. Ann Periodontol 1996;1(1):821–878

19. Cohen ME. Bursts of periodontal destruction and remission, percolation phase shifts, and chaos. J Periodontal Res 1993;28(6 Pt 1):429–436

20. Kornman KS. Mapping the pathogenesis of periodontitis: a new look. J Periodontol 2008;79(8, Suppl) 1560–1568

21. Offenbacher S, Barros SP, Singer RE, Moss K, Williams RC, Beck JD. Periodontal disease at the biofilm–gingival interface. J Periodontol 2007;78(10):1911–1925

22. Barros SP, Offenbacher S. Epigenetics: connecting environment and genotype to phenotype and disease. J Dent Res 2009;88(5):400–408

23. Offenbacher S, Barros SP, Paquette DW, et al. Gingival transcriptome patterns during induction and resolution of experimental gingivitis in humans. J Periodontol 2009;80(12):1963–1982

24. Kebschull M, Demmer RT, Grün B, Guarnieri P, Pavlidis P, Papapanou PN. Gingival tissue transcriptomes identify distinct periodontitis phenotypes. J Dent Res 2014;93(5):459–468

25. Michalowicz BS, Diehl SR, Gunsolley JC, et al. Evidence of a substantial genetic basis for risk of adult periodontitis. J Periodontol 2000;71(11):1699–1707

26. Noack B, Görgens H, Hempel U, et al. Cathepsin C gene variants in aggressive periodontitis. J Dent Res 2008;87(10):958–963

27. Laine ML, Crielaard W, Loos BG. Genetic susceptibility to periodontitis. Periodontol 2000 2012;58(1):37–68

28. Vieira AR, Albandar JM. Role of genetic factors in the pathogenesis of aggressive periodontitis. Periodontol 2000 2014;65(1):92–106

29. Engebretson SP, Lamster IB, Herrera-Abreu M, et al. The influence of interleukin gene polymorphism on expression of interleukin-1β and tumor necrosis factor-α in periodontal tissue and gingival crevicular fluid. J Periodontol 1999;70(6):567–573

30. Vaithilingam RD, Safi SH, Baharuddin NA, Ng CC, Cheong SC, Bartold PM, Schaefer AS, Loos BG. Moving into a new era of periodontal genetic studies: relevance of large case-control samples using severe phenotypes for genome-wide association studies. J Periodontal Res 2014;49(6):683–695

31. Schaefer AS, Bochenek G, Manke T, et al. Validation of reported genetic risk factors for periodontitis in a large-scale replication study. J Clin Periodontol 2013;40(6):563–572

32. Berglundh T, Zitzmann NU, Donati M. Are peri-implantitis lesions different from periodontitis lesions? J Clin Periodontol 2011;38(Suppl 11):188–202

# 4 Classification of Periodontal Diseases

1. Scully C. Oral and Maxillofacial Medicine: the Basis of Diagnosis and Treatment. 3 rd ed. London: Churchill Livingstone Elsevier; 2013

2. Armitage GC. Development of a classification system for periodontal diseases and conditions. Ann Periodontol 1999;4(1):1–6

3. Cota LOM, Aquino DR, Franco GCN, Cortelli JR, Cortelli SC, Costa FO. Gingival overgrowth in subjects under immunosuppressive regimens based on cyclosporine, tacrolimus, or sirolimus. J Clin Periodontol 2010;37 (10):894–902

4. Taichman LS, Eklund SA. Oral contraceptives and periodontal diseases: rethinking the association based upon analysis of National Health and Nutrition Examination Survey data. J Periodontol 2005;76(8):1374–1385

5. Häkkinen L, Csiszar A. Hereditary gingival fibromatosis: characteristics and novel putative pathogenic mechanisms. J Dent Res 2007;86(1):25–34

6. Doufexi A, Mina M, Ioannidou E. Gingival overgrowth in children: epidemiology, pathogenesis, and complications. A literature review. J Periodontol 2005;76 (1):3–10

7. Al-Hashimi I, Schifter M, Lockhart PB, et al. Oral lichen planus and oral lichenoid lesions: diagnostic and therapeutic considerations. Oral Surg Oral Med Oral Pathol Radiol Endod 2007; 103(Suppl): S 25.e1–12

8. Lindhe J, Ranney R, Lamster I, et al. Consensus report: chronic periodontitis. Ann Periodontol 1999;4:38-38

9. Lang N, Bartold PM, Cullinan M, et al. Consensus report: aggressive periodontitis. Ann Periodontol 1999;4:53-53

10. Armitage GC, Cullinan MP. Comparison of the clinical features of chronic and aggressive periodontitis. Periodontol 2000 2010;53:12–27

11. van der Velden U. Purpose and problems of periodontal disease classification. Periodontol 2000 2005;39:13–21

12. Flemmig TF. Periodontitis. Ann Periodontol 1999;4 (1):32–38

13. Armitage GC, Cullinan MP, Seymour GJ. Comparative biology of chronic and aggressive periodontitis: introduction. Periodontol 2000 2010;53:7–11

14. Albandar JM. Aggressive and acute periodontal diseases. Periodontol 2000 2014;65(1):7–12

15. Baelum V, Lopez R. Defining and classifying periodontitis: need for a paradigm shift? Eur J Oral Sci 2003;111(1):2–6

# 5 Epidemiology of Periodontal Diseases

1. Benamghar L, Penaud J, Kaminsky P, Abt F, Martin J. Comparison of gingival index and sulcus bleeding index as indicators of periodontal status. Bull World Health Organ 1982;60(1):147–151

2. Massler M. The P-M-A index for the assessment of gingivitis. J Periodontol 1967;38(6, Suppl)592–601

3. Löe H, Silness J. Periodontal disease in pregnancy. I. Prevalence and severity. Acta Odontol Scand 1963;21:533–551

4. Mühlemann HR, Son S. Gingival sulcus bleeding—a leading symptom in initial gingivitis. Helv Odontol Acta 1971;15(2):107–113

5. Saxer UP, Mühlemann HR. Motivation und Aufklärung. Schweiz Mschr Zahnheilk 1975;85:905–919

6. Ainamo J, Bay I. Problems and proposals for recording gingivitis and plaque. Int Dent J 1975;25(4):229–235

7. Greene JC, Vermillion JR. The oral hygiene index: A method for classifying oral hygiene status. J Am Dent Assoc 1960;61:172–179

8. Greene JC, Vermillion JR. The simplified oral hygiene index. J Am Dent Assoc 1964;68:7–13

9. Quigley GA, Hein JW. Comparative cleansing efficiency of manual and power brushing. J Am Dent Assoc 1962;65:26–29

10. Turesky S, Gilmore ND, Glickman I. Reduced plaque formation by the chloromethyl analogue of vitamin C. J Periodontol 1970;41(1):41–43

11. Silness J, Löe H. Periodontal disease in pregnancy. II. Correlation between oral hygiene and periodontal condition. Acta Odontol Scand 1964;22:121–135

12. O'Leary TJ, Drake RB, Naylor JE. The plaque control record. J Periodontol 1972;43(1):38–39

13. Russell AL. A system of classification and scoring for prevalence surveys of periodontal disease. J Dent Res 1956;35(3):350–359

14. Ramfjord SP. Indices for prevalence and incidence of periodontal disease. J Periodontol 1959;30:51–59

15. Ainamo J, Barmes D, Beagrie G, Cutress T, Martin J, Sardo-Infirri J. Development of the World Health Organization (WHO) community periodontal index of treatment needs (CPITN). Int Dent J 1982;32(3):281–291

16. World Health Organization. Oral Health Surveys: Basic Methods. 4th ed. Geneva: WHO; 1997

17. Carlos JP, Wolfe MD, Kingman A. The extent and severity index: a simple method for use in epidemiologic studies of periodontal disease. J Clin Periodontol 1986;13(5):500–505

18. Okamoto H, Yoneyama T, Lindhe J, Haffajee A, Socransky S. Methods of evaluating periodontal disease data in epidemiological research. J Clin Periodontol 1988;15(7):430–439

19. Page RC, Eke PI. Case definitions for use in population-based surveillance of periodontitis. J Periodontol 2007; 78(7, Suppl)1387–1399

20. Eke PI, Page RC, Wei L, Thornton-Evans G, Genco RJ. Update of the case definitions for population-based surveillance of periodontitis. J Periodontol 2012;83 (12):1449–1454

21. Tonetti MS, Claffey N; European Workshop in Periodontology group C. Advances in the progression of periodontitis and proposal of definitions of a periodontitis case and disease progression for use in risk factor research. Group C consensus report of the 5th European Workshop in Periodontology. J Clin Periodontol 2005;32(Suppl 6):210–213

22. Demmer RT, Papapanou PN. Epidemiologic patterns of chronic and aggressive periodontitis. Periodontol 2000 2010;53:28–44

23. Levin L, Baev V, Lev R, Stabholz A, Ashkenazi M. Aggressive periodontitis among young Israeli army personnel. J Periodontol 2006;77(8):1392–1396

24. Holtfreter B, Schwahn C, Biffar R, Kocher T. Epidemiology of periodontal diseases in the Study of Health in Pomerania. J Clin Periodontol 2009;36(2):114–123

25. Matsson L. Development of gingivitis in pre-school children and young adults. A comparative experimental study. J Clin Periodontol 1978;5(1):24–34

26. Massler M, Cohen A, Schour I. Epidemiology of gingivitis in children. J Am Dent Assoc 1952;45(3):319–324

27. Marshall-Day CD, Stephens RG, Quigley LF Jr. Periodontal disease: prevalence and incidence. J Periodontol 1955;26:185–203

28. Löe H, Anerud A, Boysen H, Morrison E. Natural history of periodontal disease in man. Rapid, moderate and no loss of attachment in Sri Lankan laborers 14 to 46 years of age. J Clin Periodontol 1986;13(5):431–445

29. Albandar JM, Brunelle JA, Kingman A. Destructive periodontal disease in adults 30 years of age and older in the United States, 1988–1994. J Periodontol 1999;70(1):13–29

30. Dye BA, Tan S, Smith V, et al. Trends in oral health status: United States, 1988–1994 and 1999–2004. Vital Health Stat 11 2007;11(248):1–92

31. Albandar JM. Underestimation of periodontitis in NHANES surveys. J Periodontol 2011;82(3):337–341

32. Eke PI, Dye BA, Wei L, Thornton-Evans GO, Genco RJ; CDC Periodontal Disease Surveillance workgroup: James Beck (University of North Carolina, Chapel Hill, USA), Gordon Douglass (Past President, American Academy of Periodontology), Roy Page (University of Washington). Prevalence of periodontitis in adults in the United States: 2009 and 2010. J Dent Res 2012;91 (10):914–920

33. Sheiham A, Netuveli GS. Periodontal diseases in Europe. Periodontol 2000 2002;29:104–121

34. Dye BA. Global periodontal disease epidemiology. Periodontol 2000 2012;58(1):10–25

35. Skudutyte-Rysstad R, Eriksen HM, Hansen BF. Trends in periodontal health among 35-year-olds in Oslo, 1973–2003. J Clin Periodontol 2007;34(10):867–872

36. Micheelis W, Schiffner U, eds. Vierte Deutsche Mundgesundheitsstudie (DMS IV). Cologne: Deutscher Zahnärzteverlag; 2006

37. Hermann P, Gera I, Borbély J, Fejérdy P, Madléna M. Periodontal health of an adult population in Hungary: findings of a national survey. J Clin Periodontol 2009;36(6):449–457

38. Löe H, Brown LJ. Early onset periodontitis in the United States of America. J Periodontol 1991;62(10):608–616

39. Susin C, Haas AN, Albandar JM. Epidemiology and demographics of aggressive periodontitis. Periodontol 2000 2014;65(1):27–45

40. Löe H, Anerud A, Boysen H. The natural history of periodontal disease in man: prevalence, severity, and

extent of gingival recession. J Periodontol 1992;63 (6):489–495

41. Albandar JM, Kingman A. Gingival recession, gingival bleeding, and dental calculus in adults 30 years of age and older in the United States, 1988–1994. J Periodontol 1999;70(1):30–43

42. Atieh MA, Alsabeeha NHM, Faggion CM Jr, Duncan WJ. The frequency of peri-implant diseases: a systematic review and meta-analysis. J Periodontol 2013;84 (11):1586–1598

## 6 Diagnosis of Periodontal Diseases

1. Peacock ME, Carson RE. Frequency of self-reported medical conditions in periodontal patients. J Periodontol 1995;66(11):1004–1007

2. Roed-Petersen B, Renstrup G. A topographical classification of the oral mucosa suitable for electronic data processing. Its application to 560 leukoplakias. Acta Odontol Scand 1969;27(6):681–695

3. Armitage GC. Periodontal diseases: diagnosis. Ann Periodontol 1996;1(1):37–215

4. Müller HP, Eger T. Furcation diagnosis. J Clin Periodontol 1999;26(8):485–498

5. Hamp SE, Nyman S, Lindhe J. Periodontal treatment of multirooted teeth. Results after 5 years. J Clin Periodontol 1975;2(3):126–135

6. Müller HP, Barrieshi-Nusair KM. Gingival bleeding on repeat probing after different time intervals in plaque-induced gingivitis. Clin Oral Investig 2005;9 (4):278–283

7. Meredith N. Assessment of implant stability as a prognostic determinant. Int J Prosthodont 1998;11 (5):491–501

8. Müller HP, Schaller N, Eger T. Ultrasonic determination of thickness of masticatory mucosa: a methodologic study. Oral Surg Oral Med Oral Pathol Oral Radiol Endod 1999;88(2):248–253

9. De Rouck T, Eghbali R, Collys K, De Bruyn H, Cosyn J. The gingival biotype revisited: transparency of the periodontal probe through the gingival margin as a method to discriminate thin from thick gingiva. J Clin Periodontol 2009;36(5):428–433

10. Müller HP, Eger T. Masticatory mucosa and periodontal phenotype: a review. Int J Periodont Restor Dent 2002;22(2):172–183

11. Müller HP, Könönen E. Variance components of gingival thickness. J Periodontal Res 2005;40(3):239–244

12. Miller PD Jr. A classification of marginal tissue recession. Int J Periodont Restor Dent 1985;5(2):8–13

13. Seibert JS. Reconstruction of deformed, partially edentulous ridges, using full thickness onlay grafts. Part I. Technique and wound healing. Compend Contin Educ Dent 1983;4(5):437–453

14. American Dental Association. US Department of Human Health and Services (2012). Dental radiographic examinations: recommendations for patient selection and limiting radiation exposure. http://www.ada.org/en/member-center/oral-health-topics/x-rays (Retrieved July 28, 2014)

15. White SC, Pharoah MJ, eds. Oral Radiology. Principles and Interpretations. 7th ed. St. Louis: Elsevier Mosby; 2014

16. Tarnow D, Fletcher P. Classification of the vertical component of furcation involvement. J Periodontol 1984;55(5):283–284

17. Murray PA, French CK. DNA probe detection of periodontal pathogens. In: Myers HM, ed. New Biotechnology in Oral Research. Basel: Karger; 1989: 33–53

18. Macheleidt A, Müller HP, Eger T, Putzker M, Fuhrmann A, Zöller L. Absence of an especially toxic clone among isolates of *Actinobacillus actinomycetemcomitans* recovered from army recruits. Clin Oral Investig 1999;3 (4):161–167

19. Slots J. Rapid identification of important periodontal microorganisms by cultivation. Oral Microbiol Immunol 1986;1(1):48–57

20. Mombelli A, Casagni F, Madianos PN. Can presence or absence of periodontal pathogens distinguish between subjects with chronic and aggressive periodontitis? A systematic review. J Clin Periodontol 2002;29 (Suppl 3):10–21, discussion 37–38

21. Listgarten MA, Loomer PM. Microbial identification in the management of periodontal diseases. A systematic review. Ann Periodontol 2003;8(1):182–192

22. Nikolopoulos GK, Dimou NL, Hamodrakas SJ, Bagos PG. Cytokine gene polymorphisms in periodontal disease: a meta-analysis of 53 studies including 4,178 cases and 4,590 controls. J Clin Periodontol 2008;35 (9):754–767

23. Karimbux NY, Saraiya VM, Elangovan S, et al. Interleukin-1 gene polymorphisms and chronic periodontitis in adult whites: a systematic review and meta-analysis. J Periodontol 2012;83(11):1407–1419

24. Huynh-Ba G, Lang NP, Tonetti MS, Salvi GE. The association of the composite IL-1 genotype with periodontitis progression and/or treatment outcomes: a systematic review. J Clin Periodontol 2007;34 (4):305–317

25. Ozmeric N. Advances in periodontal disease markers. Clin Chim Acta 2004;343(1-2):1–16

26. Gursoy UK, Könönen E, Pussinen PJ, et al. Use of host- and bacteria-derived salivary markers in detection of periodontitis: a cumulative approach. Dis Markers 2011;30(6):299–305

27. Hyvärinen K, Laitinen S, Paju S, et al. Detection and quantification of five major periodontal pathogens by single copy gene-based real-time PCR. Innate Immun 2009;15(4):195–204

28. Meisel P, Schwahn C, Gesch D, Bernhardt O, John U, Kocher T. Dose-effect relation of smoking and the interleukin-1 gene polymorphism in periodontal disease. J Periodontol 2004;75(2):236–242

## 7 Prevention of Periodontal Diseases

1. Axelsson P, Lindhe J, Nyström B. On the prevention of caries and periodontal disease. Results of a 15-year longitudinal study in adults. J Clin Periodontol 1991;18(3):182–189

2. Axelsson P, Nyström B, Lindhe J. The long-term effect of a plaque control program on tooth mortality, caries and periodontal disease in adults. Results after 30 years of maintenance. J Clin Periodontol 2004;31 (9):749–757

3. Guyatt GH, Oxman AD, Vist GE, et al; GRADE Working Group. GRADE: an emerging consensus on rating quality of evidence and strength of recommendations. BMJ 2008;336(7650):924–926

4. Hujoel PP, DeRouen TA. A survey of endpoint characteristics in periodontal clinical trials published 1988–1992, and implications for future studies. J Clin Periodontol 1995;22(5):397–407

5. Hujoel PP, del Aguila MA, DeRouen TA, Bergström J. A hidden periodontitis epidemic during the 20th century? Community Dent Oral Epidemiol 2003;31(1):1–6

6. Hujoel PP, Leroux BG, Selipsky H, White BA. Non-surgical periodontal therapy and tooth loss. A cohort study. J Periodontol 2000;71(5):736–742

7. Tomar SL, Asma S. Smoking-attributable periodontitis in the United States: findings from NHANES III. National Health and Nutrition Examination Survey. J Periodontol 2000;71(5):743–751

8. Do LG, Slade GD, Roberts-Thomson KF, Sanders AE. Smoking-attributable periodontal disease in the Australian adult population. J Clin Periodontol 2008;35 (5):398–404

9. Haffajee AD, Socransky SS, Lindhe J, Kent RL, Okamoto H, Yoneyama T. Clinical risk indicators for periodontal attachment loss. J Clin Periodontol 1991;18(2):117–125

10. American Academy of Periodontology. Position paper: Tobacco use and the periodontal patient. Research, Science and Therapy Committee of the American Academy of Periodontology. J Periodontol 1999;70 (11):1419–1427

11. American Academy of Periodontology. Diabetes and periodontal disease. J Periodontol 2000;71(4):664–678

12. World Health Organization. WHO Report on the Global Tobacco Epidemic: Implementing Smoke-free Environments. Geneva: WHO; 2009

13. Centers for Disease Control and Prevention. National diabetes fact sheet: National estimates and general information on diabetes and prediabetes in the United States, 2011. Atlanta: US Department of Health and Human Services, Centers for Disease Control and Prevention; 2011

14. Hujoel PP, Cunha-Cruz J, Loesche WJ, Robertson PB. Personal oral hygiene and chronic periodontitis: a systematic review. Periodontol 2000 2005;37:29–34

15. Watt RG, Marinho VC. Does oral health promotion improve oral hygiene and gingival health? Periodontol 2000 2005;37:35–47

16. Sheiham A. Public health aspects of periodontal diseases in Europe. J Clin Periodontol 1991;18(6):362–369

# 8 General Medical Implications

1. Nokta M. Oral manifestations associated with HIV infection. Cur HIV/AIDS Rep 2008; 5: 5–12.

2. Wilson W, Taubert KA, Gewitz M, et al; American Heart Association Rheumatic Fever, Endocarditis, and Kawasaki Disease Committee; American Heart Association Council on Cardiovascular Disease in the Young; American Heart Association Council on Clinical Cardiology; American Heart Association Council on Cardiovascular Surgery and Anesthesia; Quality of Care and Outcomes Research Interdisciplinary Working Group. Prevention of infective endocarditis. Circulation 2007;116(15):1736–1754

3. Pallasch TJ, Slots J. Antibiotic prophylaxis and the medically compromised patient. Periodontol 2000 1996;10:107–138

4. Academy of Orthopaedic Surgeons, American Dental Association. Prevention of orthopedic implant infection in patients undergoing dental procedures (2012). Evidence-based guideline and evidence report. http://www.aaos.org/Research/guidelines/PUDP/PUDP_guideline.pdf (Accessed May 2, 2015)

5. Danesh J. Coronary heart disease, Helicobacter pylori, dental disease, Chlamydia pneumoniae, and cytomegalovirus: meta-analyses of prospective studies. Am Heart J 1999;138(5 Pt 2):S434–S437

6. Khader YS, Albashaireh ZSM, Alomari MA. Periodontal diseases and the risk of coronary heart and cerebrovascular diseases: a meta-analysis. J Periodontol 2004;75(8):1046–1053

7. Bahekar AA, Singh S, Saha S, Molnar J, Arora R. The prevalence and incidence of coronary heart disease is significantly increased in periodontitis: a meta-analysis. Am Heart J 2007;154(5):830–837

8. Humphrey LL, Fu R, Buckley DI, Freeman M, Helfand M. Periodontal disease and coronary heart disease incidence: a systematic review and meta-analysis. J Gen Intern Med 2008;23(12):2079–2086

9. Lockhart PB, Bolger AF, Papapanou PN, et al; American Heart Association Rheumatic Fever, Endocarditis, and Kawasaki Disease Committee of the Council on Cardiovascular Disease in the Young, Council on Epidemiology and Prevention, Council on Peripheral Vascular Disease, and Council on Clinical Cardiology. Periodontal disease and atherosclerotic vascular disease: does the evidence support an independent association? A scientific statement from the American Heart Association. Circulation 2012;125(20):2520–2544

10. Dietrich T, Sharma P, Walter C, Weston P, Beck J. The epidemiological evidence behind the association between periodontitis and incident atherosclerotic cardiovascular disease. J Clin Periodontol 2013;40(Suppl 14):S70–S84

11. Teeuw WJ, Slot DE, Susanto H, et al. Treatment of periodontitis improves the atherosclerotic profile: a systematic review and meta-analysis. J Clin Periodontol 2014;41(1):70–79

12. US Preventive Services Task Force. Using nontraditional risk factors in coronary heart disease risk assessment: US Preventive Services Task Force Recom-

mendation Statement. Ann Intern Med 2009;151(7): 474–482

13. Buckley DI, Fu R, Freeman M, Rogers K, Helfand M. C-reactive protein as a risk factor for coronary heart disease: a systematic review and meta-analyses for the US Preventive Services Task Force. Ann Intern Med 2009;151(7):483–495

14. Paraskevas S, Huizinga JD, Loos BG. A systematic review and meta-analyses on C-reactive protein in relation to periodontitis. J Clin Periodontol 2008;35 (4):277–290

15. Beck J, Garcia R, Heiss G, Vokonas PS, Offenbacher S. Periodontal disease and cardiovascular disease. J Periodontol 1996;67(10, Suppl)1123–1137

16. Chen HH, Almontashiri NAM, Antoine D, Stewart AFR. Functional genomics of the 9p21.3 locus for atherosclerosis: clarity or confusion? Curr Cardiol Rep 2014;16(7):502

17. Schaefer AS, Richter GM, Groessner-Schreiber B, et al. Identification of a shared genetic susceptibility locus for coronary heart disease and periodontitis. PLoS Genet 2009;5(2):e1000378

18. Tonetti MS, D'Aiuto F, Nibali L, et al. Treatment of periodontitis and endothelial function. N Engl J Med 2007;356(9):911–920

19. Azarpazhooh A, Leake JL. Systematic review of the association between respiratory diseases and oral health. J Periodontol 2006;77(9):1465–1482

20. Hujoel PP, Drangsholt M, Spiekerman C, Weiss NS. An exploration of the periodontitis-cancer association. Ann Epidemiol 2003;13(5):312–316

21. Mealey BL, Oates TW; American Academy of Periodontology. Diabetes mellitus and periodontal diseases. J Periodontol 2006;77(8):1289–1303

22. Löe H. Periodontal disease. The sixth complication of diabetes mellitus. Diabetes Care 1993;16(1):329–334

23. Borgnakke WS, Ylöstalo PV, Taylor GW, Genco RJ. Effect of periodontal disease on diabetes: systematic review of epidemiologic observational evidence. J Clin Periodontol 2013;40(Suppl 14):S135 –S152

24. Engebretson S, Kocher T. Evidence that periodontal treatment improves diabetes outcomes: a systematic review and meta-analysis. J Clin Periodontol 2013;40 (Suppl 14):S153 –S163

25. Simpson TC, Needleman I, Wild SH, Moles DR, Mills EJ. Treatment of periodontal disease for glycaemic control in people with diabetes. Cochrane Database Syst Rev 2010; (5):CD004 714

26. Teeuw WJ, Gerdes VE, Loos BG. Effect of periodontal treatment on glycemic control of diabetic patients: a systematic review and meta-analysis. Diabetes Care 2010;33(2):421–427

27. Engebretson SP, Hyman LG, Michalowicz BS, et al. The effect of nonsurgical periodontal therapy on hemoglobin A1 c levels in persons with type 2 diabetes and chronic periodontitis: a randomized clinical trial. JAMA 2013;310(23):2523–2532

28. Raman RP, Taiyeb-Ali TB, Chan SP, Chinna K, Vaithilingam RD. Effect of nonsurgical periodontal therapy verses oral hygiene instructions on type 2 diabetes sub-

jects with chronic periodontitis: a randomised clinical trial. BMC Oral Health 2014;14:79

29. Shepler B, Nash C, Smith C, Dimarco A, Petty J, Szewciw S. Update on potential drugs for the treatment of diabetic kidney disease. Clin Ther 2012;34(6):1237–1246

30. Chaffee BW, Weston SJ. Association between chronic periodontal disease and obesity: a systematic review and meta-analysis. J Periodontol 2010;81(12):1708–1724

31. Nibali L, Tatarakis N, Needleman I, et al. Clinical review: Association between metabolic syndrome and periodontitis: a systematic review and meta-analysis. J Clin Endocrinol Metab 2013;98(3):913–920

32. Morita T, Yamazaki Y, Mita A, et al. A cohort study on the association between periodontal disease and the development of metabolic syndrome. J Periodontol 2010;81(4):512–519

33. Goldenberg RL, Culhane JF, Iams JD, Romero R. Epidemiology and causes of preterm birth. Lancet 2008;371 (9606):75–84

34. Ide M, Papapanou PN. Epidemiology of association between maternal periodontal disease and adverse pregnancy outcomes—systematic review. J Clin Periodontol 2013;40(Suppl 14):S181–S194

35. Polyzos NP, Polyzos IP, Zavos A, et al. Obstetric outcomes after treatment of periodontal disease during pregnancy: systematic review and meta-analysis. BMJ 2010;341:c7017

36. Uppal A, Uppal S, Pinto A, et al. The effectiveness of periodontal disease treatment during pregnancy in reducing the risk of experiencing preterm birth and low birth weight: a meta-analysis. J Am Dent Assoc 2010;141(12):1423–1434

37. Chambrone L, Pannuti CM, Guglielmetti MR, Chambrone LA. Evidence grade associating periodontitis with preterm birth and/or low birth weight: II: a systematic review of randomized trials evaluating the effects of periodontal treatment. J Clin Periodontol 2011;38(10):902–914

38. Michalowicz BS, Gustafsson A, Thumbigere-Math V, Buhlin K. The effects of periodontal treatment on pregnancy outcomes. J Clin Periodontol 2013;40 (Suppl 14):S195–S208

39. Jeffcoat M, Parry S, Sammel M, Clothier B, Catlin A, Macones G. Periodontal infection and preterm birth: successful periodontal therapy reduces the risk of preterm birth. BJOG 2011;118(2):250–256

40. Martínez-Maestre MÁ, González-Cejudo C, Machuca G, Torrejón R, Castelo-Branco C. Periodontitis and osteoporosis: a systematic review. Climacteric 2010;13 (6):523–529

41. Davison S, Davis SR. Hormone replacement therapy: current controversies. Clin Endocrinol (Oxf) 2003;58 (3):249–261

42. Agaku IT, King BA, Dube SR; Centers for Disease Control and Prevention (CDC). Current cigarette smoking among adults - United States, 2005–2012. MMWR Morb Mortal Wkly Rep 2014;63(2):29–34 http://www.cdc.gov/mmwr/preview/mmwrhtml/

mm6302a2.htm?s_cid=mm6302a2_w#tab (Accessed August 1, 2014

43. Müller HP, Stadermann S, Heinecke A. Longitudinal association between plaque and gingival bleeding in smokers and non-smokers. J Clin Periodontol 2002;29 (4):287–294

44. Bergström J. Tobacco smoking and chronic destructive periodontal disease. Odontology 2004;92(1):1–8

45. Shchipkova AY, Nagaraja HN, Kumar PS. Subgingival microbial profiles of smokers with periodontitis. J Dent Res 2010;89(11):1247–1253

46. Thomson WM, Broadbent JM, Welch D, Beck JD, Poulton R. Cigarette smoking and periodontal disease among 32-year-olds: a prospective study of a representative birth cohort. J Clin Periodontol 2007;34 (10):828–834

47. Tomar SL, Asma S. Smoking-attributable periodontitis in the United States: findings from NHANES III. National Health and Nutrition Examination Survey. J Periodontol 2000;71(5):743–751

48. Do LG, Slade GD, Roberts-Thomson KF, Sanders AE. Smoking-attributable periodontal disease in the Australian adult population. J Clin Periodontol 2008;35 (5):398–404

49. Heasman L, Stacey F, Preshaw PM, McCracken GI, Hepburn S, Heasman PA. The effect of smoking on periodontal treatment response: a review of clinical evidence. J Clin Periodontol 2006;33(4):241–253

50. Labriola A, Needleman I, Moles DR. Systematic review of the effect of smoking on nonsurgical periodontal therapy. Periodontol 2000 2005;37:124–137

51. Chambrone L, Preshaw PM, Rosa EF, et al. Effects of smoking cessation on the outcomes of non-surgical periodontal therapy: a systematic review and individual patient data meta-analysis. J Clin Periodontol 2013;40(6):607–615

52. Fowler G. Smoking cessation: The role of general practitioners, nurses, and pharmacists. In: Bollinger CT, Fagerström KO, eds. Progress in Respiratory Research, vol 28: The Tobacco Epidemic. Basel: Karger; 1997: 165–177

53. Yudkin PL, Jones L, Lancaster T, Fowler GH. Which smokers are helped to give up smoking using transdermal nicotine patches? Results from a randomized, double-blind, placebo-controlled trial. Br J Gen Pract 1996;46(404):145–148

54. Harrell PT, Simmons VN, Correa JB, Padhya TA, Brandon TH. Electronic nicotine delivery systems ("e-cigarettes"): review of safety and smoking cessation efficacy. Otolaryngol Head Neck Surg 2014;151(3):381–393

55. Tezal M, Grossi SG, Ho AW, Genco RJ. Alcohol consumption and periodontal disease. The Third National Health and Nutrition Examination Survey. J Clin Periodontol 2004;31(7):484–488

56. Linden GJ, Lyons A, Scannapieco FA. Periodontal systemic associations: review of the evidence. J Clin Periodontol 2013;40(Suppl 14):S8–S19

57. Jeffcoat MK, Jeffcoat RL, Gladowski PA, Bramson JB, Blum JJ. Impact of periodontal therapy on general health: evidence from insurance data for five systemic conditions. Am J Prev Med 2014;47(2):166–174

## 9 Emergency Treatment

1. Herrera D, Alonso B, de Arriba L, Santa Cruz I, Serrano C, Sanz M. Acute periodontal lesions. Periodontol 2000 2014;65(1):149–177

2. Topoll HH, Lange DE, Müller RF. Multiple periodontal abscesses after systemic antibiotic therapy. J Clin Periodontol 1990;17(4):268–272

3. Harrington GW, Steiner DR, Ammons WF Jr. The periodontal–endodontic controversy. Periodontol 2000 2002;30:123–130

## 10 Phase I—Cause-Related Therapy

1. Drisko CL. Periodontal debridement: still the treatment of choice. J Evid Based Dent Pract 2014;14 (Suppl):33–41.e1

2. Yaacob M, Worthington HV, Deacon SA, et al. Powered versus manual toothbrushing for oral health. Cochrane Database Syst Rev 2014;6(6):CD002281

3. Van der Weijden FA, Campbell SL, Dörfer CE, González-Cabezas C, Slot DE. Safety of oscillating-rotating powered brushes compared to manual toothbrushes: a systematic review. J Periodontol 2011;82(1):5–24

4. Van Strydonck DA, Timmerman MF, van der Velden U, van der Weijden GA. Plaque inhibition of two commercially available chlorhexidine mouthrinses. J Clin Periodontol 2005;32(3):305–309

5. Gunsolley JC. Clinical efficacy of antimicrobial mouthrinses. J Dent 2010;38(Suppl 1):S6–S10

6. Stoeken JE, Paraskevas S, van der Weijden GA. The long-term effect of a mouthrinse containing essential oils on dental plaque and gingivitis: a systematic review. J Periodontol 2007;78(7):1218–1228

7. Van Leeuwen MPC, Slot DE, Van der Weijden GA. Essential oils compared to chlorhexidine with respect to plaque and parameters of gingival inflammation: a systematic review. J Periodontol 2011;82(2):174–194

8. Van Leeuwen MP, Slot DE, Van der Weijden GA. The effect of an essential-oils mouthrinse as compared to a vehicle solution on plaque and gingival inflammation: a systematic review and meta-analysis. Int J Dent Hyg 2014;12(3):160–167

9. McCullough MJ, Farah CS. The role of alcohol in oral carcinogenesis with particular reference to alcohol-containing mouthwashes. Aust Dent J 2008;53 (4):302–305

10. Mystikos C, Yoshino T, Ramberg P, Birkhed D. Effect of post-brushing mouthrinse solutions on salivary fluoride retention. Swed Dent J 2011;35(1):17–24

11. Albert-Kiszely A, Pjetursson BE, Salvi GE, et al. Comparison of the effects of cetylpyridinium chloride with an essential oil mouth rinse on dental plaque and gingivitis—a six-month randomized controlled clinical trial. J Clin Periodontol 2007;34(8):658–667

12. Mustafa M, Wondimu B, Yucel-Lindberg T, Kats-Hallström AT, Jonsson AS, Modéer T. Triclosan reduces microsomal prostaglandin E synthase-1 expression in human gingival fibroblasts. J Clin Periodontol 2005;32 (1):6–11

13. Müller HP, Barrieshi-Nusair KM, Könönen E, Yang M. Effect of triclosan/copolymer-containing toothpaste on the association between plaque and gingival bleeding: a randomized controlled clinical trial. J Clin Periodontol 2006;33(11):811–818

14. Rosling B, Dahlén G, Volpe A, Furuichi Y, Ramberg P, Lindhe J. Effect of triclosan on the subgingival microbiota of periodontitis-susceptible subjects. J Clin Periodontol 1997;24(12):881–887

15. Riley P, Lamont T. Triclosan/copolymer containing toothpastes for oral health. Cochrane Database Syst Rev 2013;12:CD010514

16. Bedoux G, Roig B, Thomas O, Dupont V, Le Bot B. Occurrence and toxicity of antimicrobial triclosan and by-products in the environment. Environ Sci Pollut Res Int 2012;19(4):1044–1065

17. Marsh PD. Microbiological aspects of the chemical control of plaque and gingivitis. J Dent Res 1992;71(7):1431–1438

18. Addy M, Moran J, Newcombe RG. Meta-analyses of studies of 0.2% delmopinol mouth rinse as an adjunct to gingival health and plaque control measures. J Clin Periodontol 2007;34(1):58–65

19. Cartwright RB. Dentinal hypersensitivity: a narrative review. Community Dent Health 2014;31(1):15–20

20. Malamed SF. Handbook of Local Anesthesia. 6th ed. Edinburgh: Mosby Elsevier; 2012

21. Pattison AM, Pattison GL. Scaling and root planing. In: Newman MG, Takei HH, Klokkevold PR, Carranza FA. Carranza's Clinic Periodontology. 11th ed. St. Louis: Saunders Elsevier; 2012

22. Petersilka GJ. Subgingival air-polishing in the treatment of periodontal biofilm infections. Periodontol 2000 2011;55(1):124–142

23. Meissner G, Kocher T. Calculus-detection technologies and their clinical application. Periodontol 2000 2011;55(1):189–204

24. Tunkel J, Heinecke A, Flemmig TF. A systematic review of efficacy of machine-driven and manual subgingival debridement in the treatment of chronic periodontitis. J Clin Periodontol 2002;29(Suppl 3):72–81, discussion 90–91

25. Van der Weijden GA, Timmerman MF. A systematic review on the clinical efficacy of subgingival debridement in the treatment of chronic periodontitis. J Clin Periodontol 2002;29(Suppl 3):55–71, discussion 90–91

26. Hujoel PP, Leroux BG, Selipsky H, White BA. Non-surgical periodontal therapy and tooth loss. A cohort study. J Periodontol 2000;71(5):736–742

27. Badersten A, Nilvéus R, Egelberg J. Effect of nonsurgical periodontal therapy. II. Severely advanced periodontitis. J Clin Periodontol 1984;11(1):63–76

28. Haffajee AD, Cugini MA, Dibart S, Smith C, Kent RL Jr, Socransky SS. The effect of SRP on the clinical and microbiological parameters of periodontal diseases. J Clin Periodontol 1997;24(5):324–334

29. Eberhard J, Jepsen S, Jervøe-Storm PM, Needleman I, Worthington HV. Full-mouth disinfection for the treatment of adult chronic periodontitis. Cochrane Database Syst Rev 2008;1(1):CD004622

30. Azarpazhooh A, Shah PS, Tenenbaum HC, Goldberg MB. The effect of photodynamic therapy for periodontitis: a systematic review and meta-analysis. J Periodontol 2010;81(1):4–14

31. Slot DE, Kranendonk AA, Paraskevas S, Van der Weijden F. The effect of a pulsed Nd:YAG laser in non-surgical periodontal therapy. J Periodontol 2009;80(7):1041–1056

# 11 Phase II—Corrective Procedures

1. Brown R, Arany P. Mechanism of drug-induced gingival overgrowth revisited: a unifying hypothesis. Oral Dis 2015;21(1):e51–e61

2. Goldberg PV, Higginbottom FL, Wilson TG. Periodontal considerations in restorative and implant therapy. Periodontol 2000 2001;25:100–109

3. Kirkland O. The suppurative periodontal pus pocket; its treatment by the modified flap operation. J Am Dent Assoc 1931;18:1462–1470

4. Friedman N. Periodontal osseous surgery: osteoplasty and ostectomy. J Periodontol 1955;26:257–269

5. Nabers CL. Repositioning the attached gingiva. J Periodontol 1954;25:38–39

6. Friedman N. Mucogingival surgery. The apically repositioned flap. J Periodontol 1962;33:328–340

7. Takei HH, Han TJ, Carranza FA Jr, Kenney EB, Lekovic V. Flap technique for periodontal bone implants. Papilla preservation technique. J Periodontol 1985;56(4):204–210

8. Cortellini P, Prato GP, Tonetti MS. The modified papilla preservation technique. A new surgical approach for interproximal regenerative procedures. J Periodontol 1995;66(4):261–266

9. Cortellini P, Prato GP, Tonetti MS. The simplified papilla preservation flap. A novel surgical approach for the management of soft tissues in regenerative procedures. Int J Periodont Restor Dent 1999;19(6):589–599

10. Cortellini P, Tonetti MS. Improved wound stability with a modified minimally invasive surgical technique in the regenerative treatment of isolated interdental intrabony defects. J Clin Periodontol 2009;36(2):157–163

11. Ramfjord SP, Nissle RR. The modified Widman flap. J Periodontol 1974;45(8):601–607

12. Westfelt E, Bragd L, Socransky SS, Haffajee AD, Nyman S, Lindhe J. Improved periodontal conditions following therapy. J Clin Periodontol 1985;12(4):283–293

13. Magnusson I, Runstad L, Nyman S, Lindhe J. A long junctional epithelium—a locus minoris resistentiae in plaque infection? J Clin Periodontol 1983;10(3):333–340

14. Rosling B, Nyman S, Lindhe J. The effect of systematic plaque control on bone regeneration in infrabony pockets. J Clin Periodontol 1976;3(1):38–53

15. Heitz-Mayfield LJ. How effective is surgical therapy compared with nonsurgical debridement? Periodontol 2000 2005;37:72–87

16. Hynes K, Menicanin D, Gronthos S, Bartold PM. Clinical utility of stem cells for periodontal regeneration. Periodontol 2000 2012;59(1):203–227

17. Mariotti A. Efficacy of chemical root surface modifiers in the treatment of periodontal disease. A systematic review. Ann Periodontol 2003;8(1):205–226

18. Karring T, Lindhe J. Concepts in periodontal tissue regeneration. In: Lindhe J, Karring T, Lang NP, ed. Textbook of Clinical Periodontology and Implant Dentistry. 5th ed. Oxford: Wiley-Blackwell; 2008

19. Kiritsy CP, Lynch AB, Lynch SE. Role of growth factors in cutaneous wound healing: a review. Crit Rev Oral Biol Med 1993;4(5):729–760

20. Yukna RA, Carr RL, Evans GH. Histologic evaluation of an Nd:YAG laser-assisted new attachment procedure in humans. Int J Periodont Restor Dent 2007;27(6):577–587

21. Nevins ML, Camelo M, Schüpbach P, Kim SW, Kim DM, Nevins M. Human clinical and histologic evaluation of laser-assisted new attachment procedure. Int J Periodont Restor Dent 2012;32(5):497–507

22. Lynch SE. Introduction. In: Lynch SE, Marx RE, Neins M, Wisner-Lynch LA, eds. Tissue Engineering. Applications in Maxillofacial Surgery and Periodontics. 2nd ed. Chicago: Quintessence Publishing; 2008

23. Cochran DL, Wozney JM. Biological mediators for periodontal regeneration. Periodontol 2000 1999;19:40–58

24. Del Fabbro M, Bortolin M, Taschieri S, Weinstein R. Is platelet concentrate advantageous for the surgical treatment of periodontal diseases? A systematic review and meta-analysis. J Periodontol 2011;82(8):1100–1111

25. Hammarström L. Enamel matrix, cementum development and regeneration. J Clin Periodontol 1997;24(9 Pt 2):658–668

26. Bosshardt DD. Biological mediators and periodontal regeneration: a review of enamel matrix proteins at the cellular and molecular levels. J Clin Periodontol 2008;35(8, Suppl)87–105

27. Esposito M, Grusovin MG, Papanikolaou N, Coulthard P, Worthington HV. Enamel matrix derivative (Emdogain®) for periodontal tissue regeneration in intrabony defects. Cochrane Database Syst Rev 2009;6(4): CD003875

28. Laaksonen M, Sorsa T, Salo T. Emdogain in carcinogenesis: a systematic review of in vitro studies. J Oral Sci 2010;52(1):1–11

29. Nyman S, Lindhe J, Karring T, Rylander H. New attachment following surgical treatment of human periodontal disease. J Clin Periodontol 1982;9(4):290–296

30. Laurell L, Gottlow J, Zybutz M, Persson R. Treatment of intrabony defects by different surgical procedures. A literature review. J Periodontol 1998;69(3):303–313

31. Cortellini P, Stalpers G, Mollo A, Tonetti MS. Periodontal regeneration versus extraction and prosthetic replacement of teeth severely compromised by attachment loss to the apex: 5-year results of an ongoing randomized clinical trial. J Clin Periodontol 2011;38(10):915–924

32. Cortellini P, Pini Prato G, Tonetti MS. Periodontal regeneration of human intrabony defects with bioresorbable membranes. A controlled clinical trial. J Periodontol 1996;67(3):217–223

33. Needleman IG, Worthington HV, Giedrys-Leeper E, Tucker RJ. Guided tissue regeneration for periodontal infra-bony defects. Cochrane Database Syst Rev 2006;2(2):CD001724

34. Cortellini P. Minimally invasive surgical techniques in periodontal regeneration. J Evid Based Dent Pract 2012;12(3, Suppl)89–100

35. Cortellini P, Tonetti MS. Clinical and radiographic outcomes of the modified minimally invasive surgical technique with and without regenerative materials: a randomized-controlled trial in intra-bony defects. J Clin Periodontol 2011;38(4):365–373

36. Grusovin MG, Esposito M. The efficacy of enamel matrix derivative (Emdogain) for the treatment of deep infrabony defects: a placebo-controlled randomised clinical trial. Eur J Oral Implantology 2009;2(1):43–54

37. Carlsen O. Dental Morphology. Copenhagen: Munksgaard; 1987

38. Jepsen S, Eberhard J, Herrera D, Needleman I. A systematic review of guided tissue regeneration for periodontal furcation defects. What is the effect of guided tissue regeneration compared with surgical debridement in the treatment of furcation defects? J Clin Periodontol 2002;29(Suppl 3):103–116, discussion 160–162

39. Murphy KG, Gunsolley JC. Guided tissue regeneration for the treatment of periodontal intrabony and furcation defects. A systematic review. Ann Periodontol 2003;8(1):266–302

40. Kinaia BM, Steiger J, Neely AL, Shah M, Bhola M. Treatment of Class II molar furcation involvement: meta-analyses of reentry results. J Periodontol 2011;82(3):413–428

41. Huynh-Ba G, Kuonen P, Hofer D, Schmid J, Lang NP, Salvi GE. The effect of periodontal therapy on the survival rate and incidence of complications of multirooted teeth with furcation involvement after an observation period of at least 5 years: a systematic review. J Clin Periodontol 2009;36(2):164–176

42. Mörmann W, Bernimoulin JP, Schmid MO. Fluorescein angiography of free gingival autografts. J Clin Periodontol 1975;2(4):177–189

43. Grupe J, Warren R. Repair of gingival defects by a sliding flap operation. J Periodontol 1956;37:92–95

44. Bernimoulin JP, Lüscher B, Mühlemann HR. Coronally repositioned periodontal flap. Clinical evaluation after one year. J Clin Periodontol 1975;2(1):1–13

45. Langer B, Langer L. Subepithelial connective tissue graft technique for root coverage. J Periodontol 1985;56(12):715–720

46. Müller HP, Schaller N, Eger T, Heinecke A. Thickness of masticatory mucosa. J Clin Periodontol 2000;27(6):431–436

47. Müller HP, Eger T, Schorb A. Alteration of gingival dimensions in a complicated case of gingival recession. Int J Periodont Restor Dent 1998;18(4):345–353

48. Harris RJ. The connective tissue and partial thickness double pedicle graft: a predictable method of obtaining root coverage. J Periodontol 1992;63(5):477–486
49. Tarnow DP. Semilunar coronally repositioned flap. J Clin Periodontol 1986;13(3):182–185
50. Raetzke PB. Covering localized areas of root exposure employing the "envelope" technique. J Periodontol 1985;56(7):397–402
51. Müller HP, Eger T, Schorb A. Gingival dimensions after root coverage with free connective tissue grafts. J Clin Periodontol 1998;25(5):424–430
52. Allen AL. Use of the supraperiosteal envelope in soft tissue grafting for root coverage. I. Rationale and technique. Int J Periodont Restor Dent 1994;14(3):216–227
53. Chambrone L, Sukekava F, Araújo MG, Pustiglioni FE, Chambrone LA, Lima LA. Root-coverage procedures for the treatment of localized recession-type defects: a Cochrane systematic review. J Periodontol 2010;81 (4):452–478
54. Gottlow J, Laurell L, Lundgren D, et al. Periodontal tissue response to a new bioresorbable guided tissue regeneration device: a longitudinal study in monkeys. Int J Periodont Restor Dent 1994;14(5):436–449
55. Müller HP, Stahl M, Eger T. Dynamics of mucosal dimensions after root coverage with a bioresorbable membrane. J Clin Periodontol 2000;27(1):1–8
56. Buti J, Baccini M, Nieri M, La Marca M, Pini-Prato GP. Bayesian network meta-analysis of root coverage procedures: ranking efficacy and identification of best treatment. J Clin Periodontol 2013;40(4):372–386
57. Cheng GL, Fu E, Tu YK, et al. Root coverage by coronally advanced flap with connective tissue graft and/or enamel matrix derivative: a meta-analysis. J Periodontal Res 2015;50(2):220–230
58. Lindhe J, Ericsson I. Trauma from occlusion. Periodontal tissues. In: Lindhe J, Lang NP, eds. Clinical Periodontology and Implant Dentistry, 6th ed. Oxford: Wiley-Blackwell: 2015
59. Harrel SK, Nunn ME. The effect of occlusal discrepancies on periodontitis. II. Relationship of occlusal treatment to the progression of periodontal disease. J Periodontol 2001;72(4):495–505
60. Harrel SK, Nunn ME. The association of occlusal contacts with the presence of increased periodontal probing depth. J Clin Periodontol 2009;36(12):1035–1042
61. Mühlemann HR. Periodontometry, a method for measuring tooth mobility. Oral Surg Oral Med Oral Pathol 1951;4(10):1220–1233
62. Ash MM Jr, Ramfjord SP. Reflections on the Michigan splint and other intraocclusal devices. J Mich Dent Assoc 1998;80(8):32–35, 41–46
63. Nyman SR, Lang NP. Tooth mobility and the biological rationale for splinting teeth. Periodontol 2000 1994;4:15–22
64. Käyser AF. Limited treatment goals—shortened dental arches. Periodontol 2000 1994;4:7–14
65. Ong CTT, Ivanovski S, Needleman IG, et al. Systematic review of implant outcomes in treated periodontitis subjects. J Clin Periodontol 2008;35(5):438–462
66. Esposito M, Grusovin MG, Felice P, Karatzopoulos G, Worthington HV, Coulthard P. Interventions for replacing missing teeth: horizontal and vertical bone augmentation techniques for dental implant treatment. Cochrane Database Syst Rev 2009;4(4): CD003607
67. Esposito M, Grusovin MG, Rees J, et al. Interventions for replacing missing teeth: augmentation procedures of the maxillary sinus. Cochrane Database Syst Rev 2010;3(3):CD008397
68. Telleman G, Raghoebar GM, Vissink A, den Hartog L, Huddleston Slater JJR, Meijer HJA. A systematic review of the prognosis of short (< 10 mm) dental implants placed in the partially edentulous patient. J Clin Periodontol 2011;38(7):667–676
69. Lang NP, Wilson TG, Corbet EF. Biological complications with dental implants: their prevention, diagnosis and treatment. Clin Oral Implants Res 2000;11 (Suppl 1):146–155
70. Esposito M, Grusovin MG, Worthington HV. Interventions for replacing missing teeth: treatment of peri-implantitis. Cochrane Database Syst Rev 2012;1: CD004970

# 12 Phase III—Supportive Periodontal Therapy

1. Renvert S, Persson GR. Supportive periodontal therapy. Periodontol 2000 2004;36:179–195
2. Lang NP, Tonetti MS. Periodontal diagnosis in treated periodontitis. Why, when and how to use clinical parameters. J Clin Periodontol 1996;23(3 Pt 2):240–250
3. Armitage GC. Periodontal diseases: diagnosis. Ann Periodontol 1996;1(1):37–215
4. Wang HL, Burgett FG, Shyr Y, Ramfjord S. The influence of molar furcation involvement and mobility on future clinical periodontal attachment loss. J Periodontol 1994;65(1):25–29
5. Pretzl B, Kaltschmitt J, Kim TS, Reitmeir P, Eickholz P. Tooth loss after active periodontal therapy. 2: Tooth-related factors. J Clin Periodontol 2008;35(2):175–182
6. Papapanou PN, Wennström JL. The angular bony defect as indicator of further alveolar bone loss. J Clin Periodontol 1991;18(5):317–322
7. Eickholz P, Kaltschmitt J, Berbig J, Reitmeir P, Pretzl B. Tooth loss after active periodontal therapy. 1: Patient-related factors for risk, prognosis, and quality of outcome. J Clin Periodontol 2008;35(2):165–174
8. Müller HP, Barrieshi-Nusair KM. Site-specific gingival bleeding on probing in a steady-state plaque environment: influence of polymorphisms in the interleukin-1 gene cluster. J Periodontol 2010;81(1):52–61
9. Tonetti MS. Cigarette smoking and periodontal diseases: etiology and management of disease. Ann Periodontol 1998;3(1):88–101
10. Lang NP, Tonetti MS. Periodontal risk assessment (PRA) for patients in supportive periodontal therapy (SPT). Oral Health Prev Dent 2003;1(1):7–16

11. Garcia RI, Nunn ME, Dietrich T. Risk calculation and periodontal outcomes. Periodontol 2000 2009;50:65–77

## 13 Medication and Supplements

1. Mombelli A, Cionca N, Almaghlouth A, Décaillet F, Courvoisier DS, Giannopoulou C. Are there specific benefits of amoxicillin plus metronidazole in *Aggregatibacter actinomycetemcomitans*-associated periodontitis? Double-masked, randomized clinical trial of efficacy and safety. J Periodontol 2013;84(6):715–724
2. Socransky SS, Haffajee AD. Dental biofilms: difficult therapeutic targets. Periodontol 2000 2002;28:12–55
3. Müller HP, Heinecke A, Borneff M, Kiencke C, Knopf A, Pohl S. Eradication of *Actinobacillus actinomycetemcomitans* from the oral cavity in adult periodontitis. J Periodontal Res 1998;33(1):49–58
4. Müller HP, Lange DE, Müller RF. Failure of adjunctive minocycline-HCl to eliminate oral *Actinobacillus actinomycetemcomitans*. J Clin Periodontol 1993;20(7):498–504
5. Cortelli SC, Costa FO, Kawai T, et al. Diminished treatment response of periodontally diseased patients infected with the JP2 clone of *Aggregatibacter (Actinobacillus) actinomycetemcomitans*. J Clin Microbiol 2009;47(7):2018–2025
6. Griffiths GS, Ayob R, Guerrero A, et al. Amoxicillin and metronidazole as an adjunctive treatment in generalized aggressive periodontitis at initial therapy or retreatment: a randomized controlled clinical trial. J Clin Periodontol 2011;38(1):43–49
7. Gordon JM, Walker CB, Murphy JC, Goodson JM, Socransky SS. Tetracycline: levels achievable in gingival crevice fluid and in vitro effect on subgingival organisms. Part I. Concentrations in crevicular fluid after repeated doses. J Periodontol 1981;52(10):609–612
8. Sakellari D, Goodson JM, Kolokotronis A, Konstantinidis A. Concentration of 3 tetracyclines in plasma, gingival crevice fluid and saliva. J Clin Periodontol 2000;27(1):53–60
9. Müller HP, Holderrieth S, Burkhardt U, Höffler U. In vitro antimicrobial susceptibility of oral strains of *Actinobacillus actinomycetemcomitans* to seven antibiotics. J Clin Periodontol 2002;29(8):736–742
10. Herrera D, Sanz M, Jepsen S, Needleman I, Roldán S. A systematic review on the effect of systemic antimicrobials as an adjunct to scaling and root planing in periodontitis patients. J Clin Periodontol 2002;29(Suppl 3):136–159, discussion 160–162
11. Haffajee AD, Socransky SS, Gunsolley JC. Systemic anti-infective periodontal therapy. A systematic review. Ann Periodontol 2003;8(1):115–181
12. Zandbergen D, Slot DE, Cobb CM, Van der Weijden FA. The clinical effect of scaling and root planing and the concomitant administration of systemic amoxicillin and metronidazole: a systematic review. J Periodontol 2013;84(3):332–351

13. Mombelli A, Cionca N, Almaghlouth A. Does adjunctive antimicrobial therapy reduce the perceived need for periodontal surgery? Periodontol 2000 2011;55(1):205–216
14. Tonetti MS. The topical use of antibiotics in periodontal pockets. In: Lang NP, Karring T, Lindhe J, eds. Proceedings of the 2nd European Workshop on Periodontics. Berlin: Quintessence; 1996
15. Hallmon WW, Rees TD. Local anti-infective therapy: mechanical and physical approaches. A systematic review. Ann Periodontol 2003;8(1):99–114
16. Paolantonio M, D'Ercole S, Pilloni A, et al. Clinical, microbiologic, and biochemical effects of subgingival administration of a Xanthan-based chlorhexidine gel in the treatment of periodontitis: a randomized multicenter trial. J Periodontol 2009;80(9):1479–1492
17. Tonetti MS, Lang NP, Cortellini P, et al. Effects of a single topical doxycycline administration adjunctive to mechanical debridement in patients with persistent/recurrent periodontitis but acceptable oral hygiene during supportive periodontal therapy. J Clin Periodontol 2012;39(5):475–482
18. Lauenstein M, Kaufmann M, Persson GR. Clinical and microbiological results following nonsurgical periodontal therapy with or without local administration of piperacillin/tazobactam. Clin Oral Investig 2013;17(7):1645–1660
19. Gonzales JR, Harnack L, Schmitt-Corsitto G, et al. A novel approach to the use of subgingival controlled-release chlorhexidine delivery in chronic periodontitis: a randomized clinical trial. J Periodontol 2011;82(8):1131–1139
20. Oringer RJ, Al-Shammari KF, Aldredge WA, et al. Effect of locally delivered minocycline microspheres on markers of bone resorption. J Periodontol 2002;73(8):835–842
21. Hanes PJ, Purvis JP. Local anti-infective therapy: pharmacological agents. A systematic review. Ann Periodontol 2003;8(1):79–98
22. Bonito AJ, Lux L, Lohr KN. Impact of local adjuncts to scaling and root planing in periodontal disease therapy: a systematic review. J Periodontol 2005;76(8):1227–1236
23. Hung HC, Douglass CW. Meta-analysis of the effect of scaling and root planing, surgical treatment and antibiotic therapies on periodontal probing depth and attachment loss. J Clin Periodontol 2002;29(11):975–986
24. Pavia M, Nobile CG, Angelillo IF. Meta-analysis of local tetracycline in treating chronic periodontitis. J Periodontol 2003;74(6):916–932
25. Pavia M, Nobile CGA, Bianco A, Angelillo IF. Meta-analysis of local metronidazole in the treatment of chronic periodontitis. J Periodontol 2004;75(6):830–838
26. Rudney JD, Chen R, Sedgewick GJ. *Actinobacillus actinomycetemcomitans*, *Porphyromonas gingivalis*, and *Tannerella forsythensis* are components of a polymicrobial intracellular flora within human buccal cells. J Dent Res 2005;84(1):59–63
27. Reddy MS, Geurs NC, Gunsolley JC. Periodontal host modulation with antiproteinase, anti-inflammatory,

and bone-sparing agents. A systematic review. Ann Periodontol 2003;8(1):12–37

28. Serhan CN, Chiang N, Van Dyke TE. Resolving inflammation: dual anti-inflammatory and pro-resolution lipid mediators. Nat Rev Immunol 2008;8(5):349–361

29. El-Sharkawy H, Aboelsaad N, Eliwa M, et al. Adjunctive treatment of chronic periodontitis with daily dietary supplementation with omega-3 fatty acids and low-dose aspirin. J Periodontol 2010;81(11):1635–1643

30. Neiva RF, Al-Shammari K, Nociti FH Jr, Soehren S, Wang HL. Effects of vitamin-B complex supplementation on periodontal wound healing. J Periodontol 2005;76(7):1084–1091

31. Dietrich T, Nunn M, Dawson-Hughes B, Bischoff-Ferrari HA. Association between serum concentrations of 25-hydroxyvitamin D and gingival inflammation. Am J Clin Nutr 2005;82(3):575–580

32. Zhan Y, Samietz S, Holtfreter B, et al. Prospective study of serum 25-hydroxy vitamin D and tooth loss. J Dent Res 2014;93(7):639–644

33. Bashutski JD, Eber RM, Kinney JS, et al. The impact of vitamin D status on periodontal surgery outcomes. J Dent Res 2011;90(8):1007–1012

34. Garcia MN, Hildebolt CF, Miley DD, et al. One-year effects of vitamin D and calcium supplementation on chronic periodontitis. J Periodontol 2011;82(1):25–32

35. Nishida M, Grossi SG, Dunford RG, Ho AW, Trevisan M, Genco RJ. Dietary vitamin C and the risk for periodontal disease. J Periodontol 2000;71(8):1215–1223

36. Nishida M, Grossi SG, Dunford RG, Ho AW, Trevisan M, Genco RJ. Calcium and the risk for periodontal disease. J Periodontol 2000;71(7):1057–1066

37. Kaye EK. Nutrition, dietary guidelines and optimal periodontal health. Periodontol 2000 2012;58(1):93–111

38. Bonifait L, Chandad F, Grenier D. Probiotics for oral health: myth or reality? J Can Dent Assoc 2009;75 (8):585–590

39. Stensson M, Koch G, Coric S, et al. Oral administration of *Lactobacillus reuteri* during the first year of life reduces caries prevalence in the primary dentition at 9 years of age. Caries Res 2014;48(2):111–117

40. Iniesta M, Herrera D, Montero E, et al. Probiotic effects of orally administered *Lactobacillus reuteri*-containing tablets on the subgingival and salivary microbiota in patients with gingivitis. A randomized clinical trial. J Clin Periodontol 2012;39(8):736–744

# Subject Index

Note: Page numbers in *italics* refer to illustrations, tables, or boxes.